SURGERY OF THE MANDIBLE

Published Volumes

Proportions of the Aesthetic Face
Powell and Humphreys

Facial Reconstruction with Local and Regional Flaps
Becker

Rhinoplasty: Emphasizing the External Approach
Anderson

Forthcoming Volumes

Blepharoplasty
Thomas and Cook

Photography in Facial Plastic Surgery
Tardy

Rejuvenation of the Aging Face
Brennan

Psychology of Facial Plastic Surgery
Wright

Dermabrasion and Chemical Peel
McCullough

Myocutaneous Flaps
Hayden

Lasers in Skin Surgery
Wheeland

Microsurgical Reconstruction
Panje and Moran

Hair Replacement Surgery
Fleming and Mayer

The American Academy of Facial Plastic and Reconstructive Surgery

Series Editor: James D. Smith, M.D.

SURGERY OF THE MANDIBLE

Edited by

Byron J. Bailey, M.D.
Wiess Professor and Chairman
Department of Otolaryngology
University of Texas Medical Branch
Galveston, Texas

G. Richard Holt, M.D.
Division of Otorhinolaryngology
University of Texas Health Science
  Center
San Antonio, Texas

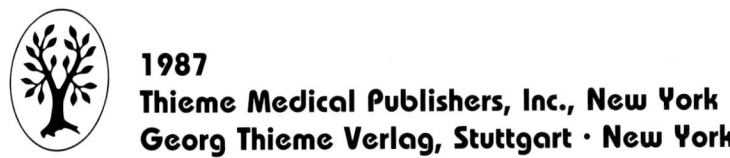

1987
Thieme Medical Publishers, Inc., New York
Georg Thieme Verlag, Stuttgart · New York

Thieme Inc.
381 Park Avenue South
New York, New York 10016

Series sponsored by the educational committee of The American Academy of Facial Plastic and Reconstructive Surgery.

SURGERY OF THE MANDIBLE
Byron J. Bailey

Library of Congress Cataloging in Publication Data
Bailey, Byron J., 1934–
  Surgery of the mandible.
  (The American Academy of Facial Plastic and
Reconstructive Surgery)
  Includes index.
  1. Mandible—Surgery. I. Holt, G. Richard.
II. Title. III. Series: American Academy of Facial
Plastic and Reconstructive Surgery (Series).
[DNLM: 1. Mandible—surgery. WU 600 B1538s]
RD526.B35   1987   617'.522   86-23175

Typeset by Maple-Vail Book Mfg. Group, Binghamton, NY, USA.
Printed and bound by Maple-Vail Book Mfg. Group, Binghamton, NY, USA.
Printed in the United States of America.

TMP ISBN 0-86577-239-8
GTV ISBN 3-13-691601-8

TMP (series) 0-86577-137-5
GTV (series) 3-13-656501-0

Important Note: Medicine is an ever-changing science. Research and clinical experience are continually broadening our knowledge, in particular our knowledge of proper treatment and drug therapy. Insofar as this book mentions any dosage or application, readers may rest assured that the authors, editors, and publishers have made every effort to ensure that such references are strictly in accordance with the state of knowledge at the time of production of the book. Nevertheless, every user is requested to carefully examine the manufacturers' leaflets accompanying each drug to check on his own responsibility whether the dosage schedules recommended therein or the contraindications stated by the manufacturers differ from the statements made in the present book. Such examination is particularly important with drugs that are either rarely used or have been newly released on the market.

Some of the product names, patents and registered designs referred to in this book are in fact registered trademarks or proprietary names even though specific reference to this fact is not always made in the text. Therefore, the appearance of a name without designation as proprietary is not to be construed as a representation by the publisher that it is in the public domain.

Copyright © 1987 by Thieme Medical Publishers, Inc. This book, including all parts thereof, is legally protected by copyright. Any use, exploitation or commercialization outside the narrow limits set by copyright legislation, without the publisher's consent, is illegal and liable to prosecution. This applies in particular to photostat reproduction, copying, mimeographing or duplication of any kind, translating, preparation of microfilms, and electronic data processing and storage.

5 4 3 2 1

Preface

The field of mandibular surgery has been characterized by numerous innovations and advances during the past two decades. Clinicians from many disciplines within medicine and dentistry have contributed significantly to this field, and the relevant information is spread throughout a broad range of journals and books. The rapidity with which change has taken place and the diversity of the sources wherein it is reported have made it difficult to follow this field. The purpose of this book is to organize and summarize material that is of great clinical importance in regard to mandibular surgery, to draw from many sources within several disciplines, and to present the distillate clearly and succinctly.

Our target audience is primarily residents and graduate trainees who are somewhat familiar with this area, but who are seeking more depth in terms of scientific information and at the same time are looking for helpful clinical hints. We have set about this task by inviting authors who have been carefully chosen from a number of surgical fields. We have arranged the material by topics that will deal with specific, focused subject matter in a way that will be immediately useful to residents and to others who wish to learn more about this complex area.

This volume deemphasizes detailed research data and tables and emphasizes the practical application of important new scientific information in daily clinical practice.

When we were invited to undertake this project, we were impressed by the unevenness and by the contradictory reports that were available from library sources. It seemed to us, therefore, that our objectives would be useful if they could be attained. We believe that we have achieved our goal of balanced reporting of differing views, while offering practical solutions and observations within the constraints of the modest size of this book.

We hope that you find the information contained in *Surgery of the Mandible* to be useful to you in your daily practice and to be of value in terms of enhancing your understanding of this difficult, interdisciplinary area of surgery.

Byron J. Bailey
G. Richard Holt

Contributors

Curtis Chilcoat, D.D.S.
Department of Oral and Maxillofacial Surgery
University of Texas, Health Science Center
San Antonio, Texas

William D. Clark, D.D.S., M.D.
Clinical Assistant Professor of Otolaryngology
University of Texas Medical Branch
Galveston, Texas

Donald L. Steed, D.D.S., M.S.
Associate Professor, Department of Surgery
Texas A & M University, College of Medicine
Professor, Department of Surgery
Division of Oral and Maxillofacial Surgery
University of Texas Medical School
San Antonio, Texas

Charles M. Stiernberg, M.D.
Assistant Professor
Department of Otolaryngology
University of Texas Medical Branch
Galveston, Texas

Victor V. Strelzow, M.D., F.R.C.S.(C)., F.A.C.S.
Director, Facial Plastic and Reconstructive Surgery
Division of Otolaryngology, Head and Neck Surgery
University of California
Irvine, California

Joseph E. Van Sickels, D.D.S.
Associate Professor
Department of Oral and Maxillofacial Surgery
University of Texas, Health Science Center
San Antonio, Texas

Contents

1. Embryology and Anatomy of the Mandible 1
   Charles M. Stiernberg

2. Principles of Bone Healing and Grafting 7
   Charles M. Stiernberg

3. Mandibular Osteotomy 11
   Byron J. Bailey

4. Stabilization and Fixation of the Mandible 25
   William D. Clark

5. Surgical Treatment of Benign and Low-Grade Malignant Lesions of the Mandible 39
   William D. Clark

6. Surgical Management of Malignant Tumors: Considerations of Mandibular Invasion 45
   Byron J. Bailey

7. Management of Mandibular Fractures 61
   Byron J. Bailey

8. Bone Plate Osteosynthesis in the Treatment of Mandibular Fractures 87
   Victor V. Strelzow

9. The Mandible: Its Role in Facial Balance 107
   Joseph E. Van Sickels and Curtis Chilcoat

10. Surgery of the Chin 117
    Donald L. Steed

11. Augmentation Mentoplasty 139
    G. Richard Holt

12. Reconstruction of the Mandible 149
    G. Richard Holt

13. Principles and Preferences in Mandibular Reconstruction 173
    Byron J. Bailey

14. Complications of Mandibular Surgery 211
    G. Richard Holt

    Index 227

1 Embryology and Anatomy of the Mandible

Charles M. Stiernberg, M.D.

Any discussion of embryology and anatomy of the mandible presumes an understanding of basic structure and composition of bone. Bone is classified by the way it forms as *membranous* or *endochondral*. *Periosteum* is a soft tissue sheet that surrounds bone and subdivides into an outer fibrous layer and an inner cambium layer. The inner layer plays an active role in fracture healing. The core of bone (marrow cavity) is also lined with a fibrous sheet, the *endosteum*, which is actively involved in fracture healing. The *haversian canal system*, or *osteon*, is the basic unit of mature bone and is composed of a central canal containing one or more blood vessels surrounded by lamellae. Small cavities knows as *lacunae* are located between the lamellae. Each lacuna contains an *osteocyte* that has cytoplasmic processes extending through canaliculi to communicate with haversian canal vessels. The size of osteons is limited because bone cells cannot survive farther than 0.1 mm away from a capillary.[1]

Mature lamellar bone consists of 8% water and 92% solids, the solid portion being 21% organic and 71% inorganic. The matrix is organic and supplies form and support for the deposition and crystallization of inorganic salts. It is composed of 98% collagen and 2% ground substance, the latter being mostly glycosaminoglycans and proteoglycans. The main inorganic component of bone is a salt known as hydroxyapatite, $Ca_{10}(PO_4)_6(OH)_2$.[2] Three principal bone cells are the *osteoblast*, the *osteocyte*, and the *osteoclast*. The roles of these cells will be discussed in Chapter 2.

EMBRYOLOGY

In early embryonic development of the head and neck, a series of distinct bilateral mesenchymal swellings appear on the ventral aspect of the embryo just caudal to the head fold. These swellings are pharyngeal, or branchial, arches that form most of the structures of the head and neck. Initially, they are separated by grooves externally and pouches internally. Each arch has a central cartilaginous rod for skeletal support and its own artery and nerve. The nerve normally passes ventral and superficial to the artery in each arch except for the fifth. The arteries come from a ventral aorta and pass through the arches to join dorsal aortas on each side (Fig. 1). Arteries of the first two arches rapidly degenerate; a stapedial artery, which remains as the only vestige of a second arch artery, is occasionally seen during ear surgery. Arteries of the third arch become carotid arteries, while those of the fourth become the aortic arch and proximal right subclavian artery.[3]

The first pharyngeal arch is the anlage of the jaws. Its cartilage is Meckel's cartilage, which provides the template for the developing mandible and also gives rise to parts of the malleus, incus, and spine of the sphenoid bone (Fig. 2). The membranous bone of the mandible forms by ossification of an osteogenic membrane which first appears at 36 gestational days. The mandible is one of the first bones in the body to begin to ossify. The mental area is the only portion of the mandible that forms by endochondral ossification of Meckel's cartilage. Initial separation of the two halves of the mandible is gradually eliminated between the 4th and 12th postnatal months, when ossification at the symphysis converts the syndesmosis into a synostosis. The neurovascular bundle of the mandible exists before ossification begins, thereby assuring formation of the mandibular canal and mental foramen. The sphenomandibular and anterior malleolar ligaments represent fibrous remnants of Meckel's cartilage.

Secondary accessory cartilages appear between the 10th and 14th gestational weeks and eventually form the head of the condyle, part of the coronoid process, and the mental protuberance. Condylar cartilage plays two roles: first, as a growth cartilage similar to an epiphyseal plate in a long bone and, second, as an articular cartilage in the temporomandibular joint. Any damage to condylar cartilage will restrict growth potential and normal downward and forward displacement of the developing man-

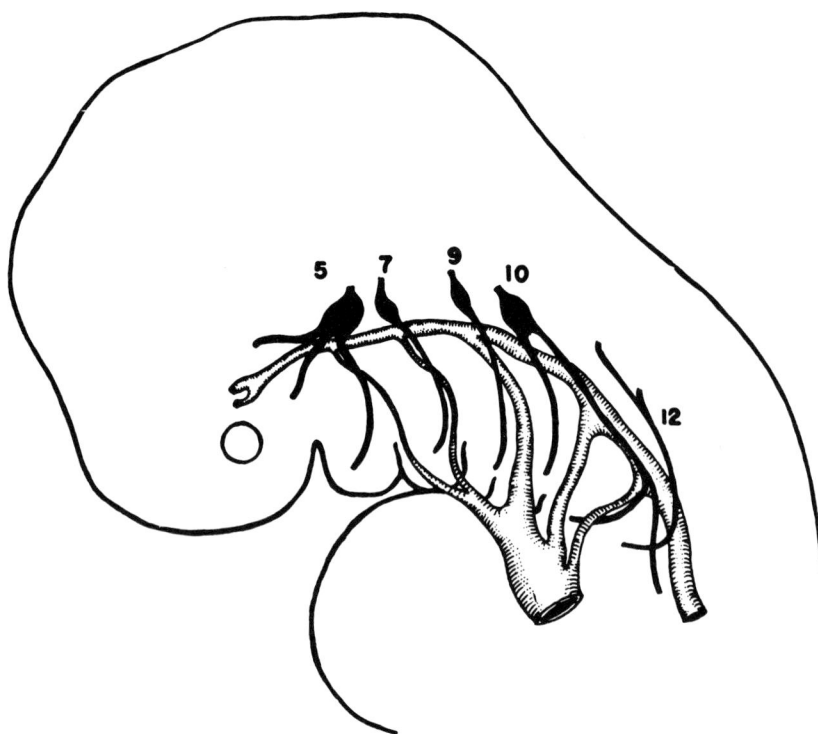

Figure 1. Human fetus at fourth gestational week. [From Davies J: Embryology of the Head and Neck in Relation to the Practice of Otolaryngology—A Manual prepared for the Use of Graduates in Medicine (Continuing Education Programs). Washington, DC: American Academy of Ophthalmology and Otolaryngology, 1957. With permission.]

dible. Growth of the horizontally oriented infant condyles increases length rather than height of the mandible (Fig. 3).

The alveolar process is the part of the mandibular body that houses the teeth. It will not develop in the absence of tooth development, which begins during the sixth gestational week as an epithelial thickening arising along the upper border of the developing mandible. This thickening is the dental lamina that serves as the primordium of the ectodermal parts of the teeth. Toothbuds begin as swellings along the dental lamina and their locations correspond to the future position of deciduous teeth. A toothbud consists of three parts: an enamel organ,

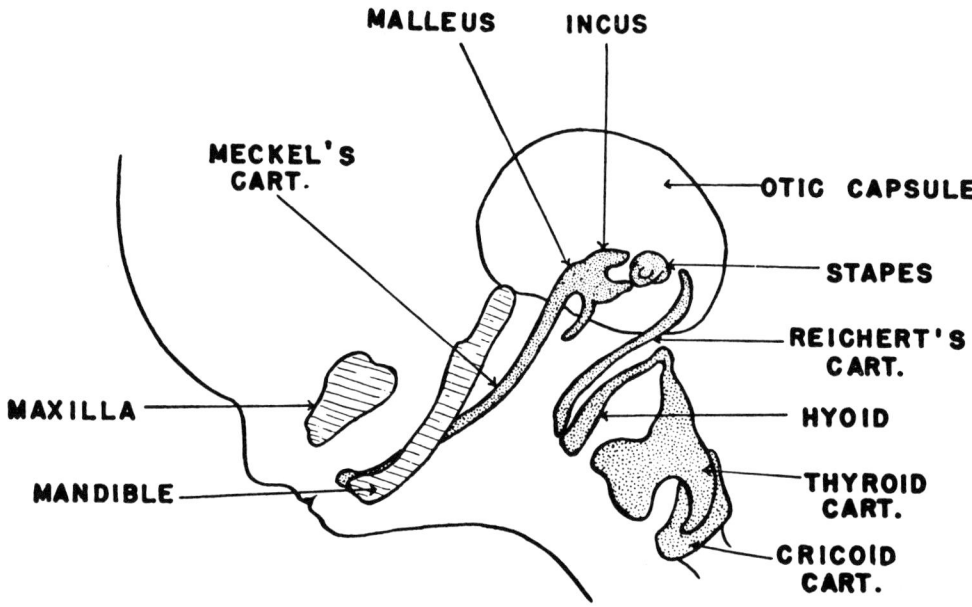

Figure 2. Development of branchial arch cartilages. [From Davies J: Embryology of the Head and Neck in Relation to the Practice of Otolaryngology—A Manual Prepared for the Use of Graduates in Medicine (Continuing Education Programs). Washington, DC: American Academy of Ophthalmology and Otolaryngology, 1957. With permission.]

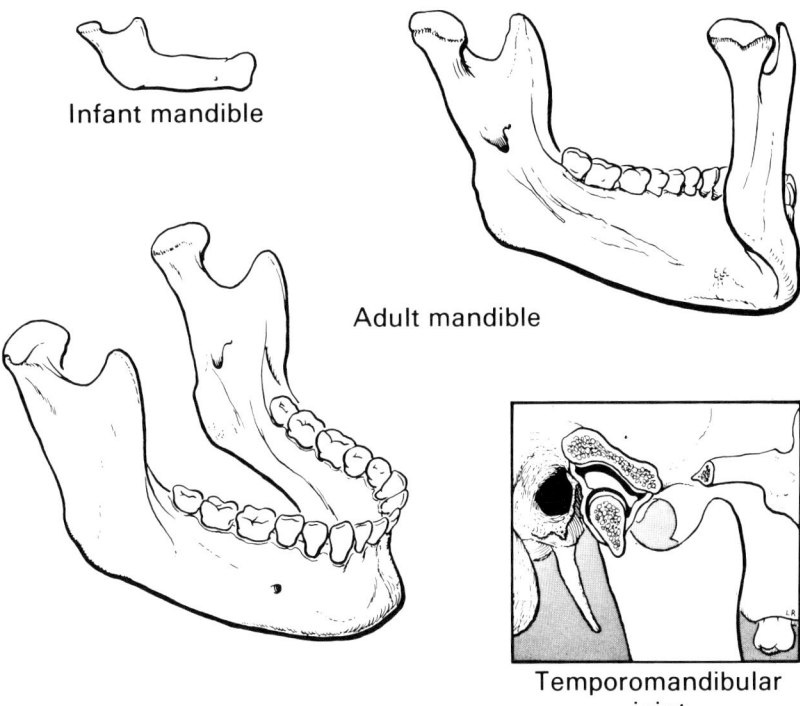

Figure 3. The edentulous infant mandible, the adult mandible with full set of permanent dentition, and a saggital section of the temporomandibular joint.

a dental papilla, and a dental sac. The enamel organ derives from oral ectoderm and is the anlage of tooth enamel. The dental papilla and dental sac derive from mesenchyme; the former produces pulp and dentin, and the latter produces cementum and the periodontal ligaments of teeth.

The chin, or mental protuberance, is formed from an accessory cartilage and the ventral end of Meckel's cartilage. Although it is poorly developed in infancy, sexual and specific genetic factors later influence its growth. Sexual differences in the chin do not appear until secondary sex characteristics begin to develop. Generally, males develop more prominent chins. The protrusive chin is a uniquely human trait, absent in all other primates.[4]

At the time of birth, the mandible tends to be retrognathic to the maxilla; this is normally corrected early in postnatal life by rapid mandibular growth and forward displacement that establishes an orthognathic or an angle Class 1 relationship. Inadequate mandibular growth will result in a Class 2 relationship, whereas overgrowth of the mandible will produce a Class 3 relationship.

The mandible is susceptible to many congenital anomalies that affect the first pharyngeal arch. Agnathia denotes a grossly deficient or absent mandible. Micrognathia means a small mandible, which is characteristic of several congenital defects including the Pierre Robin syndrome, cri du chat syndrome, Treacher-Collins syndrome, progeria, Down's syndrome (trisomy 21), and Turner's syndrome.

ANATOMY

The largest and strongest facial bone, the mandible, consists of a U-shaped body and two broad flat rami (see Fig. 3). Each ramus is attached to the body posteriorly and is oriented nearly perpendicular to it. In addition to the physiologic functions of mastication, articulation, and deglutition, the mandible also has an important facial cosmetic role. Disruption of mandibular integrity can compromise its functions, and the degree of compromise depends on which sections of the mandible are involved. For example, absence of the anterior arch of the mandible causes loss of tongue support, loss of laryngeal support, and inability to approximate the lips. Debilitation of this severity can result from surgery for a large floor of mouth cancer or from such trauma as a gunshot.

Body of the Mandible

The body of the mandible has inner and outer cortices composed of dense, compact bone. Between these cortices is a core of spongy bone, through which pass blood vessels, nerves, and lymphatics. The inferior half of the mandibular body strengthens the mandible and changes little during life. The alveolar process is mostly spongy bone and has an inner (oral) lingual plate and outer (labiobuccal) vestibular plate. Unlike the lower half of the mandible, the alveolar process changes markedly during life. Accounting for most of the mandibular body at the time of birth, the alveolar process occupies progressively less of the bone's vertical height as growth and development occur. After extraction of teeth, the alveolar process undergoes marked atrophy.

Embryologically, each half of the mandible develops separately and fuses in the midline at the symphysis. A prominent ridge at the lower end of the symphysis on the outer cortex forms the mental protuberance. Just lateral to it on each side are smaller mental tubercles, to which muscles of the chin and lower lip are attached. Also, on each side of the mandible an oblique line starts at the mental tubercle and becomes more prominent as it runs posteriorly and superiorly to join the anterior border of the ramus. This line serves as origin for the depressor labii inferioris and depressor anguli oris muscles.

A mental foramen exists on the outer cortex of each side of the mandibular body. In the adult, this opening is located below the second premolar tooth, but its position relative to the vertical height of the body depends on age. The foramen is near the inferior edge of the mandibular body in the newborn, 8 to 10 mm from the inferior edge in the fully developed mandible, and near or on the superior border in the older edentulous mandible (see Fig. 3).

Several landmarks can be found on the inner cortex of the mandibular body. The mental spine is situated in the midline near the inferior border. The genioglossus muscle attaches to the upper part of this spine and the geniohyoid muscle to its smaller, lower part. Lateral and superior to this spine is a slight concavity, the sublingual fossa, which contains the anterior end of the sublingual gland. Also, lateral to the spine and close to the inferior edge of the body is a digastric fossa, where the anterior belly of the digastric muscle attaches. The mylohyoid muscle originates along a ridge known as the *mylohyoid line,* which begins at the digastric fossa and runs obliquely as far posteriorly as the third molar tooth. Immediately below this ridge, a large fossa called the *submandibular fossa* contains the submaxillary gland.

Ramus

The mandibular ramus joins the body at an angle of 100 to 120 degrees. This angle is more obtuse in infants and elderly adults. Each broad, flat, quadrilateral ramus is composed of dense bone. Superiorly, the anterior border of each ramus terminates at the coronoid process where the tendon of the temporalis muscle inserts, and the posterior border of each ends at the condylar process that articulates with the temporomandibular joint. The crescent-shaped border of the ramus between the coronoid and condylar processes is known as the mandibular notch. The outer cortex of the ramus provides oblique ridges to which the strong masseter muscle inserts. On the medial surface of the ramus, the inferior alveolar nerve and vessels enter the mandibular canal through the mandibular foramen. Inferior to this opening, a small groove called the *mylohyoid groove* contains the mylohyoid nerve and vessels. The *lingula,* which is the site of attachment for the sphenomandibular ligament, projects upward from the anterior border of the mandibular foramen. This large ligament provides a clinical landmark for mandibular nerve blocks.[5]

Temporomandibular Joint

The temporomandibular joint is classified as a ginglymoarthrodial joint because of its gliding and hingelike actions. The articular surfaces, which are covered by fibrocartilage, include the ovoid-shaped head of the condyle and the concave mandibular, or glenoid, fossa of the temporal bone. Just anterior to the fossa is the articular eminence (Fig. 3). When the mouth opens widely, the condylar head glides over this structure, and if the mandible protrudes too far, the condylar head dislocates anterior to the eminence. An articulating disc of fibrocartilage, interposed between the articulating surfaces, divides the joint space into two separate cavities, upper and lower. The joint capsule that surrounds the disc and cavities consists of two layers, an outer fibrous layer and an inner synovial membrane. The membrane secretes synovia, which serves as a joint lubricant. The strong outer layer forms a capsular ligament attached superiorly to margins of the articular surface of the temporal bone and affixed inferiorly around the neck of the condyle. It also attaches around the entire circumference of the articular disc. The lateral aspect of the fibrous capsule forms the thick temporomandibular (lateral) ligament, which attaches superiorly to the zygomatic arch and inferiorly to the neck of the condyle. Two smaller ligaments associated with the joint include the sphenomandibular and stylomandibular ligaments. Also, upper fibers of the lateral pterygoid muscle attach to the capsule and to the anterior border of the articulating disc.

Muscles

Although 26 muscles attach to the mandible, most mandibular movements are produced by only

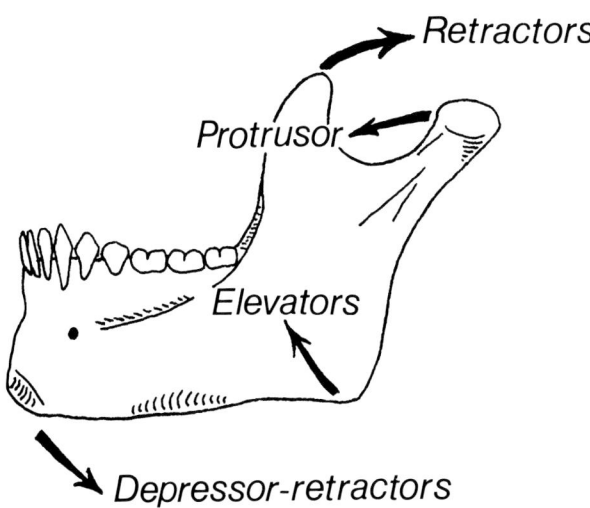

Figure 4. Four major muscle groups and their actions on the mandible. The pull of these muscles can distract the fragments of unfavorable fractures.

four muscle groups: depressor-retractors, protrusors, elevators, and retractors (Fig. 4). The pull of these muscles can either widely distract or enhance stabilization of fractured mandibular segments, depending on the direction of the fracture line. Therefore, thorough knowledge of the actions of these muscles is essential for the management of a mandibular fracture. The major muscles of mastication include the temporalis, masseter, medial pterygoid, and lateral pterygoid muscles, all of which are innervated by the mandibular division of the fifth cranial nerve.[6]

The masseter muscle has its origin on the zygomatic arch and its broad insertion on the outer aspect of the ramus. Strong tendonous attachments on the ramus provide splinting for fractures in this area. The masseteric nerve, a branch of the mandibular nerve, innervates the masseter muscle. The muscle's primary action is closure of the mouth. The parotid gland covers most of the masseter muscle, and its duct turns medially at the anterior edge of the muscle to enter the oral cavity.

The medial pterygoid muscle originates on the lateral plate of the pterygoid process and on the pyramidal process of the palatine bone. This muscle inserts on the lower half of the medial side of the ramus and angle of the mandible. Its action elevates the jaw by pulling upward, inward, and slightly forward.

The lateral pterygoid muscle attaches to the lateral surface of the lateral pterygoid plate by one head and to the infratemporal crest by another head. Its insertion is on the neck of the condyle and on the articular capsule and disc. The muscle protracts the mandible, allowing wide opening of the mouth.

The broad, fan-shaped temporal muscle originates on the side of the skull in the temporal fossa. Its strong tendon attaches to the coronoid process and medial side of the ramus, allowing this muscle to elevate and retract the mandible.

Dentition

There are 10 deciduous and 16 permanent mandibular teeth. Beginning at the midline, these teeth consist of medial and lateral incisors, a canine, two premolars, and three molars on each side. Each tooth has an enamel crown and a root composed of dentine. Molars have two roots, while all other teeth have single roots. Teeth are firmly secured to the alveolar periosteum (alveolar ligament) by cementum. The alveoli are lined by very dense bone, often called lamina dura. Each root has a central root canal, which transmits nerves and vessels into the dental pulp of the crown.

Primary functions performed by the teeth are mastication, articulation, and cosmesis. Dental occlusion is the interdigitation that occurs when the mandibular and maxillary teeth come together. Since good function depends on good occlusion, the restoration of normal occlusion following trauma is an important treatment objective. This will be covered in greater detail in later chapters.

Nerves and Vessels

The inferior alveolar and lingual nerves leave the mandibular branch of the trigeminal nerve just below the foramen ovale. Before entering the mandibular canal, the inferior alveolar nerve gives off the mylohyoid nerve, which supplies motor neurons to the mylohyoid muscle. As it courses through the canal, the inferior alveolar nerve innervates the teeth. One branch of this nerve, however, exits the canal at the mental foramen to supply sensory fibers to the lower lip and the labial gingiva. The buccal branch of the mandibular nerve innervates the buccal gingiva, while the lingual nerve supplies the lingual gingiva. Innervation to the temporomandibular joint comes from the auriculotemporal and masseteric nerves, both of which branch off from the mandibular nerve.

The main blood supply to the mandibular body and teeth comes from the inferior alveolar branch of the internal maxillary artery. This vessel joins the inferior alveolar nerve to enter the mandibular foramen on the medial side of the ramus. It also sends a mental branch through the mental foramen. Blood vessels in muscles that attach to the mandible also contribute significantly to the blood supply. The temporomandibular joint receives its vascular supply from several branches of the external carotid artery: the ascending pharyngeal, the superficial temporal, and the middle meningeal arteries. Anterior tympanic branches of the internal maxillary artery also supply the temporomandibular joint.

REFERENCES

1. Ham AW: Some histophysiological problems peculiar to calcified tissues. J Bone Joint Surg 34A:701–728, 1952
2. Heppenstall RB: Fracture healing. In Heppenstall RB (ed): Fracture Treatment and Healing. Philadelphia: WB Saunders, 1980, pp 35–64
3. Davies J: Embryology of the Head and Neck in Relation to the Practice of Otolaryngology—A Manual Prepared for the Use of Graduates in Medicine (Continuing Education Programs). Washington, DC: American Academy of Ophthalmology and Otolaryngology, 1957
4. Sperber GH (ed): Craniofacial Embryology, Ed. 2. Chicago: John Wright and Sons, Ltd. and Yearbook Medical Publishers, pp 110–120
5. Hollinshead WH: Anatomy of the jaws, teeth, and temporomandibular joint. In English GM (ed): Otolaryngology, Vol. 3. Philadelphia: Harper & Row, 1983
6. Dingman RO, Natvig P: The mandible. In Dingman RO, Natvig P (eds): Surgery of Facial Fractures. Philadelphia: WB Saunders 1964, pp 133–191

2 Principles of Bone Healing and Grafting

Charles M. Stiernberg, M.D.

Bone healing and bone grafting are similar processes because they both involve events that restore bone structure. The study of these two processes requires thorough knowledge of bone function. Generally, bone supports the human frame and provides a source of calcium. It also serves as an anchor for the origins and insertions of surrounding muscles and it protects vital soft tissue structures. The mandible, a dynamic facial bone, plays an active role in each of these functions. Fracture or extirpation of part or all of the mandible can lead to severe handicaps. The head and neck surgeon must understand bone healing to be able to restore structure and function of the mandible. Fortunately, bone resembles liver in its ability to undergo spontaneous regeneration.[1]

A patient's age and severity of injury influence the healing and grafting of bone. Although the surgeon has little control over these variables, certain principles of treatment can be applied to both bone healing and bone grafting to enhance the reparative process. These include coverage of bone with well-vascularized soft tissue, avoidance of contamination, reduction of bony fragments into their normal anatomic positions, and complete immobilization.

BONE HEALING

Similar to soft tissue, bone heals by primary or secondary intention. Primary intention healing of soft tissue wounds occurs when the defect is surgically closed and the wound edges are accurately approximated. Secondary intention healing occurs when the defect remains open and granulation tissue forms in the wound bed. This delays epithelial migration and coverage of the wound. A fundamental difference between healing of bone and all other tissues is the formation of new bone histologically the same as uninjured bone, rather than scar formation.

The mechanisms of bone formation should be reviewed before discussion of primary and secondary bone healing. Bone formation is either endochondral or membranous in nature. Endochondral bone formation occurs at the epiphyseal plate in long bones and accounts for growth. Embryologically, endochondral bone requires a preformed cartilage model that is gradually resorbed and replaced by new bone. The same sequence of events that occurs in endochondral bone formation has been described in fracture healing.[1] Membranous bone formation does not involve a cartilage model. Membranous bone forms when mesenchymal cells differentiate directly into osteoblasts, which lay down osteoid. This is followed by mineralization to form new bone. The mandible consists of both endochondral and membranous bone.

The principal bone cells involved in the process of bone healing are osteoblasts, osteocytes, and osteoclasts. Osteoblasts function primarily in matrix formation; osteoclasts are involved with bone resorption; and osteocytes function in both formation and destruction of bone. The origin of new osteoblasts is controversial, but they probably originate from fibroblasts, undifferentiated mesenchymal cells, and cells of the cambium layer of the periosteum and endosteum. Many investigators believe that periosteum contains osteogenic cells and participates in the formation of an external callus. For this reason, periosteum should be preserved during the surgical management of fractures. From his studies on bone resorption, Belanger concluded that normal resorption occurring in bone remodeling is mediated by the osteocyte, whereas pathologic resorption is mediated by the osteoclast.[2]

Three phases of bone healing are immediate reaction, reparation, and remodeling. The immediate reaction involves hematoma formation, inflammation, and induction of cells to form new bone. During the inflammatory stage, polymorphonucleocytes and monocytes debride the wound, and the fractured ends of bone undergo necrosis. During induction, cells in the periosteum, endosteum, and surrounding soft tissue are modulated to produce new osteoblasts. Although the stimulus for this modulation is unknown, it may be related to local hypoxia, acidic pH, lysosomal enzymes, or a bone morphogenic-stimulating substance as proposed by Urist.[3,4] During the reparative phase, callus formation distinguishes primary and secondary bone healing. A callus forms during secondary bone healing but not during primary bone healing. The final phase, remodeling, is a continuous process of bone resorption and deposition. This process also occurs in normal uninjured bone. Trabeculae gradually break down and new osteoid material is deposited in cancellous bone. In cortical bone, osteons (haversian canal systems) are remodeled by concentric resorption and deposition of bone around small blood vessels.[5]

Primary Bone Healing

Primary bone healing can be achieved only with absolute rigid fixation and precise anatomical alignment. Primary healing resembles normal bone remodeling except that it occurs across a fracture. Perren demonstrated that fractures treated by rigid internal fixation reveal evidence of primary bone healing without any sign of fibrous tissue or cartilage during the healing process. No evidence of external callus formation accompanies this type of treatment.[6]

Of the four distinct types of collagen, type 1 collagen is the most common and is found in bone, dermis, and fascia. Type 2 collagen is found only in cartilage and has been identified in the callus of fractures. When fractures are treated with compression plating, primary bone healing occurs and the collagen that forms is predominantly type 1.[1]

Secondary Bone Healing

Secondary bone healing occurs far more often than primary bone healing. It occurs when a gap exists between fracture fragments or when there is no rigid immobilization. Callus formation occurs in stages: a primary callus response, an external bridging callus, and a late medullary callus. The primary callus initially immobilizes the fracture. The external bridging callus forms a collar of osteogenic tissue around the fracture site that can be radiologically identified. The osteogenic cells of this callus are formed as a result of local humoral factors and, possibly, piezoelectric factors. The final stage involves a medullary callus by which cancellous bone heals. Medullary callus formation does not require preliminary cartilage formation, can bridge a fracture's gap, and will eventually replace fibrous tissue at the fracture site.[5]

Table 2–1. Graft Terminology*

Term	Donor
Autograft (autogenous)	Same individual
Homograft	Same species (live)
Alloimplant (allogenic)	Same species (dead)
Xenograft (heterograft)	Different species

*Alternative terms appear in parentheses.

BONE GRAFTING

Bone grafts are often classified according to the donor, and Table 2–1 lists terms used by head and neck and reconstructive surgeons. In addition to this classification system, bone grafts can be free or attached to a vascularized pedicle (Table 2–2). The blood supply to vascularized bone grafts is not disrupted, whereas the blood supply to revascularized bone grafts is disrupted but reconstituted by anastomosis to another vessel. Free grafts may be cancellous or cortical; mandibular defects can be reconstructed using either one or a combination of these two types. Metals, synthetic materials, and organic materials used to reconstruct the mandible are called *alloplastic implants.*

Understanding the histologic events of osseous repair by bone grafts enables the reconstructive surgeon to take steps to achieve a successful result. A bone graft undergoes the same initial processes as does fracture healing. Early stages for cortical and cancellous grafts are similar, but later stages differ considerably. Edema, inflammation, and necrosis of bone characterize the first stages. Necrotic tissue in the haversian canals and marrow spaces is removed by invading macrophages. An ingrowth of granulation, consisting of minute capillaries and primitive mesenchymal tissue, replaces the areas of resorption. This stage ends after 2 weeks. In cancellous grafts, the primitive mesenchymal cells differentiate rapidly into osteogenic cells. Osteoid is deposited along the edges of dead trabeculae. The necrotic bone is resorbed gradually through osteoclastic activity. Active new marrow cells fill the old marrow spaces to complete the reparative

Table 2–2. Types of Mandibular Bone Grafts

I. Free bone grafts.
   A. Cancellous bone and marrow.
   B. Combined cortical and cancellous bone.
      1. Iliac bone.
      2. Split rib.
II. Vascularized bone grafts.
   A. Pectoralis osteomyocutaneous.
   B. Trapezius osteomyocutaneous.
   C. Sternocleidomastoid-clavicular graft.
III. Revascularized bone grafts.
   A. Compound groin (iliac bone) flap.
   B. Compound scapular flap.

process. Cortical bone grafts take much longer to heal than do cancellous grafts. Osteoclastic resorption gradually converts the haversian canals of cortical bone into small marrow spaces, filled by invading granulation tissue and mesenchymal cells. Resorption of cortical bone grafts can be seen radiographically during this period. Finally, osteoblasts produce new osteoid tissue; the periphery of cortical bone is replaced faster than inner portions because the process does not occur at a uniform rate. Cortical bone grafts have been shown to be weaker than cancellous bone grafts for at least 1 year.[7]

Intraoperatively, the surgeon should not delay transfer of a bone graft to the recipient site. Prolonged exposure to the atmosphere decreases the number of viable cells in the graft. The recipient site should always be prepared before the bone graft is harvested. This sequence allows the procedure to be aborted if the oral cavity is inadvertently entered. If there is a delay after the graft is taken, it should be wrapped in a sponge soaked with the patient's blood. Soaking a bone graft in an antibiotic solution is unnecessary and can be detrimental to cell survival. Grafts should have maximum exposure to well-vascularized soft tissue. Dead space in the recipient site should be eliminated as much as possible. If a combined cortical and cancellous graft is used, the cancellous surface should be oriented toward the greatest vascular supply. Better results are also obtained when bone grafts are delayed rather than inserted immediately after tumor ablation. This avoids hematomas and excess dead space.[7]

The success of any bone graft depends greatly upon well-vascularized soft tissue coverage and a sterile recipient bed. Patients whose vascularity has been compromised by radiotherapy in the mandibular area are poor candidates for free bone grafts. In such cases, hyperbaric oxygen (HBO) has improved the success rate for the grafts. Marx and Ames reported a 91.6% success rate with a protocol using 30 h of preoperative HBO and 15 h of postoperative HBO in 12 patients who had received 5,500 to 7,200 rad of radiotherapy.[8] Each session used 100% oxygen for 1.5 h at 2.4 atmospheres absolute pressure. Marx and Ames used as their criteria for success (1) restoration of mandibular continuity, (2) restoration of alveolar bone height, (3) elimination of soft tissue deficiencies, (4) restoration of adequate osseous bulk, (5) maintenance of osseous quantity under function over time (18 months), and (6) restoration of acceptable facial form. With HBO, high-intermittent oxygen tension levels cause neovascularization and fibroblastic stimulation in hypoxic tissue. Fibroblasts that are otherwise suppressed in a hypoxic state begin to produce collagen, which forms the framework for the ingrowth of new capillaries.

Immobilization of the graft and remaining mandible is equally important. Choice of a fixation device depends on the type of bone graft and the presence or absence of teeth. External biphasic splints are often used for endentulous patients; intermaxillary fixation is used for patients who have enough teeth to stabilize the graft with proximal and distal mandibular segments.

Bone grafting is commonly performed today for treatment of delayed unions, nonunions, and osseous defects due to trauma or cancer surgery. Numerous methods have been developed to reconstruct mandibular defects with bone grafts. Some of these include particulate cancellous bone and marrow crib grafts, cancellous cortical grafts with dynamic bendable plates, split-rib grafts, osteomyocutaneous grafts, and cortical autografts that have been frozen or irradiated (see Table 2–2). In a landmark study, Blocker and Stout reviewed over one hundred cases of mandibular bone grafts performed during World War II. They concluded that any type of autogenous bone graft was satisfactory for reconstruction of small defects, but the use of large amounts of cancellous bone was superior for reconstruction of large defects.[9] Other studies have verified the superiority of cancellous bone grafts over cortical bone grafts. Boyne found that particulate cancellous grafts have an open structure that allows early ingress of tissue fluids and later penetration of capillaries.[10] Two donor sites for cancellous autografts are iliac bone and rib. Iliac bone can provide more cancellous bone but results in increased morbidity postoperatively with localized pain and a compromised gait from muscle spasm. An advantage of the rib donor site is its capability for bone regeneration, especially if some of the periosteum is preserved at the donor site.

SUMMARY

Adherence to the principles of bone healing and grafting enables the head and neck surgeon to restore mandibular continuity. These principles call for rigid fixation, a well-vascularized soft-tissue environment, and avoidance of contamination to enhance the probability of healing in patients with mandibular fracture or bone graft. Other factors include patient age and nutritional status, site and extent of injury, and history of radiation therapy in the mandibular area. Hyperbaric oxygen treatments improve the success rate of bone grafts in patients who have been irradiated. The three types of mandibular bone grafts are free, vascularized, and revascularized grafts. Vascularized and revascularized bone grafts maintain their own blood vessels and can be performed at the time of tumor resection. Free bone grafts with cancellous and cortical bone are best done as secondary procedures. Regardless of the type of graft used, objectives of mandibular reconstruction should include (1) restoration of bony continuity, (2) restoration of normal speech, (3) restoration of acceptable cosmetic appearance, and (4) restoration of normal mastication.

REFERENCES

1. Heppenstall RB: Fracture healing. In Heppenstall RB (ed): Fracture Treatment and Healing. Philadelphia: WB Saunders, 1980, pp 35–64
2. Belanger LF: In Bourne G (ed): Biochemistry and Physiology of Bone, Vol. 3, Ed. 2. New York: Academic Press, 1971, pp 239–270
3. Urist MR: Osteoinduction in undermineralized bone implants modified by chemical inhibitors endogenous matrix enzymes. Clin Orthop 87:132–137, 1972
4. Urist MR, Mikulski AJ, Boyd SD: A chemosterilized antigen extracted bone morphogenetic alloimplant. Arch Surg 110:416–428, 1975
5. Mattox DE: Bone healing and grafting. Ear Nose Throat J 62:409–411, 1983
6. Perren SM, Huggler A, Russenbereger M: The reaction of cortical bone to compression. Acta Orthop Scand (Suppl) 125:19–29, 1969
7. Heppenstall RB: Bone grafting in fracture treatment and healing. In Heppenstall RB (ed): Fracture Treatment and Healing. Philadelphia: WB Saunders, 1980, pp 97–112
8. Marx RE, Ames JR: The use of hyperbaric oxygen in bony reconstruction of the irradiated and tissue-deficient patient. J Oral Maxillofac Surg 40:412–420, 1982
9. Blocker TG, Stout RA: Mandibular reconstruction: World War II. Plastic Reconstr Surg 4:153–156, 1949
10. Boyne PJ: Autogenous cancellous bone marrow transplants. Clin Orthop 73:199–209, 1970

3 Mandibular Osteotomy

Byron J. Bailey, M.D., F.A.C.S.

The term "mandibular osteotomy" refers to surgical procedures that cut into or through the mandible. Surgical instruments, procedures, and indications for mandibular osteotomy vary widely. We shall summarize much of this information in this chapter as we discuss the types and techniques of mandibular osteotomies and review the issues that are important in the postoperative period.

Historically, Roux (1836) has been credited as being the first surgeon to divide the lower lip and jaw in the midline to gain surgical access to the tongue and the floor of the mouth. Sedilot (1844) improved upon the simple vertical midline transection; he divided the symphysis with a dovetail-shaped cut and added postoperative fixation of the two fragments using a custom-made gold plate and silk sutures that were anchored between the teeth. By 1902, Kocher was recommending Sedilot's operative approach for all but the smallest of tongue tumors. During this century, surgical access to cancer involving the oral cavity and oropharynx has continued to be the primary indication for mandibular osteotomy.

Bilroth (1862) was credited with the first resection of the mandible. The mandibular specimen that he described extended from the right canine tooth to the region of the left molar teeth.[1] Later, as the concept of "en bloc" resection of the oral cavity primary, adjacent mandible, and radical neck dissection specimen achieved widespread acceptance, some controversy arose over the precise indications for mandibular osteotomy versus mandibular segmental resection.

During the first two-thirds of this century, the manner in which surgeons employed osteotomy varied considerably. Some surgeons preferred anterior osteotomy for anterior oral cavity lesions and posterior (adjacent to the angle) osteotomy for lesions involving the tonsil and posterior tongue. Other surgeons held that primary tumors that were not attached to the mandible could be managed by intraoral operative procedures. More recently, we have seen a period marked by excessive concern regarding the possibility of tumor cells in the lymphatics of the mandibular periosteum; as a consequence, segmental resection may have been employed more often than necessary and even routinely in some institutions. Marchetta[2] demonstrated that unless the tumor is immediately adjacent to the mandible, there is less cause for concern about invasion of the mandibular periosteum in patients with oral cavity cancer. Newer techniques are available for reconstruction of the oral cavity, and *segmental resection* is seldom needed for surgical access, tumor exposure, or postoperative wound closure.

Trotter[3] was one of the first surgeons (1920) to popularize osteotomy rather than segmental resection for oral cavity and pharyngeal cancer surgery. He observed the possibility of performing a midline mandibular osteotomy and then incising along the lateral marginal gutter in the floor of the mouth so as to gain access to the base of the tongue and pharynx. He noted that this approach was associated with less morbidity and that it afforded good access, visibility for surgical procedure, and good long-term function. Many others have come to the same conclusion, and base the decision to preserve the mandible on the following factors:

1. Absence of tumor fixation to the mandible on physical examination.
2. Absence of x-ray or scintiscan evidence of bone involvement.
3. Absence of frozen section confirmation of tumor in the mandibular periosteum at the time of surgery.
4. Absence of mandibular involvement in patients with T1 and T2 lesions.
5. Compatibility of osteotomy with preoperative and postoperative radiation therapy.
6. Preservation of the important chewing, swallowing, and articulatory functions that may be lost with segmental resection.

RATIONALE FOR MANDIBULAR OSTEOTOMY

Mandibular osteotomy has become a popular surgical procedure because of its usefulness in gaining access to deeper structures, removing diseased tissue adjacent to the mandible, and preserving maximum mandibular function and facial appearance. Osteotomy near the angle or in the midline can provide access for the surgeon to resect various oral cancers, to remove deep lobe parotid and parapharyngeal space tumors, and to perform a variety of skull base vascular and tumor surgical procedures. The osteotomy offers numerous advantages over intraoral resection of malignant neoplasms, particularly for larger lesions and for those tumors encroaching upon the mandible. The procedure carries much less morbidity than segmental resection of the mandible and is strongly preferred to segmental resection for surgical access or as a necessary portion of the reconstruction and closure.

Median mandibulotomy and the "mandibular swing" procedure described by Shumrick[4] and popularized by Strong and Spiro[1] have been the subject of a great deal of surgical interest during the past decade. Proponents consider the midline approach advantageous to a lateral approach for most oral cavity tumors that do not invade the mandible. They base this preference on the observation that this approach achieves mandibular stabilization and solid osseous union more readily and with less morbidity.

Other surgeons prefer the lateral osteotomy, usually performed at the junction of the posterior body and the angle of the mandible, for access to posterior oral cavity and tonsil tumors. DeSanto[7] reports a dramatic increase in the tendency to substitute osteotomy for segmental mandibular resection at the Mayo Clinic. The rationale for the decision to preserve the mandible is based on several variables: the absence of roentgenographic evidence of bone involvement; the absence of tumor involvement of the periosteum (preoperative clinical impression); frozen section analysis showing no evidence of tumor in the mandibular periosteum at the time of surgery; and the statistical probability that T1, T2, and some small T3 lesions will be treated successfully by this approach. The experience at Mayo Clinic has paralleled a national movement away from segmental mandibular resection and toward marginal resection and osteotomy without bone sacrifice.

Osteotomy is also a valuable technique for mandibular mobilization and repositioning to correct traumatic and congenital deformities. When a malalignment follows mandibular fracture, osteotomy becomes a step either in recreating the injury at the same fracture site or in performing vertical sagittal osteotomies in the region of the ramus to permit repositioning of the entire mandibular arch, a procedure most often associated with complications after condylar neck fractures. Orthognathic surgery, dealt with in other chapters in this book, is based on the concept of osteotomy, mobilization, and repositioning of major mandibular segments.

OSTEOTOMY TECHNIQUES

General Principles

A common set of principles should be observed whether the surgeon employs a mallet and osteotome, a Gigli saw, or a powered sagittal saw to accomplish mandibular osteotomy. The site for osteotomy and the surgical approach to this site should be selected so as to limit the injury to vascular and neural structures that pass near and through the mandible. Design of geometric pattern of the osteotomy, the marginal resection, or the segmental resection must be consistent with requirements for postoperative stabilization and healing and with consideration of the mechanical forces that will be acting on the mandible postoperatively. Flaps, grafts, and even the healing of the simple local soft tissue closure should be considered in designing the surgical defect. For example, sharp bone edges, instability in the fixation of fragments, and the contouring and fixation of bolsters all can influence the outcome of the repair, thereby determining whether or not the postoperative period will be prolonged by complications.

Osteotomy should be accomplished without injury to adjacent soft tissue by steps that provide control of the mandibular segments and the osteotomy instruments. Careful retraction and protection of soft tissue by the use of appropriate factors is a fundamental precaution.

Anterior Mandibular Osteotomy

Osteotomy in the region of the mentum or symphysis provides a suitable surgical approach for anterior and posterior oral cavity lesions. Most of the early malignant tumors of the oral cavity will be cured by local excision or radiation therapy. When tumors have advanced to the large T2 or T3 size or when they are beginning to encroach upon the mandible, some form of cervical lymph node resection, either radical neck dissection or a modified dissection, will probably be considered. This portion of the procedure is performed first, from inferiorly to superiorly; when the surgeon reaches the inferior margin of the mandible, a midline osteotomy is performed. This can be accomplished in either a straight vertical cut, a step-cut, or a dovetail geometric configuration (Figures 5 to 7). The mandible is exposed and the periosteum is

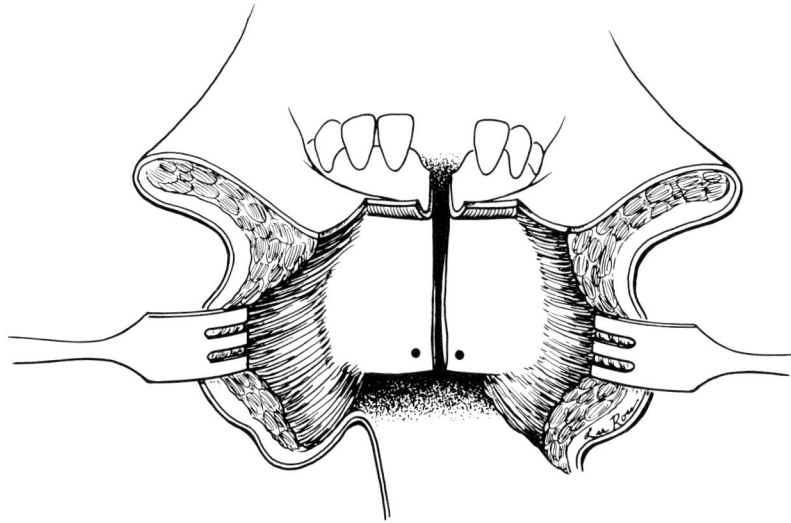

Figure 5. Anterior mandibular osteotomy; straight vertical bone cut.

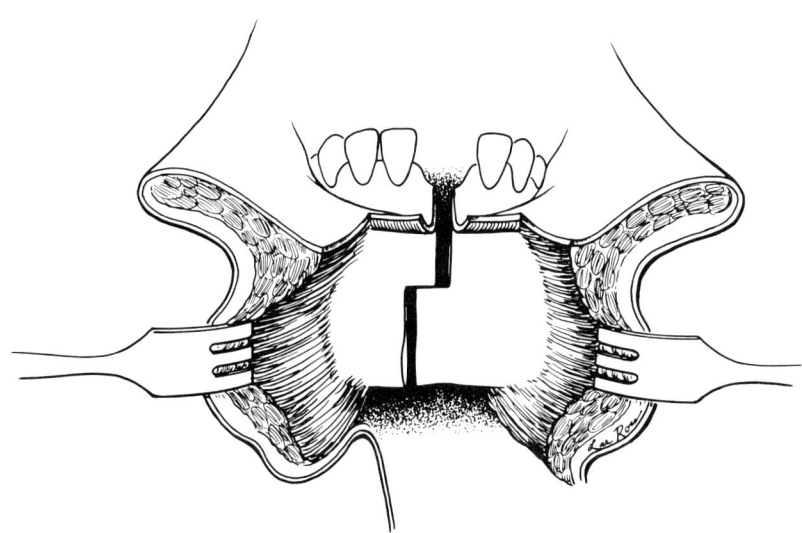

Figure 6. Anterior osteotomy; step cut through the socket of a single central incisor.

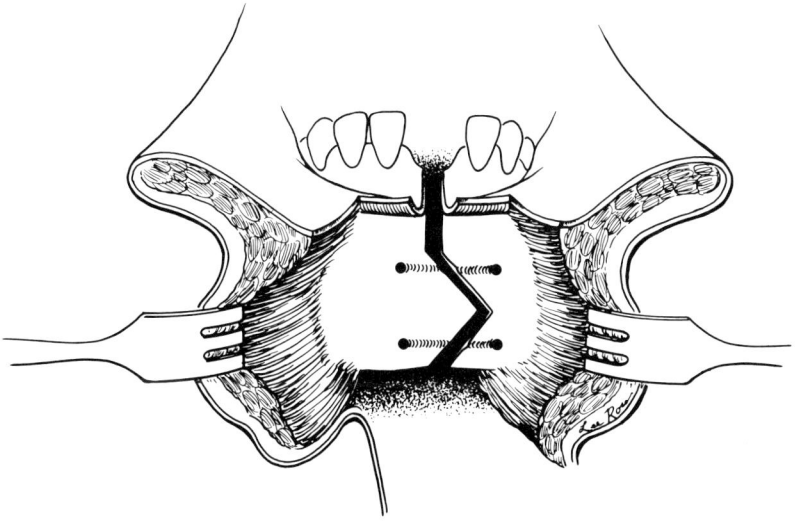

Figure 7. Anterior dove-tail osteotomy.

elevated in a manner that treats the periosteal tissues gently, avoids unnecessary elevation of the tissues of the labial-buccal surface of the mandible, and avoids traumatizing the mental nerve, the marginal branch of the facial nerve, and the muscles of the floor of the mouth. Removal of at least one central canine tooth in the region of the osteotomy so as to avoid the inadvertent late postoperative loss of two teeth is usually desirable.

The mandible can be divided with osteotomes or with the Gigli saw, but more precise cuts can be made with a powered sagittal osteotome. The floor of the mouth is dissected away from the mandible and gingiva; this incision line is extended as far posteriorly as is required by the location of the primary lesion. Alternatively, if the lesion is located more centrally in the base of the tongue, the tongue can be divided in the midline from the tip toward the base to gain exposure for ressection.

In those patients with tumors encroaching upon the mandible, careful dissection and sequential frozen section biopsy analysis will permit a determination of whether or not the mandible has been invaded. An example of this form of approach as described recently by Spiro and colleagues[1] is shown in Figures 8 to 10.

Posterior Osteotomy

Some surgeons prefer to approach primary lesions arising posteriorly in the oral cavity or in the

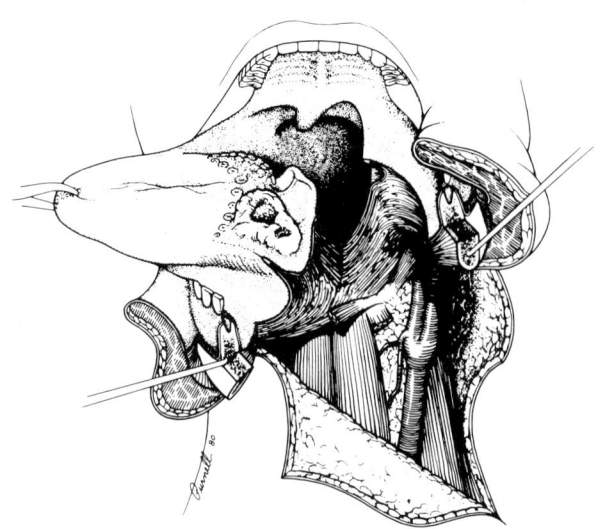

Figure 9. The paralingual incision has been extended posteriorly across the glossopalatine fold and down the lateral pharyngeal wall to expose a tumor in the base of the tongue. The hyoid bone and portions of the supraglottic larynx can be included with the specimen when necessary. (From Spiro R.H. et al.: Head Neck Surg 3:373, 1981. With permission.)

oropharynx by way of an osteotomy sited near the junction of the posterior body and the angle of the mandible. Again, the first portion of this operative sequence usually involves some form of neck dissection; when the inferior margin of the mandible is reached, the periosteum is elevated from its lingual and buccal surfaces. Periosteal elevation is usually more extensive than for anterior osteotomies (Fig. 11 to 14).

The osteotomy incision can be in the configuration of a stairstep or can be V-shaped with the point directed posterioraly (Figures 15 and 16). Retraction of the proximal and distal fragments permits visualization and surgical access for the subsequent resection of tumors on the base of the tongue and the tonsil.

Baker and Conley[5] prefer the V-shaped posterior mandibular osteotomy, finding that it facilitates the surgical excision of deep lobe tumors of the parotid (see Fig. 8). Most surgeons agree with Doyle[6] that tumors of the deep lobe of the parotid gland, including most tumors with retromandibular extension, can be excised usually without mandibular osteotomy. Even those tumors with extensive intraoral presentation can be displaced inferiorly and removed utilizing an approach from below. However, every rule has its exceptions and if the deep, retromandibular portion of the tumor extends into the nasopharynx, blunt dissection is inadvisable. In such cases, the lack of access and visibility should be overcome by proceeding with posterior mandibular osteotomy, reflection of the proximal segment laterally, and resection of the deep lobe

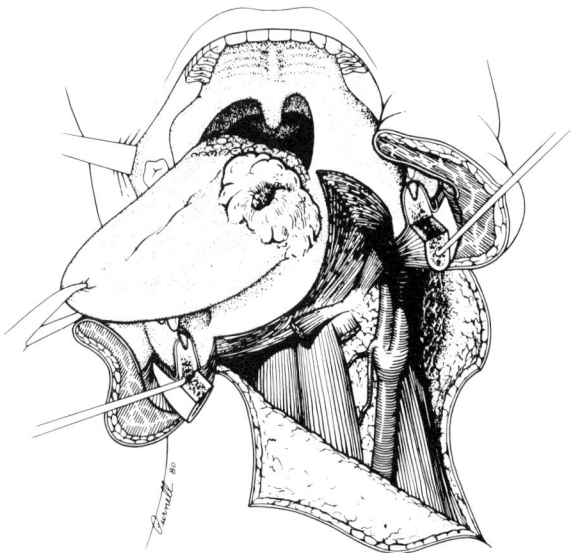

Figure 8. Once the mandible is transected, the incision is carried posteriorly in the floor of the mouth, usually dividing the mylohyoid muscle and the anterior belly of the digastric. The cut ends of the mandible are retracted laterally to expose a tumor involving the oral tongue. (From Spiro R.H. et al.: Head Neck Surg 3:373, 1981. With permission.)

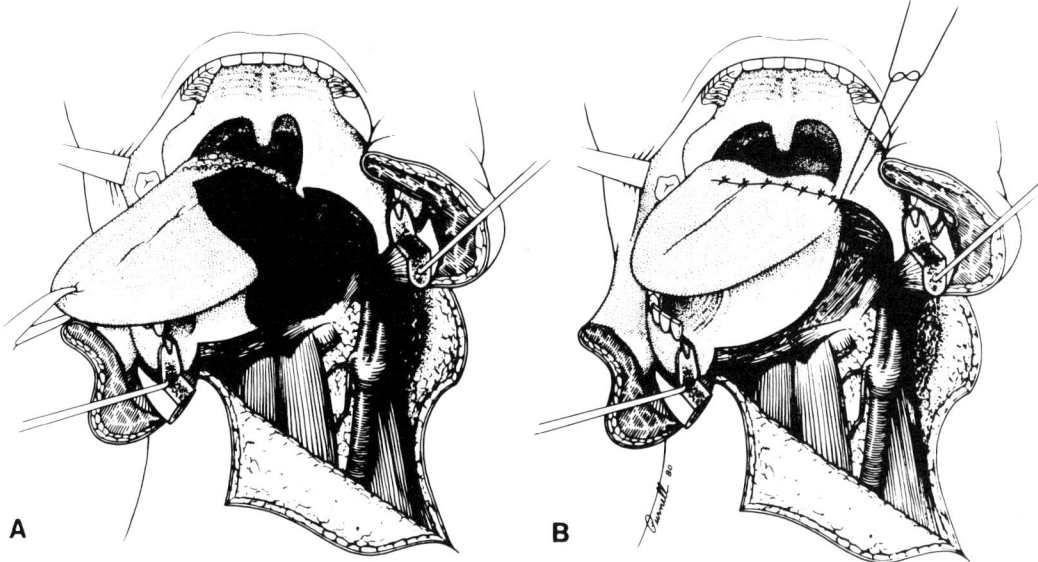

Figure 10. (A) This illustration shows the defect remaining when a tongue lesion is wedge-resected with the axis oriented transversely. (B) The defect is closed with interrupted sutures, after the remaining oral tongue is displaced posteriorly.

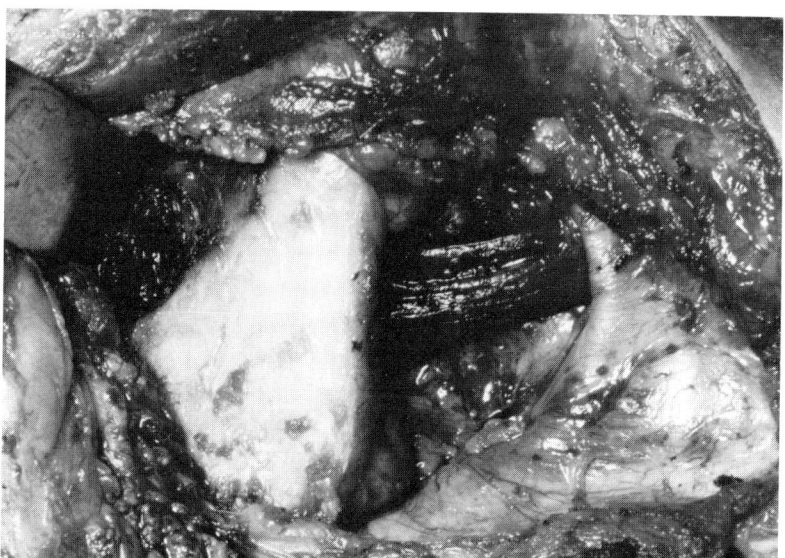

Figure 11. Site of posterior osteotomy for access and exposure of tumor of the tongue.

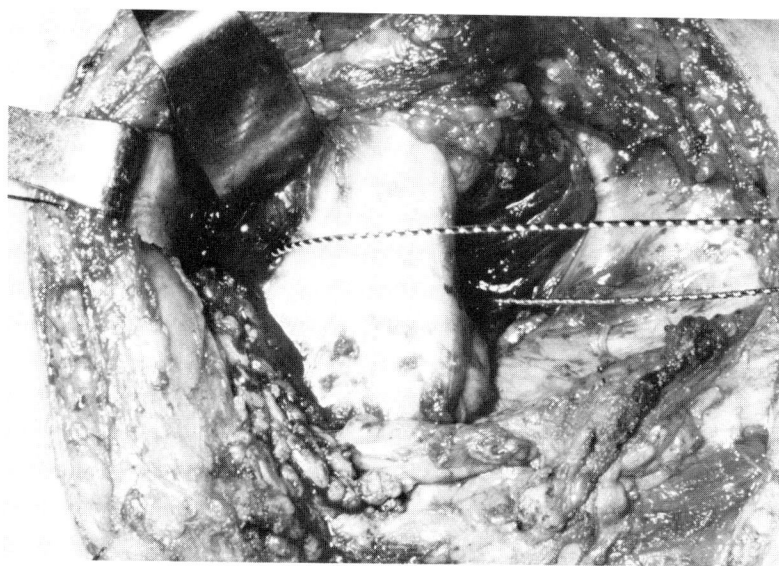

Figure 12. Osteotomy using the Gigli saw.

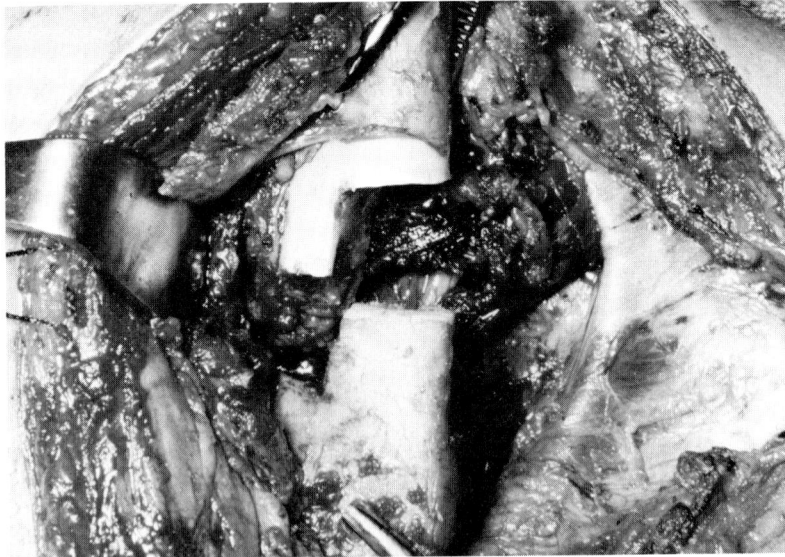

Figure 13. Step cut posterior osteotomy.

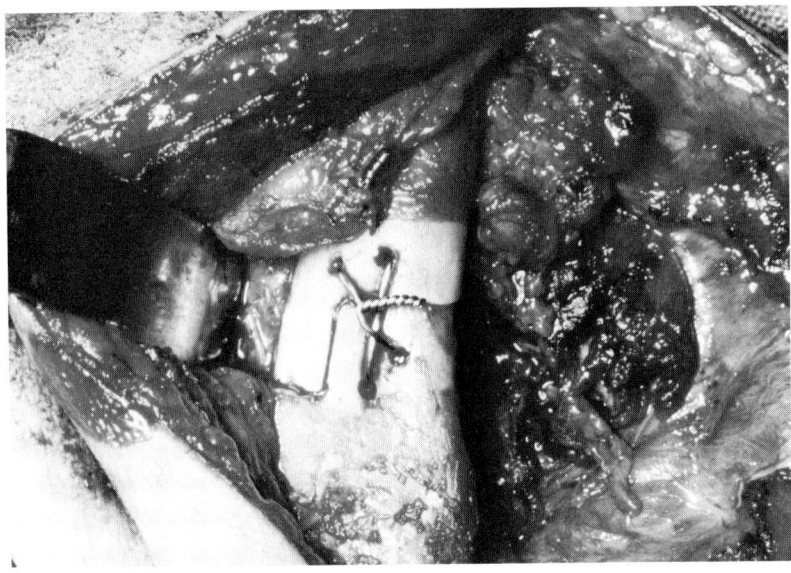

Figure 14. Closure and stabilization of the osteotomy site using 25 gauge stainless steel wire.

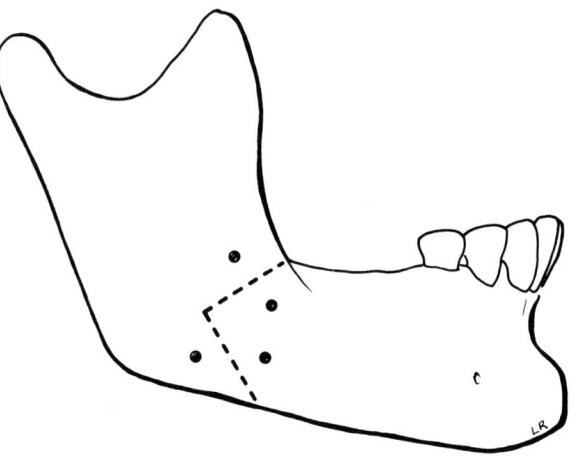

Figure 15. Mandibulotomy site exposed and V-shaped osteotomy cuts made.

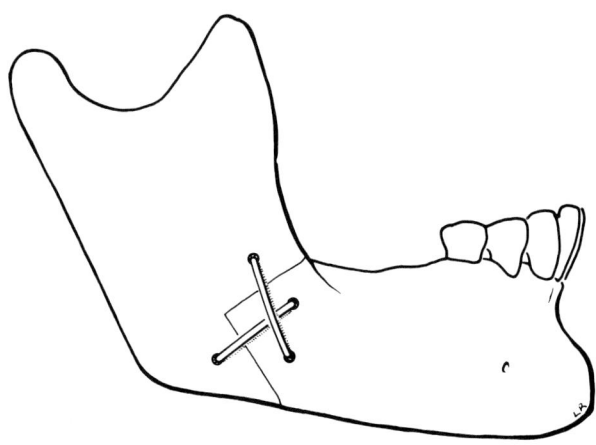

Figure 16. Figure 8 wire for stabilization.

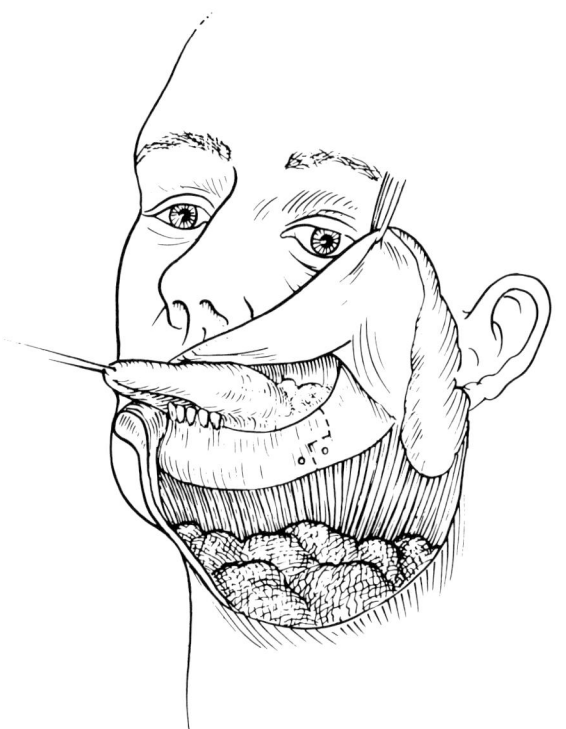

Figure 17. Stepped osteotomy incision at or near the plane of circumvallate papillae. (From DeSanto LW et al.: Arch Otolaryngol 101:654, 1975. With permission.)

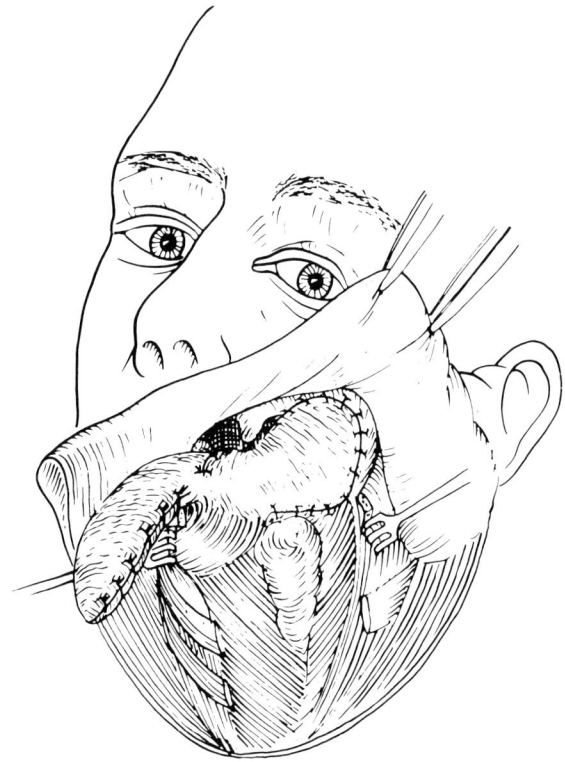

Figure 18. Laterally based tongue flap in position after unrolling free border of mobile anterior tongue and rotation of 180 degrees. (From DeSanto LW et al.: Arch Otolaryngol 101:654, 1975. With permission.)

tumor under direct vision so as not to injure the vascular and neural structures adjacent to the tumor.

Closure of the surgical defect occasionally can be accomplished by simple approximation of the wound edges. The point of concern, however, is that if this results in significant tethering of the tongue, associated functional problems with speech and swallowing will arise. In the event that primary closure would be problematic, a variety of options for reconstruction are available.

Tongue flap reconstruction techniques are gaining popularity because of their high degree of versatility and reliability. Each tongue flap must be designed carefully to sacrifice the minimum amount of normal tongue and to retain maximum tongue bulk and mobility. Despite the rich collateral and cross-circulation of the tongue, the flap must afford adequate arterial supply and venous drainage from the side contralateral to the resection because sacrifice of the ipsilateral lingual artery is frequently necessary. The description of this technique reported by DeSanto[7] provides more details of the operative sequence (Fig. 17 and 18).

Lateral Mandibulotomy

Recently, interest has been rekindled in the older concept of lateral mandibulotomy, generally a division of the mandible just anterior to the mental foramen. Either a step-cut as shown in Figures 19 and 20 and described by Dichtel and co-workers[8] or a vertical transection as proposed by McGregor and MacDonald[9] may be used (Fig. 21). This location has the advantage of avoiding injury and transection of the genioglossus, geniohyoid, and digastric muscles. Placement of the osteotomy just anterior to the mental foramen preserves the sensory innervation of the lower lip and chin, if appropriate care is taken not to traumatize the mental nerve.

The exposure from this approach affords adequate access to the mid and posterior oral cavity, the tonsil, oropharynx, and the parapharyngeal space. The proximal mandibular segment is retracted laterally, and dissection posteriorly along the mandible will provide access to the neurovascular structures in the neck. Dichtel used this approach to repair an injury to the internal carotid artery near the base of the skull and considered it useful for other skull base operations. The exposure is equivalent to that provided by osteotomy performed at the symphysis, and offers the added advantage of decreased morbidity avoiding the midline muscle complex in the floor of the mouth.

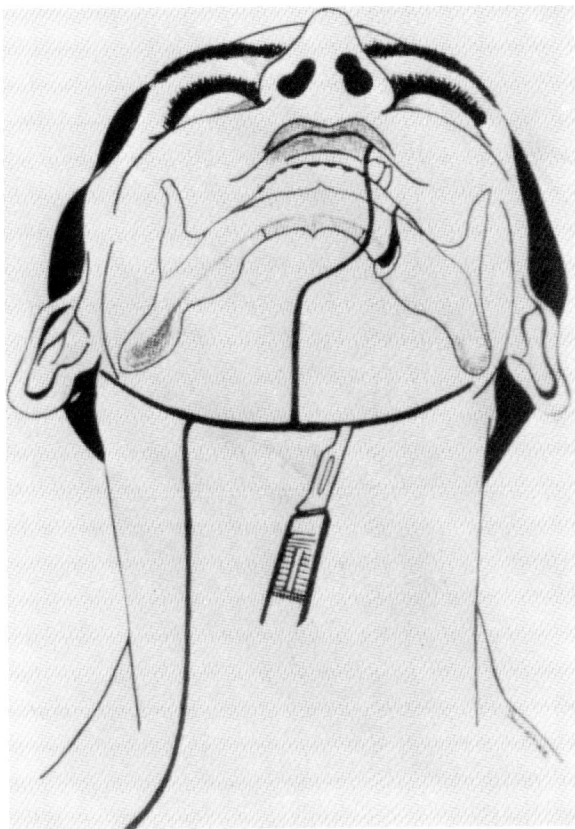

Figure 19. Lateral mandibulotomy is performed near the mental foramen with Gigli's saw. (From Mazzarella LA, Friedlander AA: Arch Otolaryngol 107:246, 1981. With permission.)

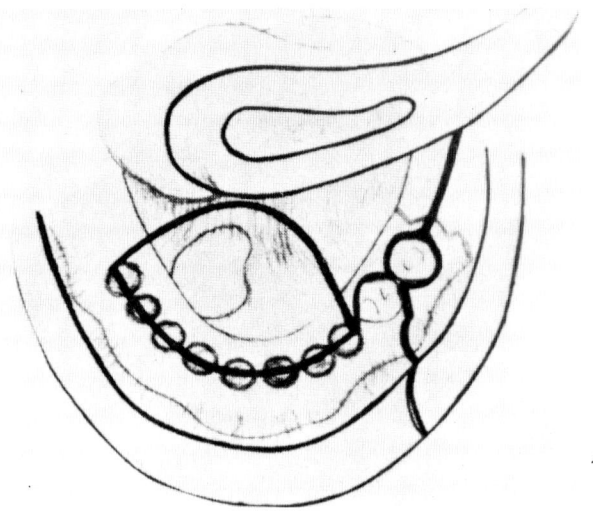

Figure 20. The digastric, mylohyoid, stylohyoid, and medial pterygoid muscles are divided. The lateral segment of the mandible is rotated upwards exposing the internal carotid artery at the skull base. (From Mazzarella LA, Friedlander AA: Arch Otolaryngol 107:246, 1981. With permission.)

Osteotomy with Marginal Resection

Carcinoma involving the mandibular alveolus is found commonly and accounts for as much as 10% of all oral malignancy in some series. Several issues regarding the management of this lesion remain

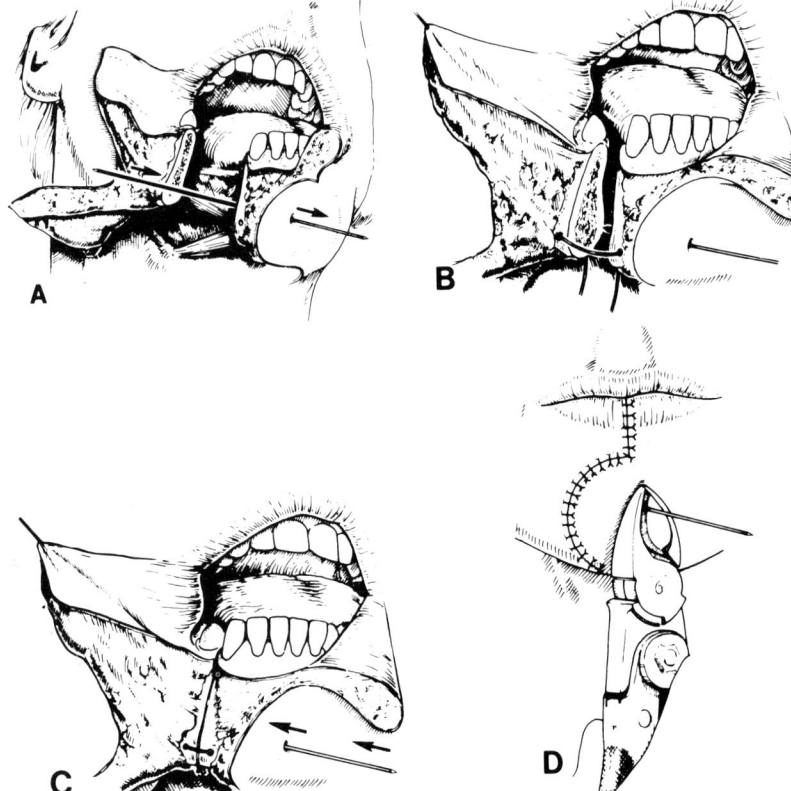

Figure 21. The use of transfixing K-wire together with direct wiring to stabilize the mandible reconstituted after osteotomy. (A) The K-wire being passed retrograde into the osteotomy site and emerging from the skin. (B) The K-wire just emerging from the bone at the osteotomy site and the direct wire inserted. (C) The bone ends held together by the direct wire and the K-wire ready to be driven across the osteotomy site to stabilize the bone. (D) The K-wire being cut, leaving the end palpable under the skin, capable of being removed subsequently if desired. (From McGregor IA, MacDonald DG: Head Neck Surg 5:459, 1985. With permission.)

controversial; the superiority of marginal versus segmental resection, the role of radiation therapy, assessment of bone invasion by tumor, and comparative studies dealing with these different issues. Wald and Calcaterra[10] note that the cure rate for alveolar ridge carcinoma increased markedly after World War II, when the problems of bone invasion were appreciated and prevailing modes of treatment underwent a transition from radiotherapy to surgery. For a while, the standard treatment consisted of en bloc resection of the primary, a segment of adjacent mandible, and radical neck dissection, with or without postoperative radiation therapy. Recently, marginal resection of the mandible has gained popularity. The technique of sagittal ostectomy for floor of mouth cancer[11] involves the en bloc removal of the primary tumor in continuity with a partial thickness of the adjacent mandible or mandibular cortex and a neck dissection specimen (Figs. 22 to 24). At least one-half of the thickness of the mandible is preserved; the objective is to leave sufficient structural support for postoperative function without interrupting the integrity of the mandibular arch. This may involve removing the superior one-half of the mandible for lesions that arise on the gingival surface. When the primary tumor arises in the floor of the mouth and adjacent to the mandible, it is sometimes more appropriate to remove an angled transection specimen for the anterior floor of the mouth or a lingual cortical specimen for the midportion of the floor of the mouth (Fig. 25). When a metastatic tumor in a lymph node adheres to the inferior margin of the mandible (usually in the region of the submandibular salivary gland or posteriorly near the angle), removal of the inferior one-half of the mandible may be appropriate.

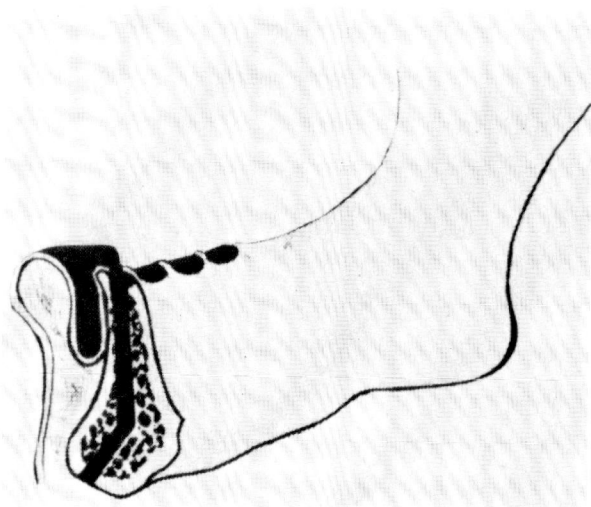

Figure 23. Angulation required to confine superior and inferior sagittal ostectomy cuts between medical and lateral cortical plates of alveolar and basal bone of mandible. (From Mazzarella LA, Friedlander AA: Arch Otolaryngol 107:247, 1981. With permission.)

Taking adequate care, the surgeon can usually preserve the neurovascular bundle within the mandible; this is important for the postoperative vitality of the distal mandibular tissue and teeth. Occasionally a question arises as to whether or not a sufficiently strong mandibular arch has been preserved. We have employed the use of reinforcing iliac crest or rib grafts to deal with this problem, as shown in Figure 26.

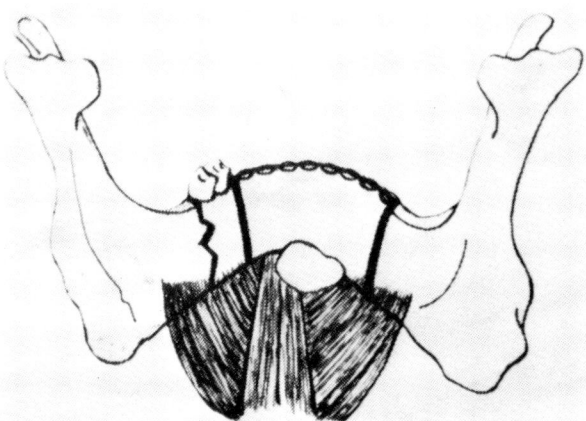

Figure 22. Relationship of alveolar ostectomy and medial ostectomies to surgical fracture site of mandible and floor of mouth. (From Mazzarella LA, Friedlander AA: Arch Otolaryngol 107:247, 1981. With permission.)

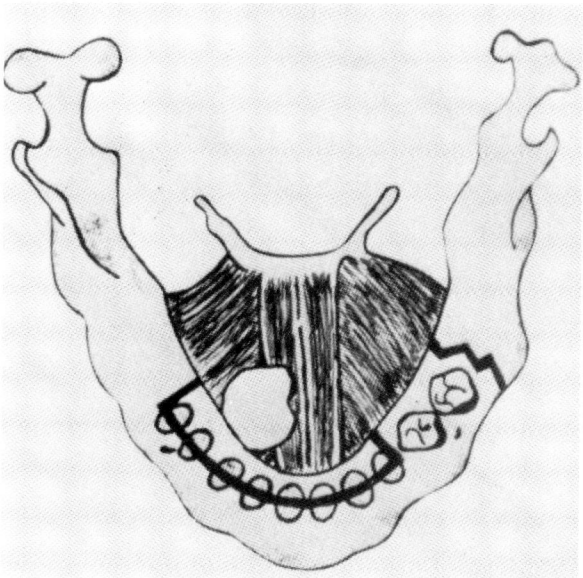

Figure 24. Medial ostectomy cuts and their relationship to alveolar sagittal ostectomy, surgical fracture site of mandible, and floor of mouth.

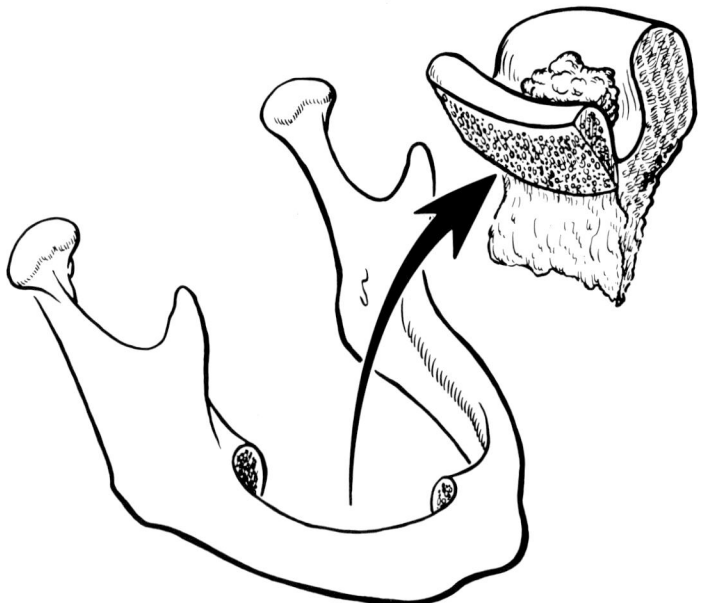

Figure 25. Marginal resection of mandible. Superior one-half of mandibular body may be resected for alveolar ridge malignancy.

Osteotomy for Surgery at the Base of the Skull

Gaining surgical access, visibility, and operating control of tumors (and other problems amenable to surgical management) is a challenge in the skull base region. Surgery in this region has advanced rapidly during the past decade, and a variety of transmandibular approaches have been devised.

One example of this type of approach is described in the report by Wood and colleagues[12] and is illustrated in Figures 27 to 37. Using this approach, the surgeon can biopsy or remove lesions of the clivus, cervicomedullary junction, or upper cervical vertebrae. The approach combines anterior mandibulotomy with a midline split of the tongue and palate.

Stabilization and Fixation of the Osteotomy Site

Considerable difference of opinion centers on the necessity for intermaxillary fixation or stabilization by externally applied metal plates. Spiessl and Tschopp[13] advocate the application of metal plates in most instances, but this is only beginning to gain popularity in the United States. Step-cut and V-shaped osteotomies often provide sufficient stability for postoperative stabilizations by direct interosseous wiring. Any evidence of instability, however, suggests the wisdom of applying dental arch bars and elastic band traction for intermaxillary fixation during the period of healing. The extra margin of safety and reassurance of healing in good position are usually worth the extra time that this

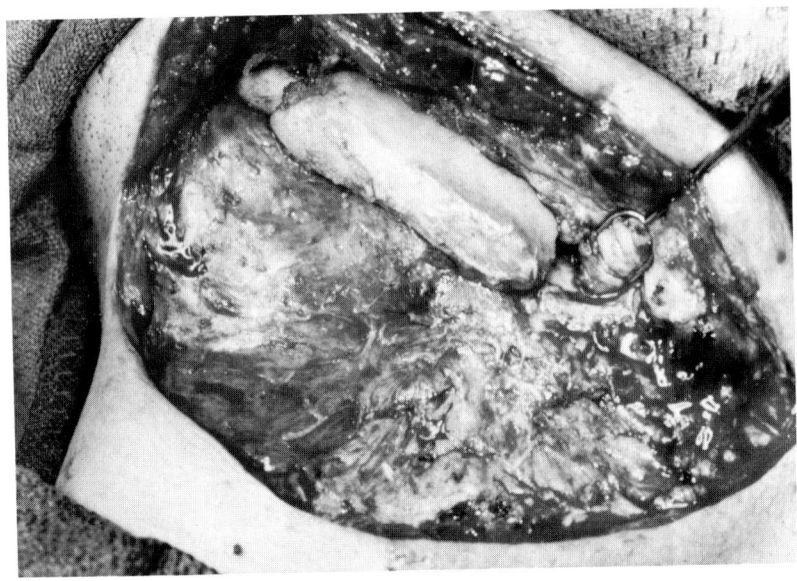

Figure 26. Reinforcing bone graft adjacent to the inferior margin of mandibular body subsequent to marginal resection of inferior half of mandible.

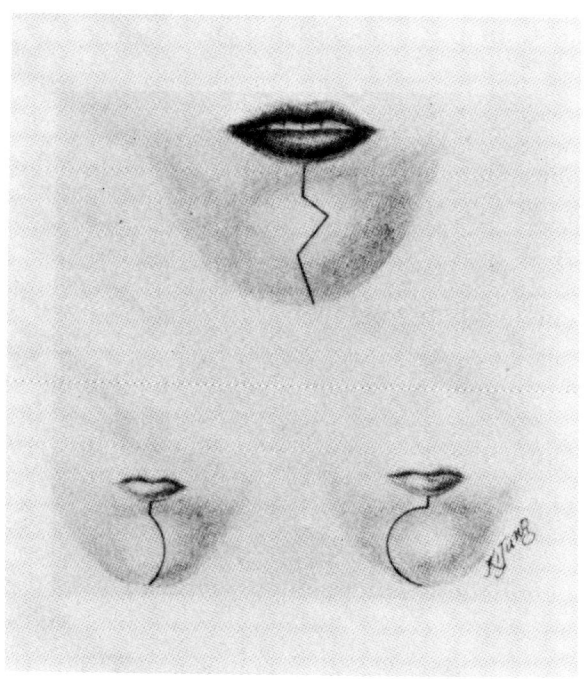

Figure 27. Various skin incisions. (From Wood BG, et al.: Arch Otolaryngol 106:2, 1980. With permission.)

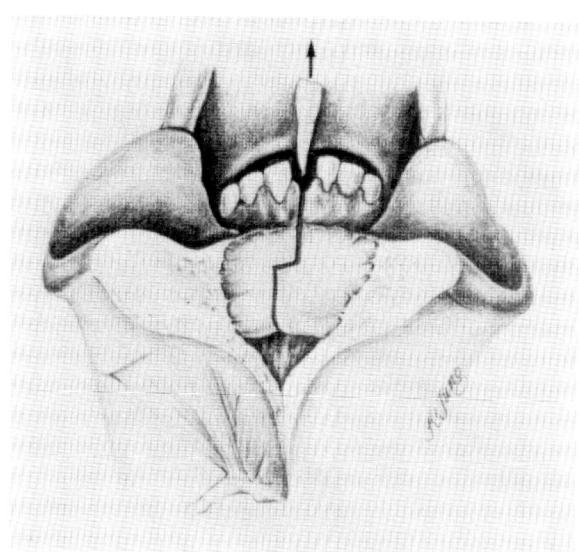

Figure 29. Step-like mandibular osteotomy, with removal of central incisor (arrow). (From Wood BG, et al.: Arch Otolaryngol 106:2, 1980. With permission.)

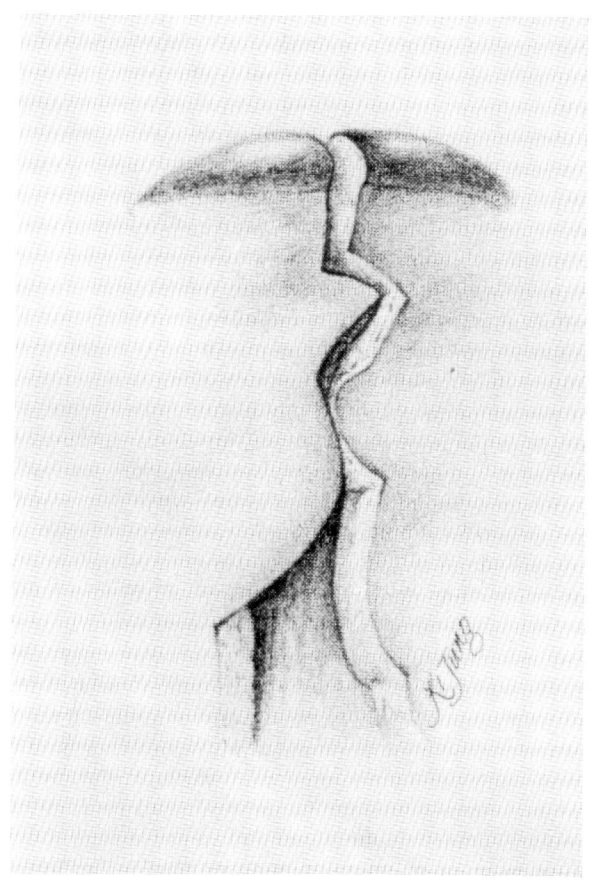

Figure 28. Lip-chin-submental incision completed. (From Wood BG, et al.: Arch Otolaryngol 106:2, 1980. With permission.)

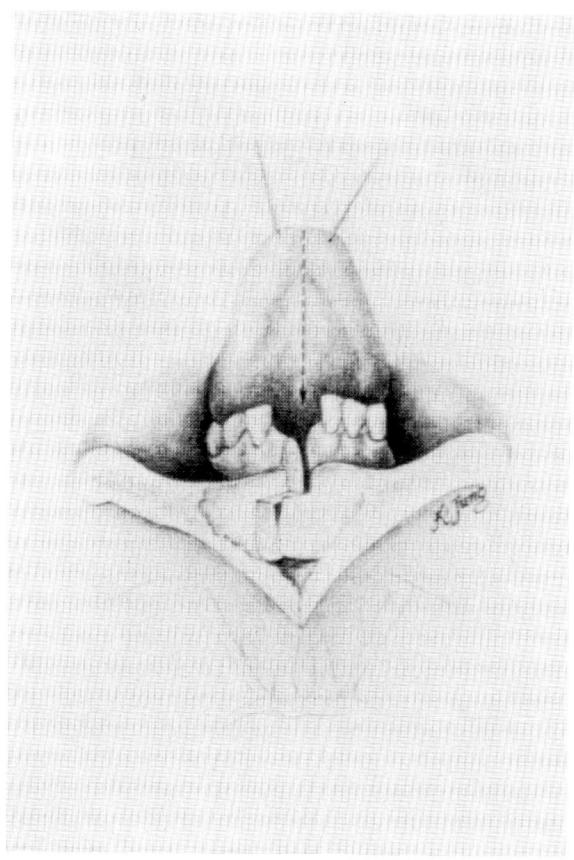

Figure 30. Entire tongue is incised in midline (arrow). (From Wood BG, et al.: Arch Otolaryngol 106:2, 1980. With permission.)

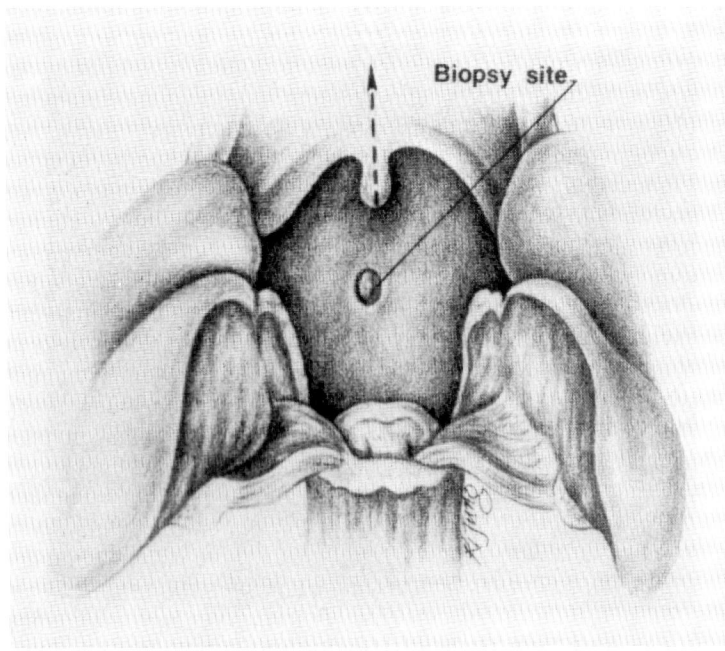

Figure 31. Mandibular-lingual halves are retracted and soft palate is split (arrow). (From Wood BG, et al.: Arch Otolaryngol 106:2, 1980. With permission.)

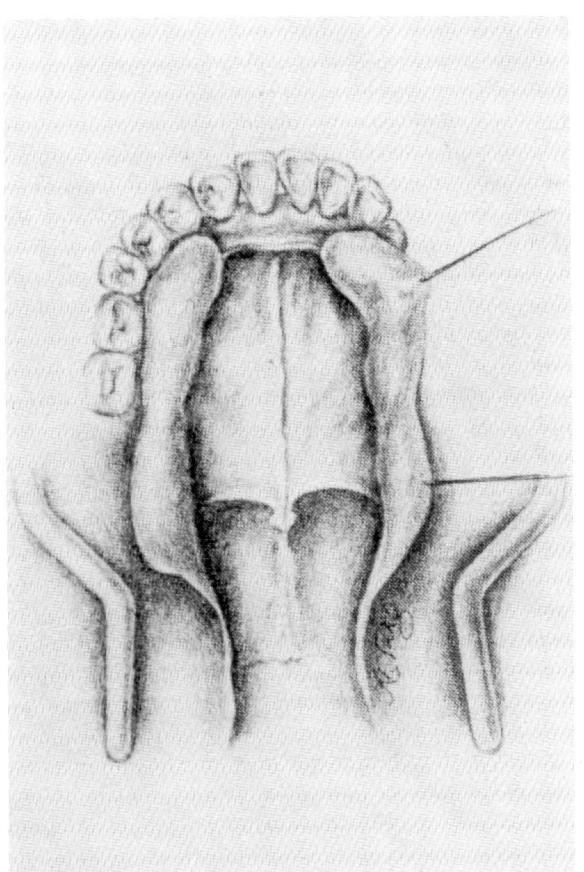

Figure 32. Bony palate flaps are elevated; soft palate is retracted and posterior vomer is visible. (From Wood BG, et al.: Arch Otolaryngol 106:2, 1980. With permission.)

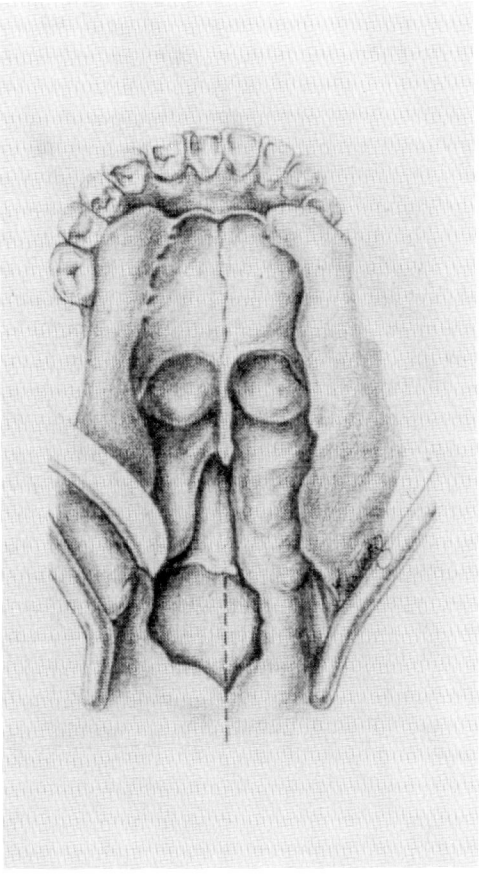

Figure 33. Posterior bony palate is removed; mucomuscular flaps are elevated in retropharyngeal space. (From Wood BG, et al.: Arch Otolaryngol 106:2, 1980. With permission.)

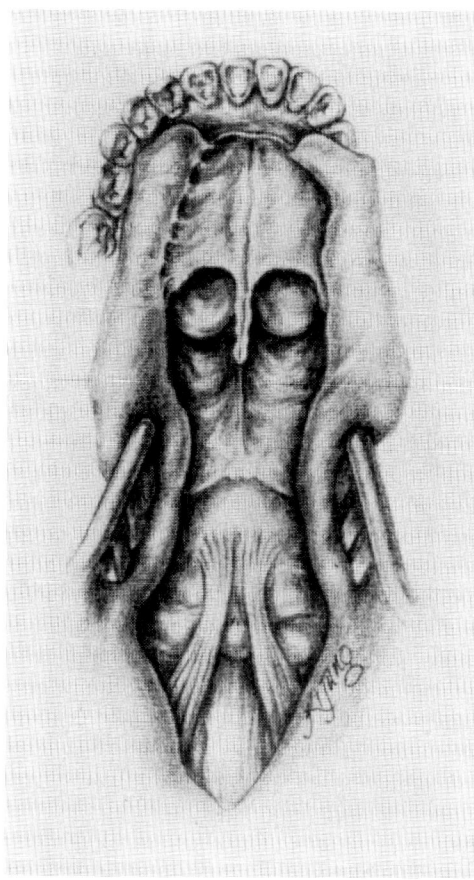

Figure 34. Ventral surface of clivus is exposed (no overlying soft tissue). (From Wood BG, et al.: Arch Otolaryngol 106:2, 1980. With permission.)

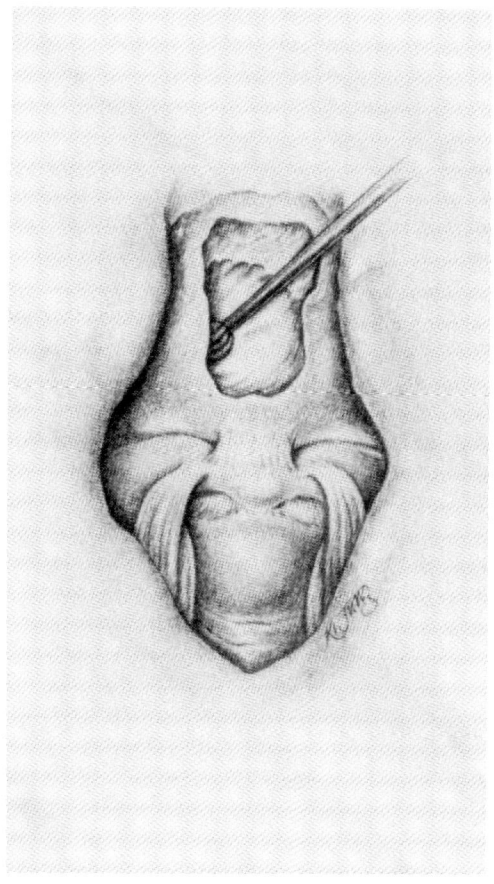

Figure 35. Removal of clivus, with exposure of dura covering brainstem. (From Wood BG, et al.: Arch Otolaryngol 106:2, 1980. With permission.)

step involves. Carroway and McGregor[14] are enthusiastic about mandibular fixation using a combination of K-wire and interosseous wire to stabilize the vertical midline symphyseal osteotomy. Their technique is similar to that illustrated in Figure 21.

COMPLICATIONS OF OSTEOTOMY

The major complications of osteotomy are similar to those of mandibular fractures. They include infection at the osteotomy site, delayed union, malunion, and nonunion. These complications may be avoided generally by appropriate alignment and stabilization of the mandibular segments and by the routine use of perioperative antibiotic therapy.

Occasional problems are prolonged pain and tenderness near the osteotomy site. Sataloff and Price[15] have reported the association of persistent pain with stylohyoid pain syndrome secondary to excessive tension or stretching of the stylomandibular ligament after osteotomy. Surgical intervention may help relieve these symptoms once this diagnosis has been clearly established. The differential diagnosis includes temporomandibular joint (TMJ) syndrome, glossopharyngeal neuralgia, dental disorders, cercival arthritis, and spendopalatine ganglia neuralgia.

Osteoradionecrosis is the most dreaded complication and osteotomy sites are always areas of concern. Recent experience with the techniques we have described suggests that osteotomy is highly compatible with preoperative and postoperative radiation therapy. Assuming other factors are properly managed, we find no contraindication to the use of mandibular osteotomy and adjuvant chemotherapy or radiation therapy.

Pathologic fractures following marginal resection are a cause for concern. When 50% or more of the mandibular diameter is retained, the patient can usually tolerate a soft diet and relatively normal daily activities. Obviously, the patient is extremely vulnerable to trauma, even relatively minor inju-

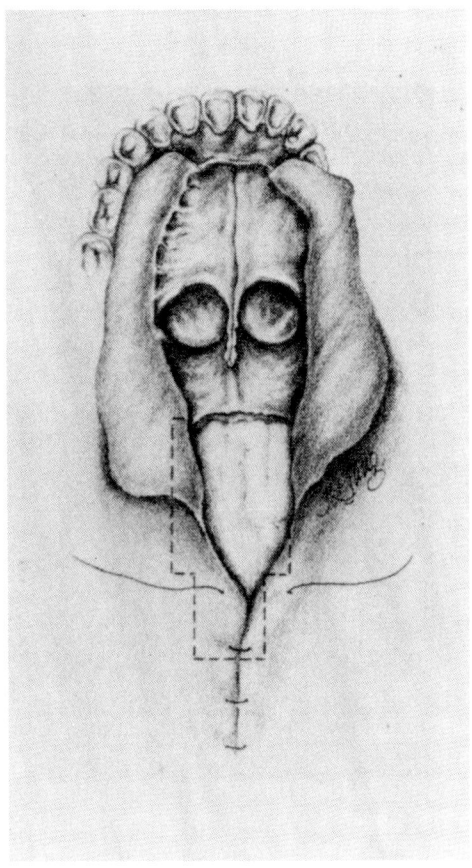

Figure 36. Closure of nasopharyngeal mucomuscular flaps. (From Wood BG, et al.: Arch Otolaryngol 106:2, 1980. With permission.)

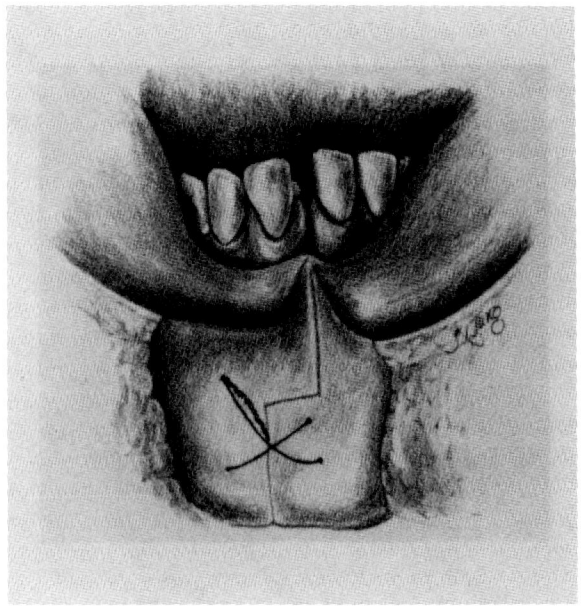

Figure 37. Fixation of mandibular osteotomy. (From Wood BG, et al.: Arch Otolaryngol 106:2, 1980. With permission.)

ries, and this must be emphasized in patient counseling.

Injury to the marginal branch of the facial nerve results in a serious lip deformity and, therefore, should be avoided. Occasionally, extention of tumor may require resection and sacrifice of the facial nerve, but these situations occur infrequently. Also, the surgeon must identify and work around the mental nerve to preserve chin and lower lip sensation.

REFERENCES

1. Spiro RH, Gerold FP, Strong EW: Mandibular "swing" approach for oral and oropharyngeal tumors. Head Neck Surg 3:371–378, 1981
2. Marchetta FC, Sako K, Murphy JB: The periosteum of the mandible and intraoral carcinoma. Am J Surg 122:711–713, 1971
3. Trotter W: Method of lateral pharyngotomy for exposure of large growths in epilaryngeal region. J Laryngol Rhinol Otol 35:289–295, 1920
4. Shumrick DA: Carcinoma of the supraglottic and tongue treated by supraglottic laryngectomy and mandibular swing. Laryngoscope 79:1443–1452, 1969
5. Baker, DC, Conley J: Surgical approach to retromandibular parotid tumors. Ann Plast Surg 3:304–314, 1979
6. Doyle PJ: Surgery for tumors of the deep lobe of the parotid gland. J. Otolaryngol 11:155–160, 1982
7. DeSanto LW, Whicker JH, Devine KD: Mandibular osteotomy and lingual flaps. Arch Otolaryngol 101:652–655, 1975
8. Dichtel WJ, Miller RH, Feliciano DV, et al.: Lateral mandibulotomy: A technique of exposure for penetrating injuries of the internal carotid artery at the base of the skull. Laryngoscope 94:1140–1144, 1984
9. McGregor IA, MacDonald DG: Mandibular osteotomy in the surgical approach to the oral cavity. Head Neck Surg 5:457–462, 1983
10. Wald, RM, Calcaterra TC: Lower alveolar carcinoma. Arch Otolaryngol 109:578–582, 1983
11. Mazzarella LA, Friedlander AA: Sagittal ostectomy of the mandible for floor of mouth cancer. Arch Otolaryngol 7:245–248, 1981
12. Wood BG, Sadar ES, Levine HL, et al.: Surgical problems of the base of the skull. Arch Otolaryngol 106:1–5, 1980
13. Spiessl B, Tschoff HM: Surgery of the jaws. In Nauman HH (ed), Stell PM (trans): Head and Neck Surgery: Indications, Techniques, Pitfalls Philadelphia: WB Saunders, 1980
14. Carraway JH, McGregor IA: Restoration of mandibular continuity after symphyseal osteotomy. Br J Plast Surg 34:392–394, 1981
15. Sataloff RT, Price DB: Mandibular osteotomy complicated by styloid pain. J Oral Surg 56:25–28, 1983

4 Stabilization and Fixation of the Mandible

William D. Clark, D.D.S., M.D.

In this chapter, *secondary bone healing* is defined as the common series of events that begins with the fracture hematoma, progresses through soft callus formation, hard callus formation, and new bone maturation, and ends with extensive remodeling at the fracture site. Primary bone union will be considered the less common process by which the fragments "weld" together without callus formation and with minimal resorption and remodeling.

In the mandible, secondary bone healing will usually take place when apposition of fragments and limitation of motion at the fracture site are reasonably good. Primary bone union requires rigid fixation and tight apposition of fragments.

STABILIZATION

Stabilization comprises supportive dressings, horizontal wiring, intermaxillary fixation (IMF), and specialized stabilizing splints. More specific descriptions of these techniques to achieve stabilization follow.

Supportive Dressings

A Barton bandage or similar supportive dressing may offer the patient with an acute mandibular fracture some comfort by minimizing fragment motion. These dressings must be applied with care, however, to avoid further fracture displacement, and the following criteria should be met prior to the application of any mouth-closing device:

1. An adequate nasal airway.
2. Means for patient to deal with liquid accumulations in the oral cavity and pharynx.
3. Patient free of nausea.
4. Patient reasonably cooperative and with stable mental status.

Our experience shows that once the patient has been placed in a bed with his head elevated 30 to 45 degrees, kept still and quiet, and given appropriate analgesics, a supportive dressing adds little to his comfort and may be perceived as a nuisance.

If definitive treatment of the fracture must be delayed beyond 24 to 48 h, temporary immobilization using a simple wiring technique should be considered.

Horizontal Wiring

Wire ligatures may be utilized to produce horizontal forces on mandibular fractures.

Simple Ligation of Teeth

Simple wire ligatures may be placed on the first sound tooth on each side of the fracture line and then twisted together to produce some reducing force and stabilization. In practice, this technique is often impractical and alternatives that yield better results are usually available.

Essig and Risdon Wiring

These techniques require the presence of a reasonable number of mandibular teeth on each side of each fracture. Comminuted fractures are a contraindication since overimpaction is likely to occur. See Figures 38 and 39 for details of these techniques.

Intermaxillary Fixation

Intermaxillary fixation is the cornerstone of mandibular fracture therapy in the United States. In most circumstances, properly applied and maintained IMF stabilizes fragments, reduces fracture motion, and insures the maintenance of preinjury dental occlusion during bone healing.

Contraindications to IMF include:

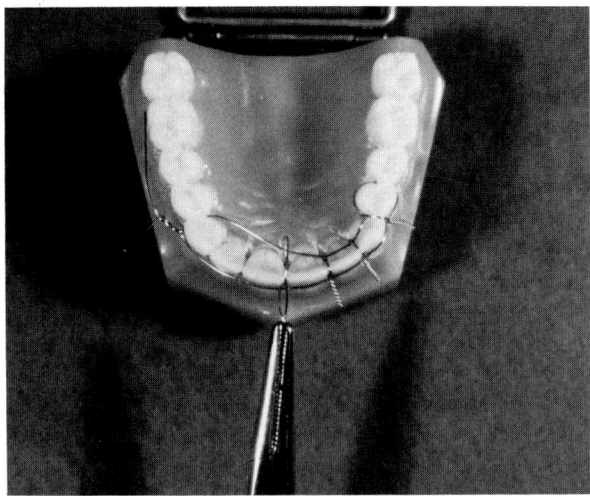

Figure 38. The Essig method of horizontal wiring.

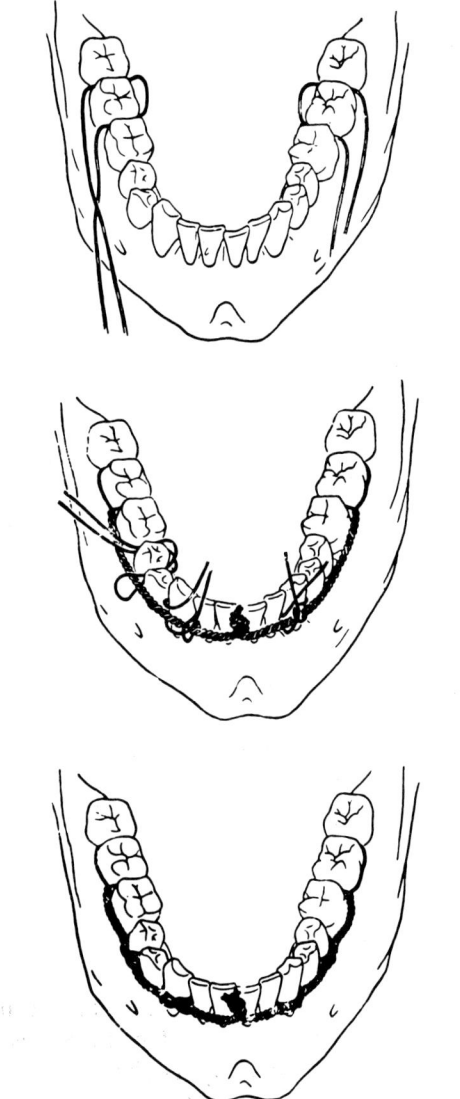

Figure 39. The Risdon method of horizontal wiring. (From Rowe NL, Killey HC: Fractures of the Facial Skeleton, Ed. 2. Baltimore: Williams & Wilkins, 1968. With permission.)

—Nausea and/or vomiting.
—Poorly controlled seizure disorder.
—Insufficient nasal airway (without tracheostomy.
—Combative patient.

Direct dental wiring, as described by Gilmer,[1] involves placing dental ligatures on mandibular and maxillary teeth, followed by simply twisting opposing ligatures together (Fig. 40). A reasonable number of sound teeth are required and there is danger of loosening and/or extracting ligated teeth. A satisfactory technique for temporarily obtaining IMF, this is especially suitable for use in primitive settings.

Noncontinuous loop wiring techniques are handy for temporary IMF and may even suffice for definitive treatment of minor fractures in the presence of a near-complete dentition. Eby/Ivy loops are shown in Figure 41. This technique of placing noncontinuous loop wires was as described by Eby[2] and Ivy.[3] Figure 42 displays Kazanjian's technique for producing wire projections that serve as attachment points for intermaxillary elastics or wires.[4]

Continuous loop wiring works well when a rigid appliance is not required. Figures 43 and 44 show the techniques of Stout[5] and Obwegeser[6] to form continuous loop wiring for each dental quadrant. These techniques require a minimum of three sound teeth in each dental quadrant.

Preformed arch bars are available in several styles. We favor the Erich type, feeling that it combines sufficient rigidity with reasonable malleability.

Arch bars should be sized and contoured for accurate fit to enhance stability and decrease the risk of unwanted tooth movement. We use 26-

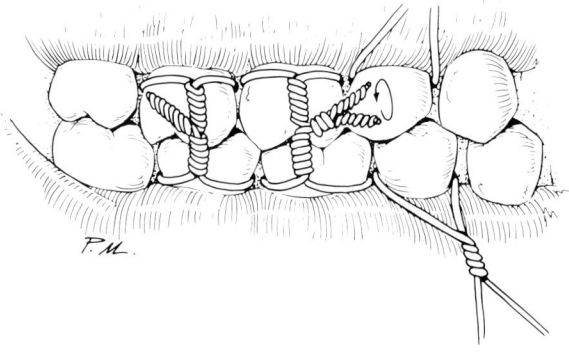

Figure 40. Gilmer's method of interdental wiring to produce intermaxillary fixation. (From Shelton DW: Fractures of the mandible. In Miller RH (ed): The Surgical Atlas of Airway and Facial Trauma, p 24. In Lee KJ (ed): Comprehensive Surgical Atlases in Otolaryngology and Head and Neck Surgery. New York: Grune Stratton, 1983. With permission.)

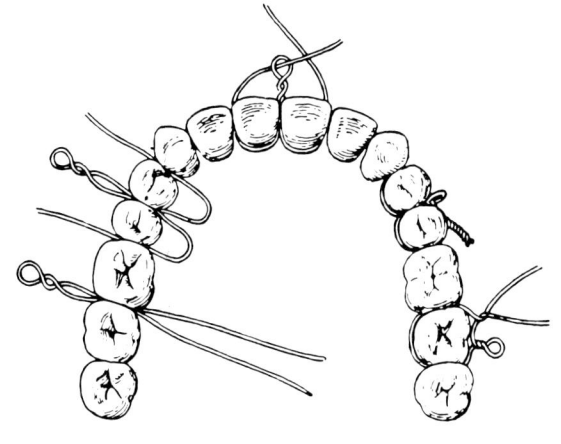

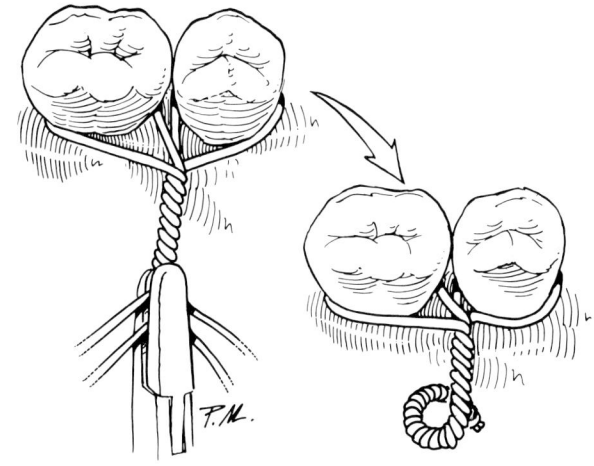

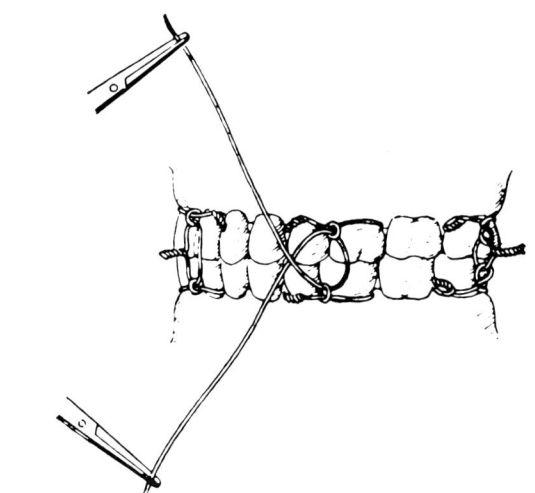

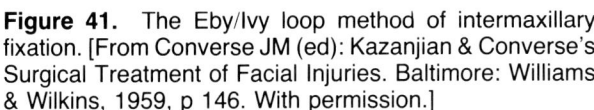

Figure 41. The Eby/Ivy loop method of intermaxillary fixation. [From Converse JM (ed): Kazanjian & Converse's Surgical Treatment of Facial Injuries. Baltimore: Williams & Wilkins, 1959, p 146. With permission.]

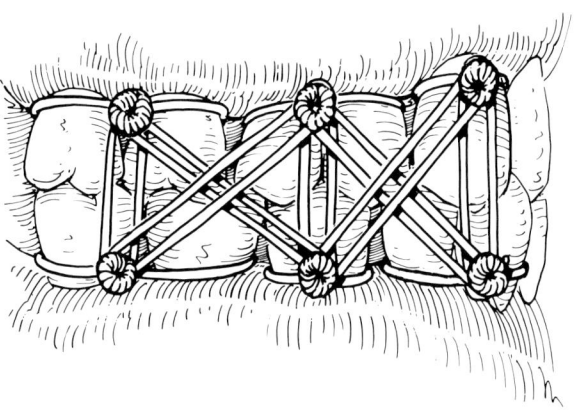

Figure 42. Kazanjian's method of producing intermaxillary fixation (From Shelton DW: Fractures of the mandible. In Miller RH (ed): The Surgical Atlas of Airway and Facial Trauma, p 25. In Lee KJ (ed): Comprehensive Surgical Atlases in Otolaryngology and Head and Neck Surgery. New York: Grune & Stratton, 1983. With permission.)

gauge stainless steel wire to ligate the cuspid (canine), bicuspid (premolar), and molar teeth securely to the arch bar. Occasionally, we ligate maxillary central incisors to achieve anterior stability. If anterior stabilization is required in the mandibular arch, we favor circum-mandibular wiring over ligation of mandibular incisors.

Cast metal can be used to make custom arch bars. Such appliances are especially useful when the teeth are mobile from periodontal disease and/or a number of teeth are missing.

The disadvantages to these appliances are the added time and expense required for their fabrication.

Splints

Splints offer a number of approaches to IMF. The four types discussed below are dentures, Gunning splints, lingual splints, and occlusal wafers.

Dentures as Splints for Intermaxillary Fixation

Full dentures make ideal splints to provide IMF. Even when fractured, they can be quickly repaired and put back into service. Once the dentures are wired to the patient, they may be fastened to each other. Several techniques may be used to hold the

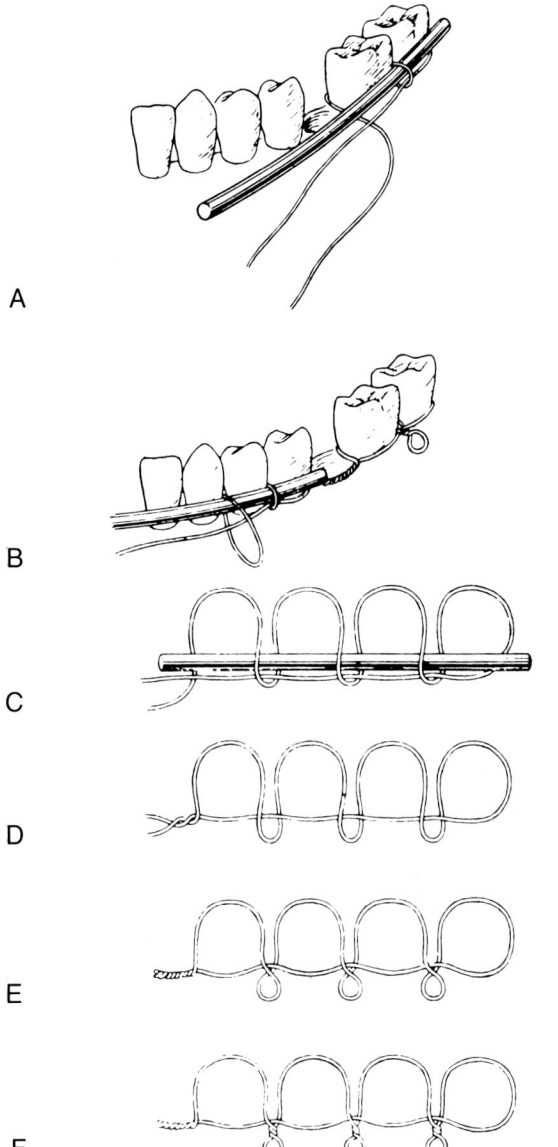

Figure 43. Stout wiring to produce intermaxillary fixation. (From Converse JM (ed): Kazajian and Converse's Surgical Treatment of Facial Injuries, 2 ed., Baltimore, Williams & Wilkins, 1959 p. 146.)

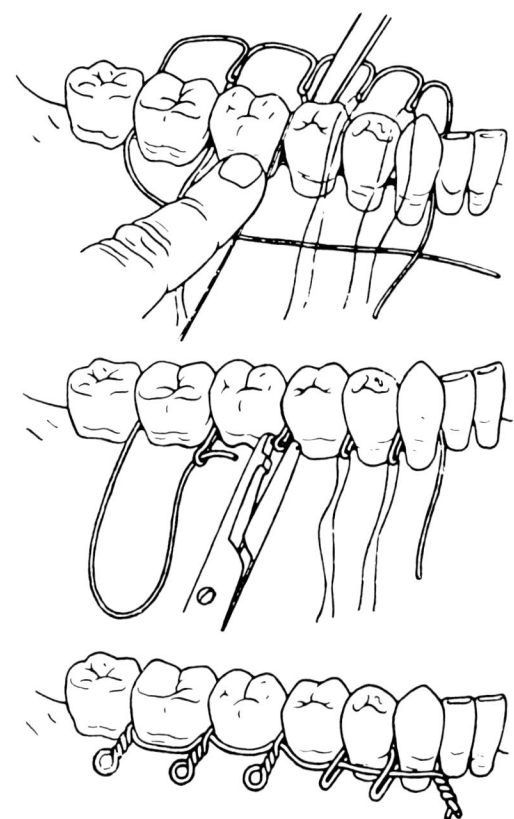

Figure 44. Continuous loop wiring by the Obwegeser technique. (From Rowe NL, Killey HC: Fractures of the Facial Skeleton, Baltimore: Williams & Wilkins, 1968, p. 47. With permission.)

dentures in occlusion, including previously applied arch bars.

Gunning Splints

Using himself as one of several case reports, Gunning described the use of splints to manage mandibular fractures in 1866.[7] Fabrication of useful Gunning splints requires skills in dental impression taking, in recording centric occlusion, and in determining proper interarch distance. Practitioners lacking a formal dental education rarely have sufficient proficiency in these areas to justify undertaking such a task.

Once the splints are fabricated, they are secured to the patient and then to each other, as described for full dentures.

Lingual Splints

Arch bars splint the mandible from its facial aspect. Circumstances in which lingual mandibular splinting may be desirable include the following:

—Symphyseal/parasymphyseal fractures when one or more fragments tend to rotate lingually.
—Symphyseal/parasymphyseal fractures combined with one or more posterior fractures when there is a tendency for posterior splaying and/or faciolingual rotation.
—Bilateral body fractures producing the "bucket handle" effect.
—Mandibular fractures in children.
—Numerous teeth missing or excessively movable.
—Inadequate posterior "stops" on one or both sides.

The fabrication of a lingual splint does not require formal dental training but does require some practice in the laboratory. Impressions of the mandibular and maxillary dental arches are obtained and plaster of paris casts are made from these. A coping saw is then used to reproduce the fracture(s) in the mandibular cast. The sections of the mandibular cast are occluded with the maxillary cast to reestablish preinjury occlusion. This relationship must be maintained as the mandibular cast is reassembled, first with wax or clay and then with plaster. The reassembled mandibular cast forms the template for a lingual splint of self-curing dental acrylic resin. Final preparation of the splint includes smoothing its external surface and drilling holes to accommodate dental ligature wires. Figure 45 shows the steps in this process.[13]

Two modifications of the lingual splint merit special mention. One combines a lingual splint with an occlusal wafer; the other replaces missing posterior teeth to provide occlusal "stops." When opposing teeth meet in occlusion, they prevent the mandible from further closing. Lacking sufficient stops, a mandibular fragment is less stable, not reduced by occlusal forces, and may be free to migrate toward the maxilla. To incorporate stops into a lingual splint, extra acrylic resin is built up on edentulous areas to the approximate height of the teeth being replaced and the maxillary cast is occluded to the mandibular cast while the resin polymerizes. When large or bilateral segments of the mandible are edentulous posteriorly, circum-mandibular wiring may be necessary to stabilize the splint

Occlusal Wafer

These devices could also be called "intermaxillary occlusal splints." A properly made occlusal wafer indexes the occlusion of opposing teeth without producing an open bite. This enhances the stabilizing effects gained by the intermeshing of teeth and a splinting of individual teeth.

Occlusal wafers should be considered under the following circumstances:

1. Periodontal disease producing severe tooth mobility.
2. Natural dentition present but occlusal surfaces worn flat.
3. Dentures to be used as splints have flat or otherwise noninterlocking occlusal surfaces.
4. Other unstable conditions of occlusion that are manifested by one dental arch sliding on the other.

In the fabrication of occlusal wafers, dental casts are prepared as described in Lingual Splints, above. A strip of self-curing acrylic resin is placed over the occlusal surfaces of one dental arch and the opposing arch is pressed into occlusion with the first. The wafer is trimmed and polished on the facial and lingual surfaces to provide comfort for the patient. Irving and co-workers have detailed a simple technique for fabricating occlusal wafers.[8]

A one-piece splint combining an occlusal wafer and lingual splint may sometimes be used advantageously. Childhood fractures of the mandibular symphysis or body are our primary indications for these splints. The fracture is reduced, the splint applied with circum-mandibular wiring, and a soft diet prescribed. As a rule, the fracture heals uneventfully and the disadvantages of IMF are avoided.

FIXATION

As used in this discussion, fixation is a relative term. Certainly, the application of a single wire ligature to a fracture site does not produce rigid fixation; however, a properly applied dynamic compression plate (DCP) may produce rigidity exceeding that of the mandible prior to injury. Techniques for achieving fixation are described below.

Direct Osseous Wiring

Direct interosseous wires should aid in reduction and close apposition of fragments while producing stability and even a mild degree of fixation. This is a time-tested and proven procedure, worthy of application to most unstable fractures of the mandible that require an open approach.

Simple, Two-Hole Wiring

Holes are drilled 5 to 7 mm from the inferior margin of the mandible and the same distance from the fracture line. A 24-gauge stainless steel wire ligature is passed through the holes and tightened as the fracture is held in reduction. These ligatures produce stability about a vertical axis (medial-lateral movement) but are limited in their ability to oppose forces about a horizontal axis (superior-inferior movement). This limitation is especially true in the angle of the mandible area, where virtually all fractures are unstable about a horizontal axis, and has led to the development of the more complex wiring techniques discussed below.

30 Surgery of the Mandible

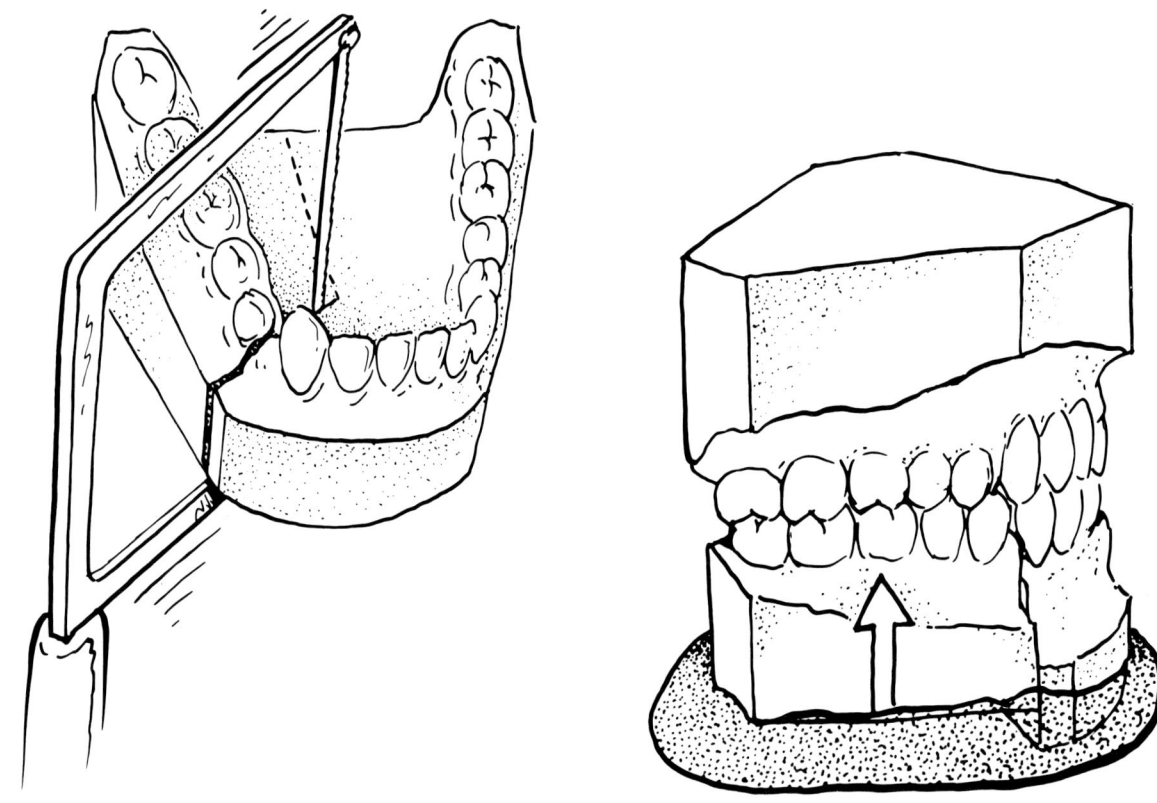

Figure 45. Shelton's steps in fabricating a lingual splint. (A) Malocclusion from mandibular fracture is evident when occluding casts of dental arches. (B) The fracture is "reproduced in plaster." (C) The sectioned mandibular cast is occluded with the maxillary cast, thus "reducing the fracture." Wax or clay can be used to maintain the position of the mandibular cast fragments once occlusion is reestablished. Plaster of paris then permanently bonds the cast fragments. (D) The repaired cast is then used as a template to form a lingual splint of self-curing dental acrylic resin. (E) The lingual splint is wired to the patient with dental ligatures. (From Shelton DW: Fractures of the mandible. In Miller RH (ed): The Surgical Atlas of Airway and Facial Trauma, pp 30–32. In Lee KJ (ed): Comprehensive Surgical Atlas in Otolaryngology and Head and Neck Surgery. New York: Grune & Stratton, 1983. With permission.)

Four-Hole Figure-of-Eight Ligature

A figure-of-eight wire ligature resists forces about both the horizontal and vertical axes. When four holes are used, however, there exists greater risk of injury to the neurovascular bundle of the mandible and the passage of wires can be technically difficult.

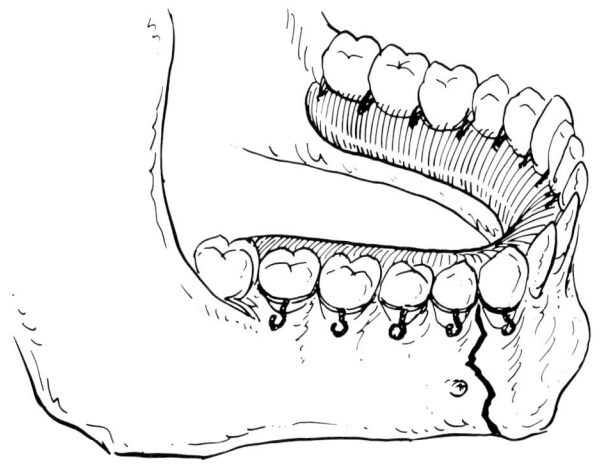

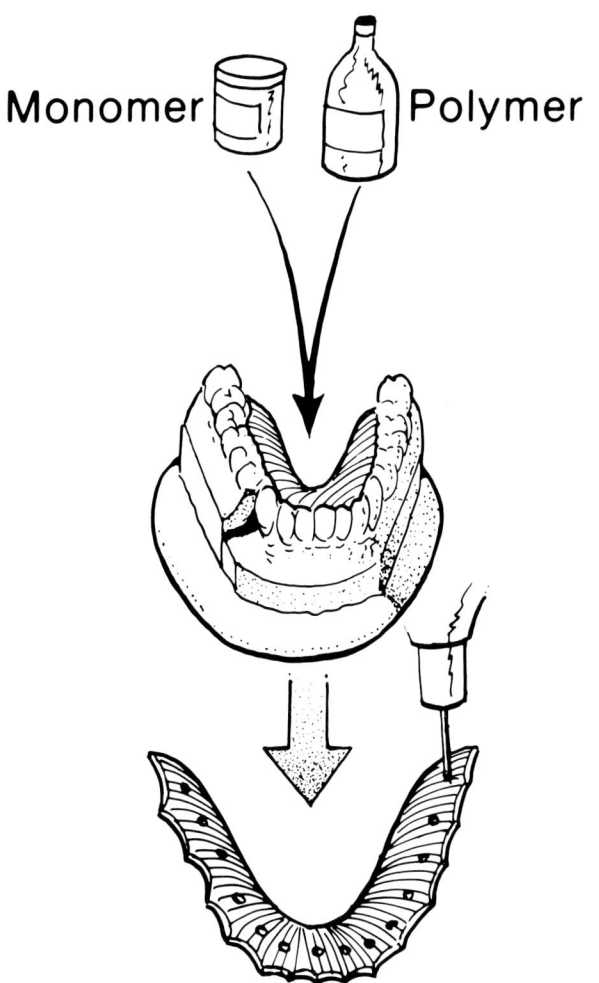

Figure 45. (Continued).

Two-Hole Figure-of-Eight

A figure-of-eight ligature can easily be made, placing two holes as described above in Simple, Two-Hole Wiring.[16] The wire is passed from lateral to medial in the first hole and then retrieved; the same end is passed from lateral to medial through the second hole. The surgeon must insure that the deeper of the two crossing segments of wire is not parallel to the fracture line. Otherwise, this segment of wire may slip into the fracture line and thereby prevent anatomic reduction (Fig. 46).

Rigid Internal Fixation

Dynamic compression plating is covered as a separate subject in Chapter 9. Discussion in the present chapter is confined to a general overall perspective of rigid internal fixation. Particular attention will be given to four types of appliances that may be used to achieve stable internal fixation:

1. Dynamic compression plates.
2. Eccentric dynamic plates (EDCP).
3. Reconstruction plates/mandibular bridging plates.
4. Lag screws.

While some proponents recommend stable internal fixation as a relatively routine approach to mandibular fractures, we feel that specific indications and contraindications should govern the use of this approach. Stable internal fixation by DCP, EDCP or reconstruction plates should be considered under the following conditions:

1. Intermaxillary fixation contraindicated (poorly controlled seizures, intolerant patient, nasal obstruction, poor state of nutrition).
2. Special need for mandibular rigidity (midface fracture combined with mandibular fracture).

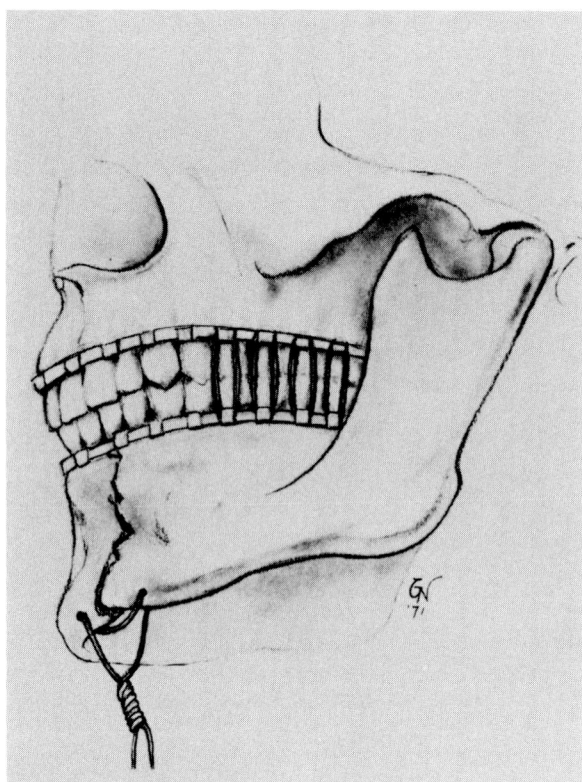

Figure 46. The two-hole figure-of-eight ligature is preferred for direct interosseous wiring. (From Clark WD, Bailey BJ; Management of fractures of the mandible. In Mathog RH (ed): Maxillofacial Trauma. Baltimore: Williams & Wilkins, 1984, p 148. With permission.)

3. Edentulous mandible without dentures for splints.
4. Special need for access to oral cavity.
5. Special need for prolonged fixation.

Contraindications to stable internal fixation by DCP or EDCP are:

1. Fracture that may be managed by less aggressive approach with a good chance of success.
2. Insufficient bone to support hardware.
3. Extensively comminuted fracture.
4. Major loss of bone (compression plates may be used with cortical bone grafts).

Inherent disadvantages to stable internal fixation are:

1. Need for wide exposure with resulting longer incisions, more extensive dissection, and reduction of local blood supply.
2. Large amount of implanted foreign material.
3. Need to remove hardware in certain instances (e.g., cold intolerance, oral exposure).
4. Longer operating times and higher costs.
5. Need for expensive, specialized instruments and supplies.
6. Higher complication rate expected when the technique is used by inexperienced practitioner.
7. No possibility for dynamic improvements in occlusion once the devices are secured in place.

Inherent advantages to the use of stable internal fixation are:

1. Patient more comfortable during the healing phase.
2. Good nutrition more easily accomplished.
3. Oral hygiene easily maintained with resulting improved dental health.
4. Primary bone union usually accomplished.
5. No compromise in oral airway or ability to clear oropharyngeal secretions.
6. Lower rates of infection, delayed union and nonunion.

Dynamic Compression Plates

Dynamic compression plates utilize the spherical gliding principle to compress bone at and around the fracture site. The screw holes form a "bent cylinder" path which forces the hemispherical screwheads to move toward the fracture line when tightened (Fig. 47). This compresses the bone while slightly stretching the plate. The DCP are designed to produce more compression that masticatory forces are likely to produce, thereby preventing relative movement between the hardware and the bone. Relative motion will loosen screws and result in loss of rigid fixation.

Dynamic compression plates produce compression primarily at the facial cortex near the inferior border of the mandible. To produce compression at the lingual cortex, the plates should be contoured so that they touch bone at their extremities but are at a slight distance away from bone at their midportion (3 to 5 degrees of overcontouring) (Fig. 48).

Dynamic compression plates need additional hardware to insure compression at the alveolus—a condition considered important by Spiessl and associates. Devices such as tension band bars, tension band plates, and special splints can be utilized to produce compression at the alveolar level. Spiessl's book and articles are recommended for further details on these devices.[9–11]

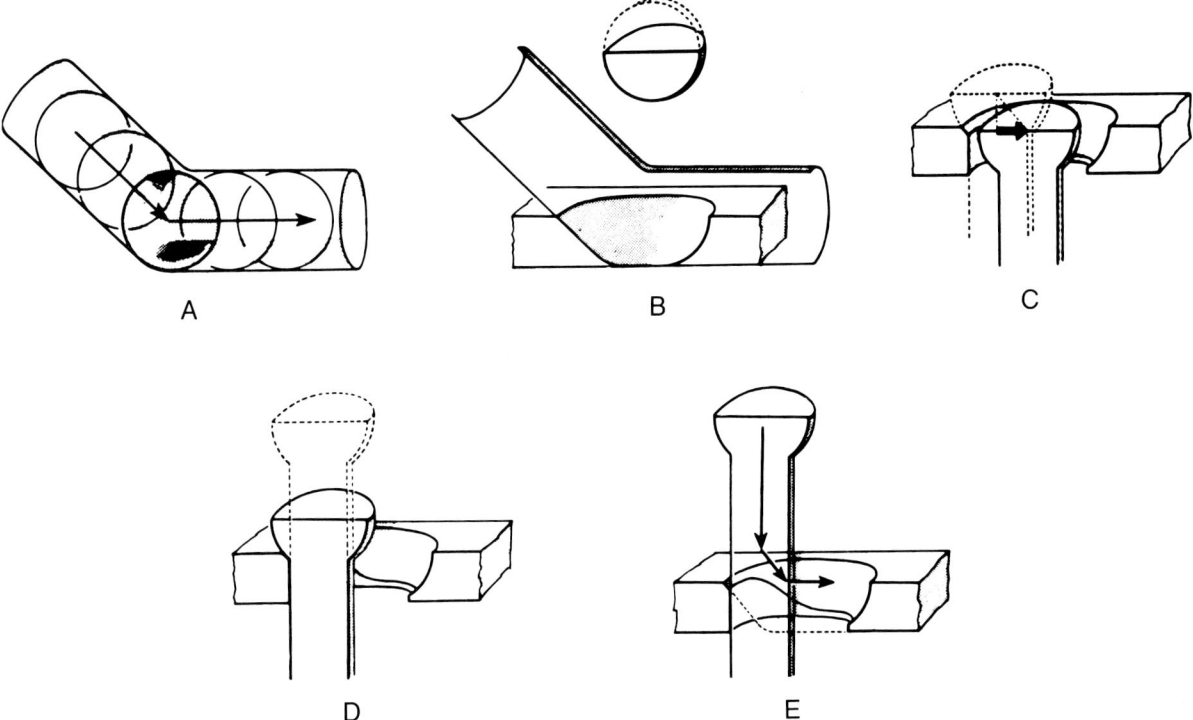

Figure 47. The pathway of a hemispherical screw head in a dynamic compression device approximates the path of a sphere traveling through a bent cylinder. (From Spiessl B: Stable internal fixation. In Mathog RH (ed): Maxillofacial Trauma. Baltimore: Williams & Wilkins, 1984, p. 167. With permission).

Eccentric Dynamic Compression Plates

Eccentric dynamic compression plates contain two sets of dynamic drill holes. The inner set of screw holes glides toward the fracture, providing compression at the inferior mandibular border, while the outer two holes glide superiorly to produce compression at the level of the alveolus (Fig. 49). Eccentric dynamic compression plates do not need intraoral devices to produce compression at the alveolus.

Reconstruction Plates/Bridging Plates

A.O. reconstruction plates are sturdy and contain screw holes at close intervals. They incorporate a special design to facilitate bending in all directions while maintaining rigidity. They can be cut to length, but at least four screws are required at each area of fixation. These plates may be used to bridge multiple fractures and areas of bone loss. The Osteo plating system available through Richards Medical Co. (Memphis, TN) includes ten lengths. These

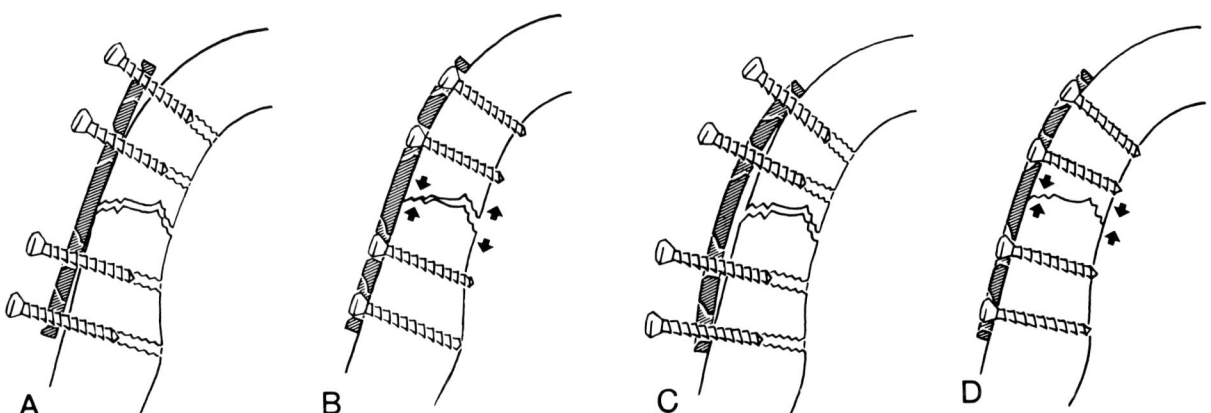

Figure 48. Overcontouring a compression plate by 3 to 5 degrees produces compression at the lingual cortex. (From Spiessl B: Stable internal fixation. In Mathog RH (ed): Maxillofacial Trauma. Baltimore: Williams & Wilkins, 1984, p. 168. With permission).

2.7 - EDCP®

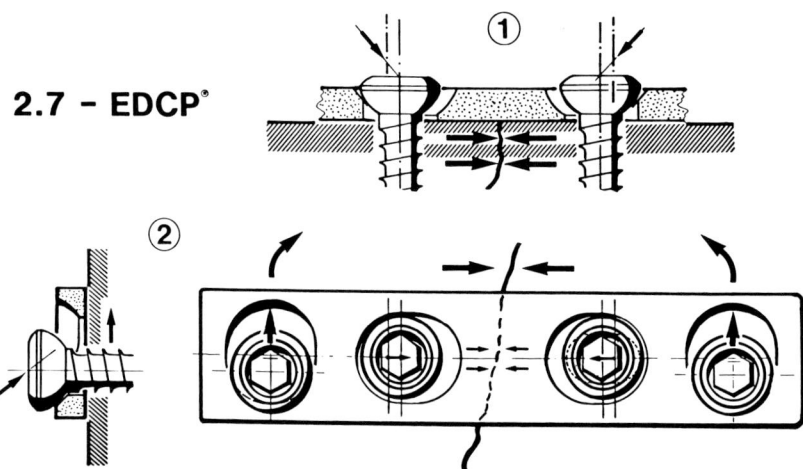

Figure 49. With the eccentric dynamic compression plate, one set of screws produces compression at the inferior border of the mandible, while the second produces compression at the alveolus. (From Spiessl B: Stable internal fixation. In Mathog RH (ed): Maxillofacial Trauma. Baltimore: Williams & Wilkins, 1984, p. 170. With permission).

plates are designed to bridge mandibular defects while supporting bone grafts. The amounts of compression vary, depending on screw hole placement.

Lag Screws

Mandibular fractures may occur with enough faciolingual obliquity to allow the use of lag screws to produce interfragmental compression. The length of reduced fracture overlap must be at least twice the thickness of the mandible for lag screw compression to be effective. The drill hole is made at 90 degrees to the plane of fragment juncture. The drill hole in the outer fragment is enlarged so that the screw will pass through it without engaging, and the hole on the deep fragment is tapped. Tightening of the lag screw pulls the deep fragment against the superficial one, producing compression.

Comment

As a general admonition, we propose that the following criteria should be met prior to undertaking new techniques of stable internal fixation:

1. The practitioner has thorough familiarity with the theories, principles, and philosophy of this approach.
2. Availability of and familiarity with a complete set of instruments and related accessories.
3. The practitioner has extensive experience in more traditional approaches to mandibular fractures.

External Pin Fixation

Rigid immobilization of mandibular segments while maintaining their spatial orientation may be accomplished with external pin fixation.[14] In early devices, two threaded pins were screwed into each segment of mandible. The relation of the pins was maintained by a series of connecting rods and joints, which could be tightened in place once the fracture was reduced.

The Morris biphase apparatus uses similar hardware, modified to allow replacement of connecting rods and joints with a bar of autopolmerizing polymethalmethacrylate (Figs. 50 to 53).[15] Further modifications of this technique use pins connected by an endotracheal tube filled with self-curing acrylic resin.

Indications for external pin fixation include the following:

—Need for long-term stabilization.
—Maintenance of space and spatial relationships after surgical or traumatic loss of bone.
—Intermaxillary fixation contraindicated or impractical.

Advantages of external pin fixation are:

1. Relatively rigid immobilization.
2. Exact spatial relationships may be maintained if device placed prior to resection of a portion of the mandible.
3. Lack of instrumentation and foreign body implantation at fracture site.
4. Intermaxillary fixation not required.

The disadvantages of external pin fixation are:

1. Not cosmetically pleasing.
2. Scars are produced at pin puncture sites in skin.
3. Possible soft tissue and bony infection around pins.
4. Requires special equipment and expertise.

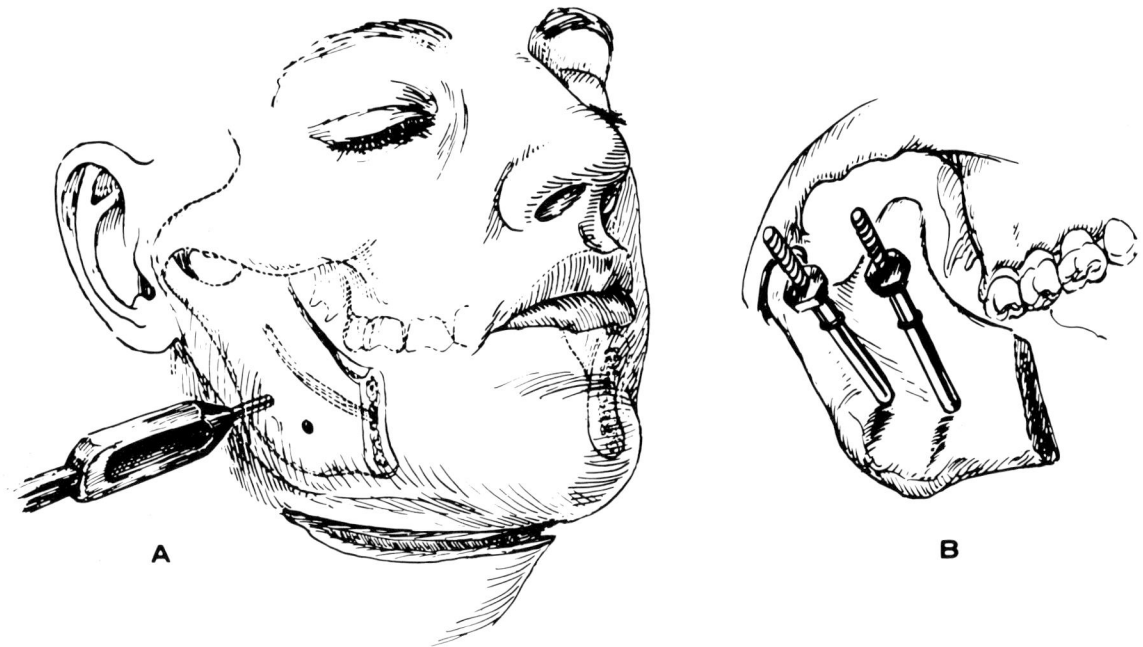

Figure 50. The Morris biphase requires two special bone screws in each fragment. (From Converse JM (ed): Kazanjian and Converse's Surgical Treatment of Facial Injuries, 3 ed. Baltimore: Williams & Wilkins, 1974, p. 217.)

Cap Splint Fixation

Cast metal splints that are cemented over the clinical crowns of mandibular teeth may be used to produce fixation of tooth-bearing mandibular fragments.[12] After a separate splint is made for each segment, the fracture is reduced and the intersplint relationship is registered utilizing plaster of paris. The relationship as recorded is then used to construct a connecting rod that will allow the splints to be joined rigidly together.

Cap splints have the following advantages over conventional techniques:

1. Buccolingual rotation is prevented.
2. Relatively rigid fixation is obtained.

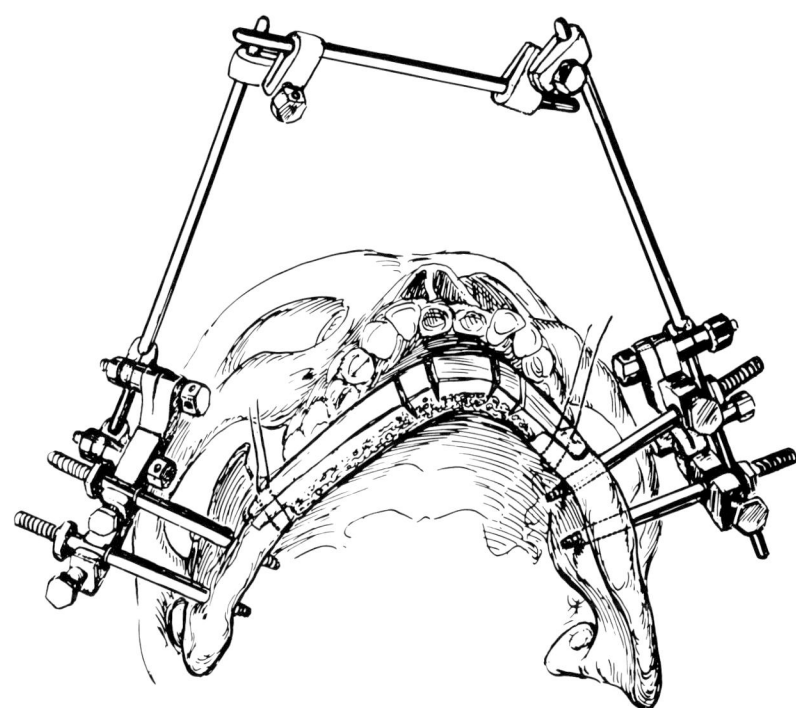

Figure 51. The first phase has been completed. (From Converse JM (ed): Kazanjian and Converse's Surgical Treatment of Facial Injuries, 3 ed. Baltimore: Williams & Wilkins, 1974, p. 217.)

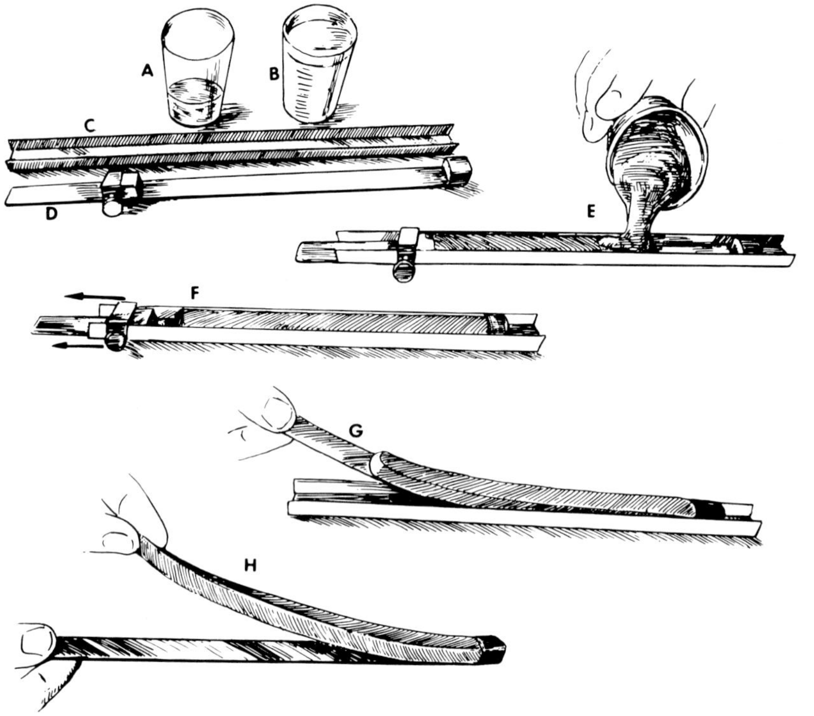

36　Surgery of the Mandible

Figure 52. Self-curing dental acrylic is mixed and applied to a special mold. When the "doughy" stage has been reached, the bar of acrylic is removed for molding to the screwheads. (From Converse JM (ed): Kazanjian and Converse's Surgical Treatment of Facial Injuries, 3 ed. Baltimore: Williams & Wilkins, 1974, p. 218.)

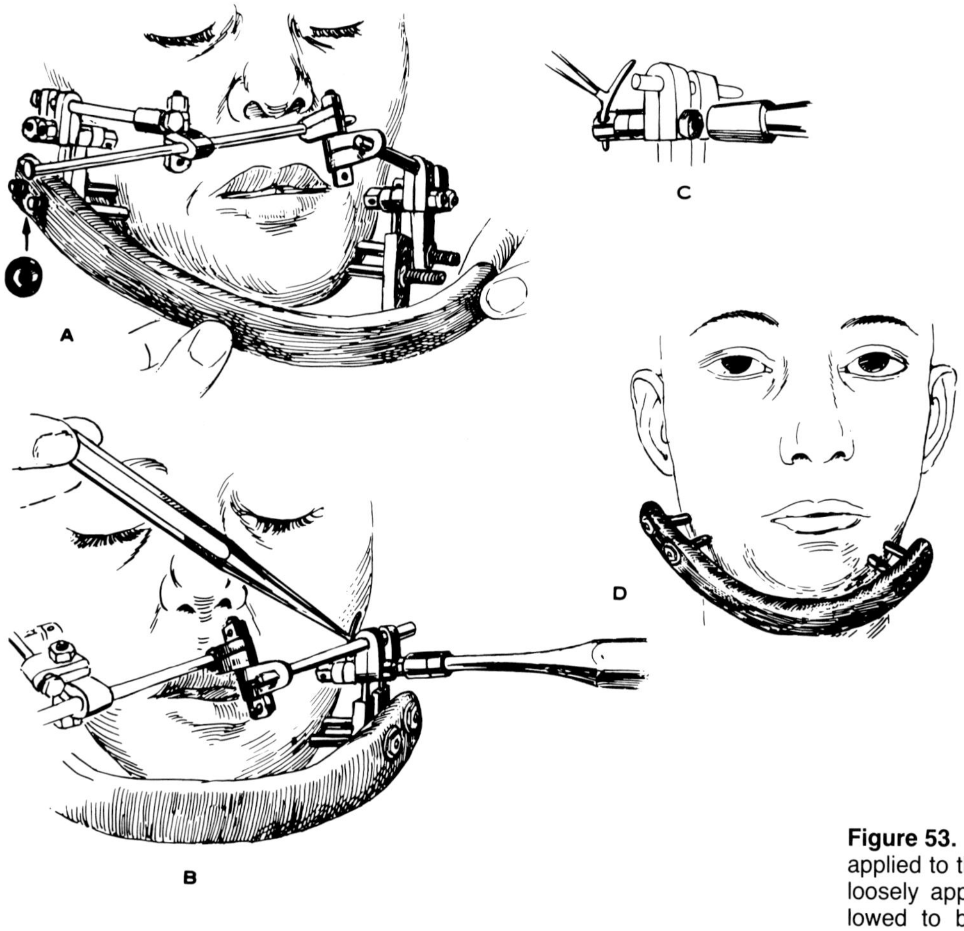

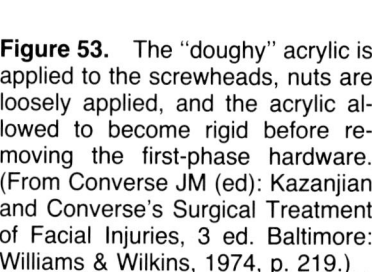

Figure 53. The "doughy" acrylic is applied to the screwheads, nuts are loosely applied, and the acrylic allowed to become rigid before removing the first-phase hardware. (From Converse JM (ed): Kazanjian and Converse's Surgical Treatment of Facial Injuries, 3 ed. Baltimore: Williams & Wilkins, 1974, p. 219.)

3. Intermaxillary fixation and attendant disadvantages are avoided.
4. Not as dependent on sound dentition.
5. Open procedures are avoided.

Cap splints have the following disadvantages:

1. Cumbersome, time-consuming, and costly.
2. Minor degrees of occlusal disharmony are routine.
3. Dental laboratory facilities to support this technique rare outside the United Kingdom.
4. Each segment must be tooth bearing.

SUMMARY

Those who treat mandibular fractures or excise portions of the mandible need to have a number of stabilization and fixation techniques available to them. Most situations can be effectively managed by the application of the basic, conventional techniques that should be familiar to all; however, familiarity with nonconventional techniques is desirable and perhaps essential if we are to provide the best care for our patients.

REFERENCES

1. Gilmer TL: Fractures of the inferior maxilla. Illinois St Dent Soc Trans 67:104, 1981
2. Eby JD: Principles of orthodontia in the treatment of maxillofacial injuries. Int J Orthod 6:273–310, 1920
3. Ivy RH: Practical method of fixation in fractures of the mandible. Surg Gynecol Obstet 22:670–673, 1934
4. Kazanjian VH: Immobilization of wartime, compound, comminuted fractures of the mandible. Am J Orthod Oral Surg 28:551–560, 1942
5. Stout R: Manual of Standard Practice of Plastic and Maxillofacial Surgery. Philadelphia: WB Saunders, 1943.
6. Obwegeser H: Uber eine Methode der friedhanisen Drahtschienung von Kieferbruchen. Osterreichischen Z Stomat 49:652, 1952
7. Gunning RB: The treatment of fractures of the lower jaw by interdental splints. NY State J Med 3:433–448; 4:11–29; 4:274–277. 1866–1867.
8. Irving SP, Costa LE, Salisbury PE III: The occlusal wafer: Simple technique for construction and its use in maxillofacial surgery. Laryngoscope 94:1036–1041, 1984
9. Spiessl B: Rigid internal fixation of fractures of the lower jaw. Reconstr Surg 7:124, 1972
10. Spiessl B (ed): New Concepts in Maxillofacial Bone Surgery. Berlin: Springer Verlag, 1976, p 12
11. Spiessl B: Stable internal fixation, In Mathog RH (ed): *Maxillofacial Trauma*. Baltimore: Williams & Wilkins, 1984, pp 162–172
12. Rowe NL, Killey HC: Fractures of the Facial Skeleton, Ed. 2. Baltimore: Williams & Wilkins, 1968
13. Shelton DW: Fractures of the mandible. In Miller RH (ed): The Surgical Atlas of Airway and Facial Trauma, pp 23–51. In Lee KJ (ed): Comprehensive Surgical Atlases in Otolaryngology and Head and Neck Surgery. New York: Grune & Stratton, 1983
14. Converse JM (ed): Kazanjian & Converse's Surgical Treatment of Facial Injuries, Ed. 3. Baltimore: Williams & Wilkins, 1974
15. Converse JM (ed): Kazanjian & Converse's Surgical Treatment of Facial Injuries, Ed. 2. Baltimore: Williams & Wilkins, 1959, p 146
16. Clark WD, Bailey BJ: Management of fractures of the mandible. In Mathog RH (ed): Maxillofacial Trauma. Baltimore: Williams & Wilkins, 1984, p 148

5 Surgical Treatment of Benign and Low-Grade Malignant Lesions of the Mandible

William D. Clark, D.D.S., M.D.

The surgical treatment of benign and low-grade malignant lesions of the mandibular bone is considered in this chapter. Lesions of overlying gingiva and alveolar mucosa will not be discussed. Carcinomas and sarcomas involving the mandible will be covered in Chapter 6.

We will not consider the diagnosis or treatment of dental periapical abscesses, granulomas, and cysts as these lesions usually respond to appropriate dental treatment such as endodontic therapy or tooth extraction with trans-socket curettage.

The treatment discussions assume that a firm diagnosis precedes definitive surgical treatment. In patients with large neoplasms, the diagnosis is usually established by an incisional biopsy. For small lesions, an excisional biopsy may serve both diagnostic and therapeutic purposes. Because of the relative rarity of the various odontogenic lesions, the general pathologist may need to consult with the oral pathology department of a dental school or the Armed Forces Institute of Pathology.

SURGICAL APPROACHES

Techniques for Benign Lesions

The techniques of exposure and removal of lesions in this group do not differ much from lesion to lesion. Exceptions will be discussed under the heading for the particular lesions to which they apply.

The intraoral route is the preferred approach to most of these lesions; however, large lesions extending into the ascending ramus may require an external approach. We prefer long horizontal incisions, placed a few millimeters below the junction of free mucosa with attached gingiva, to expose mandibular lesions from the mid-alveolus to the inferior border.

When the superior alveolus must be exposed, a higher incision is required. A no. 15 scalpel blade is placed into the facial gingival sulcus of each tooth at 90 degrees to the occlusal plane and the epithelial attachment of gingiva to tooth is severed as atraumatically as possible. Each interdental papilla is cut across to join the gingival sulcus incisions; the gingiva and oral mucosa are carefully elevated from the teeth and bone of the mandible. These incisions usually require vertical limbs at each end to facilitate inferior exposure. Suturing such wounds is difficult in tooth-bearing areas. Sutures are passed from lingual to facial, inferior to the interdental contact area; the facial half of the interdental papilla serves as a guide to suture placement. The suture is then tied over the contact area (Fig. 54).

Once the "buccal plate" of mandibular bone overlying the lesion has been adequately exposed and hemostasis is acquired, a window in the bone is made carefully by a power-driven bur or mallet and chisel. After a portion of the lesion is uncapped, various rongeurs are convenient for further bone removal. A rotating bur, used with care, can also accomplish this task. The bone removal should be adequate to expose the entire lesion, when practical.

The consistency of the lesion will dictate the technique of its removal. Well-circumscribed lesions with resilient walls or capsules can be removed intact with the usual selection of blunt elevators. Friable lesions may be removed with various elevators and curettes. After removal of a soft tissue lesion appears to be complete, a "margin" of normal bone should be removed in all directions by curettement or burring.

The bony cavity that results from excision of a benign lesion is usually irrigated and then filled with Gelfoam before wound closure. Prophylactic antibiotic coverage is used routinely in these patients.

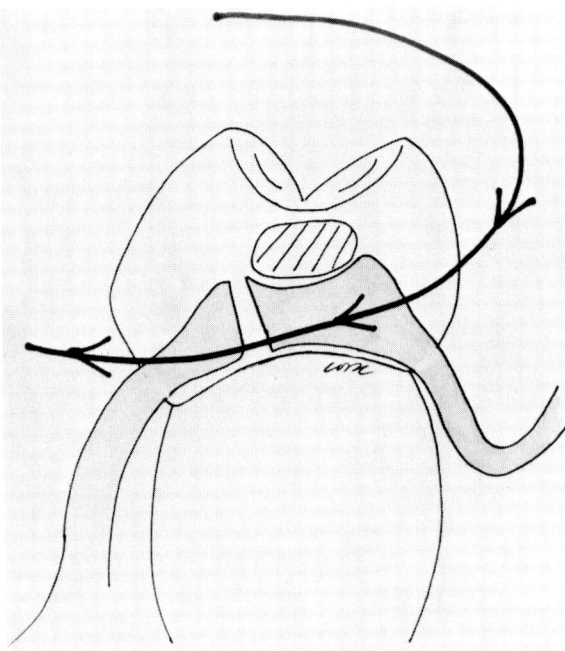

Figure 54. Contact area is shaded. Needle and suture pass inferior to the contact areas from lingual to facial. Facial interdental papilla serves as a guide for suture placement. The suture is tied around the contact area, with the knot on the facial side.

Techniques for Aggressive Benign and Low-Grade Malignant Neoplasms

Ameloblastoma, the most common of the "gray-zone" neoplasms of the mandible, typifies this group of lesions. These tumors are somewhat analogous to basal cell carcinomas of skin in that both derive from epithelial appendages, metastasize rarely, and often cause local tissue destruction. Treatment analogies between these two tumors exist also in that some authors favor treatment by conservative approaches (curettage, cautery, and limited resections) while others are strong proponents of en bloc resection.

For dealing with large and/or recurrent ameloblastomas, most surgeons agree with the use of en bloc resection techniques. For dealing with small and/or predominantly cystic lesions, some controversy continues. Occasionally, a small ameloblastoma will be found inside a cyst. If the exterior of the cyst wall is not involved and the cyst wall was not violated during enucleation, no further treatment may be required. In all other ameloblastomas, we favor resection of involved bone and overlying soft tissues, with a margin of normal tissue. Small lesions may be managed by marginal resection, while larger lesions usually require segmental resection. Massive lesions may require hemimandibulectomy or even total mandibulectomy if there is to be any hope of gaining control.

Planning for later mandibular reconstruction may call for placement of an external pin fixation device such as the Morris biphase before resecting a segment of mandible.

SPECIFIC LESIONS

The pathologic processes that affect the mandible are numerous, varied, and difficult to classify. In this chapter, we are treating all lesions with potentially aggressive behavior as Aggressive benign and low-grade malignant neoplasms, regardless of their tissue of origin.

Nonneoplastic Lesions

Odontogenic Cysts

The following classification of odontogenic cysts is modified from Thoma[1]:

I. Follicular cysts.
   A. Primordial cysts.
   B. Dentigerous cysts.
      1. Central.
      2. Lateral.
      3. Circumferential.
II. Periodontal cysts (radicular).
   A. Apical.
   B. Lateral.
   C. Gingival.
III. Residual cysts.
   A. Circumferential.
   B. Dentigerous.
   C. Periodontal.

For the most part, odontogenic cysts are removed as outlined and described in the section Surgical Approaches, subsection Techniques for Benign Lesions, above. Exceptions include eruption cysts of the primary dentition which are usually observed until eruption eliminates the problem, and eruption cysts of the permanent dentition which are often uncapped to facilitate tooth eruption.

Nonodontogenic Cysts

Nonodontogenic cysts are seen commonly in the maxilla but rarely in the mandible. The occasional median mandibular cyst is removed by enucleation.

Table 5–1. Giant Cell Reparative Granuloma Versus Giant Cell Tumor of Bone

	Giant Cell Reparative Granulomas of Bone	Giant Cell Tumor of Bone
Age of patient	Usually under 21 years	Usually over 21 years
Clinical behavior	Self-limited: may regress, seldom recurs, never metastasizes	Aggressive: no regression, recurs often, occasionally metastasizes
Histologic features	1. Giant cells group around hemorrhagic focci. 2. Stroma shows oval cells and equally large numbers of spindled fibroblasts with zones of fibrosis and relatively few giant cells. 3. Evidence of old and recent hemorrhage with hemosiderin. 4. Giant cells are generally smaller, frequently irregular, and elongated, with relatively few nuclei. 5. Foci of osteoid and new bone function in the center of lesions are frequently present.	1. Giant cells uniformly disperse and dominate the entire field. 2. Stroma is richly vascularized and is composed of plump round and oval cells. 3. Recent hemorrhage is slight to moderate; hemosiderin is rare. 4. Giant cells are generally larger and rounder with more nuclei. 5. Osteoid or new bone is not characteristically produced.
Response to therapy	Usually cured by curettage	Recurs if excision is incomplete

Source: Batsakis JG (ed). Tumors of the Head and Neck—Clinical and Pathological Considerations, Vol. 2, Ed. 2. Baltimore: Williams & Wilkins, 1979, p 399. With permission.

Giant Cell Reparative Granuloma

These granulomas must be differentiated from giant cell tumors of bone. Table 5–1 shows Batsakis's[2] modification of Hirschl's and Katz's[3] comparison of these two disease processes. Whether these lesions result from trauma is debatable. Treatment consists of thorough curettage and Gelfoam packing. Some clinicians advocate the use of caustic agents applied to surrounding bone after curettage.[1]

"Brown Tumor"

These lesions, thought to be produced by an excess of parathormone, have been associated classically with primary hyperparathyroidism. Patients with secondary hyperparathyroidism may also manifest these lesions as a result of their renal disease and long-term dialysis.

Treatment should be directed toward the underlying disorder.

Fibrous Dysplasia of Bone

Fibrous dysplasia of bone is probably a developmental aberration rather than a true neoplasm. This abnormality grows actively during childhood and usually slows or stops after skeletal growth is complete.

Complete surgical removal is rarely a practical consideration because these lesions tend to be diffuse and benign. Surgical treatment, when indicated, is limited to recontouring for functional and cosmetic reasons and is best delayed until after puberty.

Cherubism

Familial intraosseus fibrous swelling of the jaws is an inherited condition thought to result from a disturbance in osteogenesis. This autosomal-dominant disorder is characterized by variable penetrance and expression.

The lesions typically appear in the region of the angles of the mandible. Histologically, lesions have some areas that resemble fibrous dysplasia and others that simulate giant cell reparative granuloma. These lesions usually involute at puberty. When functional and/or cosmetic considerations demand, surgery may be employed to provide more nearly normal bony contours.

Aneurysmal Bone Cysts

Aneurysmal bone cysts occur rarely in the mandible. Their etiology is unknown. They usually respond well to evacuation of the contents of the "cyst" and thorough curettage of surrounding bone. The bony cavity often requires firm packing with a resilient substance such as Surgicel to control bleeding. An occasional patient may not respond to packing and may require ligation of the regional blood supply.

Hemorrhagic (Traumatic) Bone Cyst

Hemorrhagic bone cysts are thought to be related to local trauma. They usually respond well to evacuation, curettage of surrounding bone, and packing with Gelfoam.

Neoplastic Lesions

Hemangiomas

Hemangiomas of the mandible are uncommon. The first manifestation may be severe hemorrhaging after tooth extraction. Usually small lesions may be managed successfully by curettage/local excision, but larger lesions may require segmental resection with control of the regional blood supply. Preoperative Gelfoam embolization may reduce bleeding in patients with large lesions.

Tori, Exostoses, and Enostoses

These tumors consist of histologically normal bone growing in an abnormal location. *Exostoses* are bony outgrowths from the external surface of the mandible. The torus mandibularis is a specific type of extosis. *Tori* are usually multiple, spheroidal, and occur on the lingual aspect of the mandible in the bicuspid region. Tori are removed by elevating overlying soft tissues and chiseling at the line of juncture between lesion and normal mandible. Indications for removal of tori include chronic irritation from mastication and the need to fit a dental appliance. Other mandibular exostoses may be more difficult to remove, requiring the use of power drills and/or bone rasps.

Enostoses occur from the inner aspect of cortical bone and protrude into the narrow space. Often, they must be removed for the clinician to make a definitive diagnosis.

Osteomas

Osteomas are true neoplasms with a predilection for the bones of the skull and face. These uncommon lesions, often situated in the mandible, are removed only when they generate functional or cosmetic concern. Mandibular osteomas are sometimes associated with Gardner's syndrome.

Benign Odontogenic Tumors

Benign odontogenic tumors fall into three groups: odontoma, cementoma, and odontogenic fibroma.
ODONTOMA GROUP. This group consists of the following:

1. *Odontoblastoma*. Simple enucleation of odontoblastoma usually cures these lesions.
2. *Compound and complex odontomas*. Compound and complex odontomas respond well to simple enucleation.
3. *Ameloblastic odontoma*. Enucleation followed by vigorous curettage of surrounding bone usually cures these tumors. Treatment of recurrences should involve excision with a margin of normal bone.
4. *Ameloblastic fibro-odontoma*. Adequate surgical curettage usually insures against recurrence of ameloblastic fibro-odontoma. Malignant degeneration of these lesions has been reported and is heralded by rapid growth.

CEMENTOMA GROUP. This group comprises the following:
1. *Periapical cemental dysplasia*. Typically, periapical cemental dysplasia are asymptomatic; they are located about the apical ends of the roots of mandibular incisors and occur predominantly in black women older than 25 years. The associated teeth show normal vitality to electrical stimulation, a feature that rules out periapical abscess, cyst, and granuloma. The radiodensities of these lesions vary from soft tissue to bony. The condition can be diagnosed on the basis of these typical features and it requires no treatment.
2. *Cementifying fibroma*. Cementifying fibroma probably represent a variant of periapical cemental dysplasia, but they occur in the posterior mandible, about the apices of molars or bicuspids. The findings of a periapical lesion with the associated posterior teeth retaining normal viability should suggest this diagnosis. Excisional biopsy cures the condition.
3. *Benign ("true") cementoblastoma*. Rare neoplasms, benign cementoblastoma attach to the root of a molar or biscupid tooth; they are cured by enucleation with extraction of the involved tooth. A recent report details the successful retention of a tooth involved with a benign cementoblastoma by excising the lesion and performing endodontic therapy.[4]
4. *Familial multiple (gigantiform) cementoma*. Usually diagnosed in middle-aged black women, these deforming lesions are apparently inherited by an autosomal-dominant mode. Complete excision constitutes the treatment of choice for familial multiple cementoma.
ODONTOGENIC FIBROMA.   This is the final category of benign ontogenic tumors. Enucleation with curettement of surrounding bone provides sufficient treatment for these nonagressive tumors.

Aggressive Odontogenic Tumors

Some neoplasms that involve the mandible are prone to recurrences and/or extensive local tissue destruction. These comprise aggressive odontogenic tumors, adenoameloblastoma, calcifying epithelial odontogenic (Pindborg) tumor, and myxoma. Because of the similar behavior and treatment among these lesions, they will be considered together in this section.

Aggressive odontogenic tumors comprise the following:

1. *Ameloblastoma.* This lesion is discussed earlier in this chapter.
2. *Adenoameloblastoma.* Adenomeloblastoma are less aggressive than ameloblastoma. Small and cystic lesions can usually be cured by enucleation and vigorous curettage. Large, recurrent lesions deserve en bloc resection.
3. *Melanoameblastoma.* Melanoameblastoma is usually a disease of infancy. Rather than being truly odontogenic, these tumors may originate in the neural crest. Less aggressive than ameloblastoma, they respond well to local curettage and removal of involved teeth/tooth buds.
4. *Calcifying epithelial odontogenic Tumor (Pindborg tumor).* These rare tumors usually occur in the mandibular biscuid region, often in association with the follicle of an unerupted tooth. Individual tumors vary considerably in their degree of aggressiveness, but they should receive treatment similar to that recommended for an ameblastoma.
5. *Myxoma,* which are rare lesions, also have a high recurrence rate when treated nonaggressively. Therefore, they should be removed along with a small margin of normal bone.

Aggressive Nonodontogenic Tumors

1. *Giant cell tumors.* Giant cell tumors in the mandible do not usually manifest that frankly malignant behavior that appears in nonfacial skeletal locations. Nevertheless, treatment should respect the local aggressive/low-grade malignant behavior of these tumors and should be similar to that recommended for ameloblastoma.
2. *Osteoblastoma and osteoid osteoma.* Histologically and clinically similar, these neoplasms may be variants of a "basic osteoblastic tumor."[5] Complete surgical excision with a margin of normal bone is recommended because these tumors tend to recur after lesser procedures.[5]
3. *Chondroma.* While histologically benign, chondromas of the mandible exhibit low-grade malignant tendencies and may develop into chondrosarcomas, especially after multiple, noncurative surgical interventions. Therefore, excision with an en bloc technique is prudent.

REFERENCES

1. Thoma KH: Oral Surgery, Vol. 2, Ed. 5. St. Louis: CV Mosby, 1969
2. Batsakis, JG (ed): Tumors of the Head and Neck—Clinical and Pathological Considerations, Vol. 2, Ed. 2. Baltimore: Williams & Wilkins, 1979, p 399
3. Hirschl S, Katz A: Giant cell reparative granuloma outside the jaw bone: Diagnostic criteria and review of the literature with the first case described in the temporal bone. Hum Pathol 5:171–181, 1974
4. Goerig AC, Fay JT, King E: Endodontic treatment of a cementoblastoma. Oral Surg 58:133–136, 1984
5. McClatchey KD: Odontogenic lesions—tumors and cysts. In Batsakis JD (ed): Tumors of the Head and Neck—Clinical and Pathological Considerations, Vol. 2, Ed. 2. Baltimore: Williams & Wilkins, 1979, pp 531–561

6 Surgical Management of Malignant Tumors: Considerations of Mandibular Invasion

Byron J. Bailey, M.D.

Management of malignancy in the oral cavity requires careful assessment of the possibility that the patient's tumor may invade either the mandible or its periosteal covering. Mandibular involvement is most likely when the primary tumor is visually and palpably close to the mandible or when it extends to involve the alveolus or retromolar trigone. The typical patient profile is that of a 60-year-old male with a long history of tobacco and ethanol usage, some degree of malnutrition and weight loss, and *at least* mild pulmonary and cardiovascular disease.

Since primary lesions are often readily visible, most of these patients present to a physician with a T1 or T2 lesion. Most patients do not have papable cervical lymphadenopathy when they are first seen, but many of the patients with T2 lesions present with occult cervical node metastases and most of those with T3 and T4 lesions do have positive nodes. Patients with a primary tumor located in the anterior floor of the mouth are definitely at risk for the development of cervical node metastases bilaterally. This group of patients has a high incidence of second primary carcinomas.[1]

Treatment for patients with oral cavity carcinoma is selected according to the stage of the disease and some other variables that will be discussed subsequently The malignancy in most of these patients can be cured if the initial assessment and management are adequate.

REVIEW OF CANCER STAGING

The *Manual for Staging of Cancer, Second Edition* (1983), prepared by the American Joint Committee on Cancer, is an excellent standard for the staging of these patients.[2]

Sites of the oral cavity with the potential to involve the mandible include tumors arising on the lips, buccal mucosa, floor of the mouth, oral tongue, hard palate, and gingiva. These tumors (primaries) are staged as T1 when they have a greatest diameter of 2 cm or less; as T2 when they have a greatest diameter of more than 2 cm but not greater than 4 cm; as T3 when the greatest diameter is more than 4 cm; and as T4 when there is a large tumor with deep invasion to involve adjacent bony structures, the base of the tongue, or the skin of the neck. Interestingly, this staging system pays very little specific attention to the mandible even though it is presumed to be the structure involved most frequently by oral cavity primaries. Because of the frequency of mandibular invasion and the importance of dealing with the mandible correctly, the American Joint Committee on Cancer may consider directing more attention to this topic in the future.

Lesions involving the oropharynx, nasopharynx, and superior portion of the hypopharynx may also extend to involve the mandible. Staging of these primaries (T) is also based on size and follows exactly the same pattern as is used for primary lesions of the oral cavity. The sites most likely to involve the mandible are the tongue, the tonsil, and the palate.

The staging system for lymph node status (N) and for distant metastasis (M) is identical to that employed for all of the head and neck primary sites. The process of tumor staging is complete; many procedures and studies are available that can be employed to achieve higher levels of accuracy. Within the practical constraints of time, availability, and cost, certain items are considered essential for tumor staging accuracy. These include the following:

—A complete physical examination of the head and neck region, including inspection and palpation of all accessible structures.
—Indirect examination of the nasopharynx and larynx.
—Biopsy of the primary tumor.
—Appropriate radiographic studies (chest roentgenogram, sinus roentgenograms for tumors involving the palate, and at least one type of radiographic assessment for tumors that place the mandible at risk for invasion).

Considerable controversy centers around the radiographic assessment of the mandible. The panorex film is probably the most widely used in practice, but dental (occlusal) films or computed tomography (CT) have strong advocates.

Staging must be conducted with great care before the physician can proceed to the next step, that of selecting appropriate therapy. Most early lesions are treated by surgery or radiation therapy; most advanced lesions are managed by combined modalities. Selection of the appropriate therapy is crucial for preserving of optimal function and appearance and for achieving the highest possible rates of cure. Physicians who diagnose cancer in anatomic regions adjacent to the mandible must attempt to ascertain whether or not the mandible is involved, either by periosteal invasion or actual bone invasion. Mandibular involvement becomes a critical factor in treatment selection and will be the major topic of this chapter.

FACTORS ASSOCIATED WITH MANDIBULAR INVASION

Gilbert and colleagues have demonstrated some of the factors that correlate with mandibular invasion by tumor.[3] In their recent study, these investigators found that certain points of origin carry a significant prognostic implication for invasion. The sites of origin with the highest likelihood of subsequent mandibular invasion were the alveolus (39% probability), the floor of the mouth (22%), the retromolar trigone (18%), the tongue (15%), and the tonsil (11%). Other sites of primaries had less than a 10% probability of association with mandibular or periosteal invasion. Not surprisingly, progressive increases in the stage of the disease tended to be associated with increasing likelihood of mandibular involvement, except for a slight decrease in stage 4 disease. The occurrence of mandibular invasion found in each stage was stage 1 disease (7%), stage 2 (22%), stage 3 (28%), and stage 4 (23%).

These investigators also confirm the value of the clinical impression on physical examination. They noted that when the tumor seemed to be "attached" to the mandible, incidence of histologic evidence of mandibular invasion was 30%; when the tumor seemed "not attached," incidence of confirmed invasion was only 8%. Their study does not indicate a correlation between the presence or absence of clinical nodes with mandibular invasion. They also found no correlation between the degree of tumor differentiation and the probability for incidence of future invasion of the mandible.

REVIEW OF EARLIER PATTERNS OF TREATMENT

As a general rule, the continuity of the mandible should be preserved if no direct involvement can be demonstrated. Some patients, however, fall into a "gray zone" in which we are not entirely certain whether the mandible has or has not been invaded. Some patients with primaries near the mandible will be selected appropriately for treatment by surgical resection including a marginal or coronal partial mandibulectomy with preservation of the mandibular arch: Also, some of these patients will be treated appropriately by including a supraomohyoid or modified neck dissection.

Carcinoma of the floor of the mouth involves the mandible in about one of each four patients. For example, Gilbert and co-workers[3] reported an incidence of 23% and Slaughter and associates[4] reported an incidence of 29%.

Ward and Robben[5] felt that decisions regarding treatment could be based reliably on the physical examination. They proposed that the "pull-through" operation be utilized in those patients in whom the margin of the primary carcinoma was greater than 1 cm distant from the mandible. Marchetta[6,7] was a pioneer in evaluating the significance of periosteal invasion. His experience supported a surgical policy of sparing the mandible in patients where the primary lesion is "clinically separated" from the mandible.

Surgeons differ in their preferences for the specific technical modifications that they employ, but the trend favors preserving the mandible whenever possible. Whichever alternative is chosen, the decision-making process should be based upon all of the information that can reasonably be acquired.

ASSESSMENT OF MANDIBULAR INVASION

Opinion continues to differ with regard to the optimal assessment of mandibular invasion. Roentgenographic evaluation lacks sensitivity, therefore missing some instances of the involvement, but a positive roentgenogram is usually accurate. Bone scans lack specificity and may suggest tumor invasion where it is not present. Furthermore, among the proponents of radiographic evaluation, some physicians state that occlusal (dental) films should always be used anteriorly and that CT scanning should be employed posteriorly (unless there are extensive dental fillings) to obtain the most reliable evaluation; while others conclude that all radiologic studies are too imperfect for making a final plan.

Baker and colleagues[8] conducted a prospective study, comparing the sensitivity of the panorex roentgenogram and the bone scan in the detection of subclinical invasion of the mandible by squamous cell carcinoma. Their observations suggest the bone scanning technique is more sensitive in detecting early cancer involvement and may be a better indicator of the extent of involvement. In their experience, the panorex roentgenogram tended to miss or underestimate the extent of some mandibular invasion by cancer.

Noyek[9] asserts that the triphasic bone scan rules out the false negatives and shows positive findings only when the bone is actually involved. Weisman and Kimmelman[10] found a fairly high correlation between the findings generated from bone scan and radiographic studies. They noted that when a difference between the two occurred it always consisted of a positive scan and a negative radiograph. When both studies are positive or when both are negative, little doubt remains regarding the presence or absence of bone invasion. The bottom line seems to be that the scan has the advantage of showing early, and even periosteal, involvment with tumor but has the disadvantage that it could suggest tumor invasion when only periodontal infection or even an old fracture is present. Of course, the bone scan would be positive in the presence of osteomyelitis or osteoradionecrosis, but these would be rare problems at the time of the initial assessment. Gilbert and colleagues[3] also found that the bone scan was more sensitive, but their experience included false-positive findings half of the time. Sixty percent of the patients with positive radiographs had bone invasion (7% of the negatives had bone invasion), while 50% of the patients with positive scans had bone invasion (none of the patients with a positive scan had no bone invasion).

Much remains to be learned about the prognostic significance of mandibular invasion. Our understanding of the natural history of tumor spread to periosteum and into bone is quite limited. To know why bone invasion occurs in one patient but not in another, even though their primary lesions appear to be identical, would be enormously helpful. Is the periosteum an invitation or a barrier to bone invasion? Are there measurable characteristics of the primary tumor that will predict bone invasion? Has bone invasion any prognostic implication for the probability of cervical node metastasis, distant metastasis, or survival? Are we dealing with tumors that are more aggressive biologically or with host defense defects that are local or systemic? What is the correlation between bone invasion and nutritional factors, and can these be modified by nutritional therapy? The answers to these and other pressing questions await further study.

SURGICAL OPTIONS

In general, most patients with malignant tumors arising close to the mandible can be managed surgically without interrupting permanently the continuity of the mandible. In some instances, resection of any mandibular component can be avoided entirely; in others, inclusion of only a coronal or marginal portion of the mandible will be necessary. However, in patients who have advanced disease associated closely with the mandible and those who exhibit objective evidence of mandibular invasion, one of the following options must usually be selected:

1. *Segmental partial mandibulectomy.* This procedure involves resection of the primary lesion, usually in continuity with with a complete (full thickness) segment of the adjacent mandible, leaving both discontinuity and a structural defect between the two mandibular segments that remain (Fig. 55).

2. *Hemimandibulectomy.* This usually refers to the resection of one-half of the mandible but sometimes refers to resection extending from the midline to the angle of the mandible (Fig. 56).

3. *Total mandibulectomy.* This term describes excision of the mandible from angle to angle, or any more extension resection including a total excision of the entire mandible (Fig. 57). We have followed the policy of resecting limited portions of the mandible (marginal or coronal resections) when we suspect strongly that the periosteum or superficial cortex of the mandible may be invaded. When we are reasonably certain of tumor invasion on the basis of a bone scan or radiographic study, we have usually proceeded with segmental resection. Many head and neck surgeons feel that segmental resection of the mandible should be performed routinely in all patients with malignant lesions that are clinically adherent to the mandible, all lesions involving the alveolar epithelium, and all patients with cancer near the mandible and with positive bone scans or radiographs. Recently some newer possibilities have been proposed and these will be discussed in Contemporary Surgical Trends, below.

Guillamondegui and co-workers[1] reported the outcome for a group of 104 patients at M. D. Anderson Hospital who were evaluated for treatment for carcinoma involving the anterior floor of the mouth. This group of patients had received no prior treatment and the study reviews the selection of treatment and the analysis of various factors involved in treatment success and failure. The physicians chose to manage 61 of the 104 patients by surgery only; 47 required some form of mandibular resection.

Most patients who required surgical resection of

a portion of the mandible were treated by coronal resection (27 patients); the remainder received hemimandibulectomy (15), segmental partial mandibulectomy (3), or total mandibulectomy (2). Fifteen of these patients were treated by sequential surgical excision and radiotherapy. This was not a randomized protocol, and patients were selected for one form of treatment or another by the size of the primary lesion, the degree of tumor infiltration, primary tumor appearance, the extent of cervical lymph node metastasis, and other individual and variable factors. Primary tumor resection interorally with defect repair by skin grafts or local flaps was employed in many patients.

After analyzing their long-term results, Guillamondegui and colleagues concluded that surgical

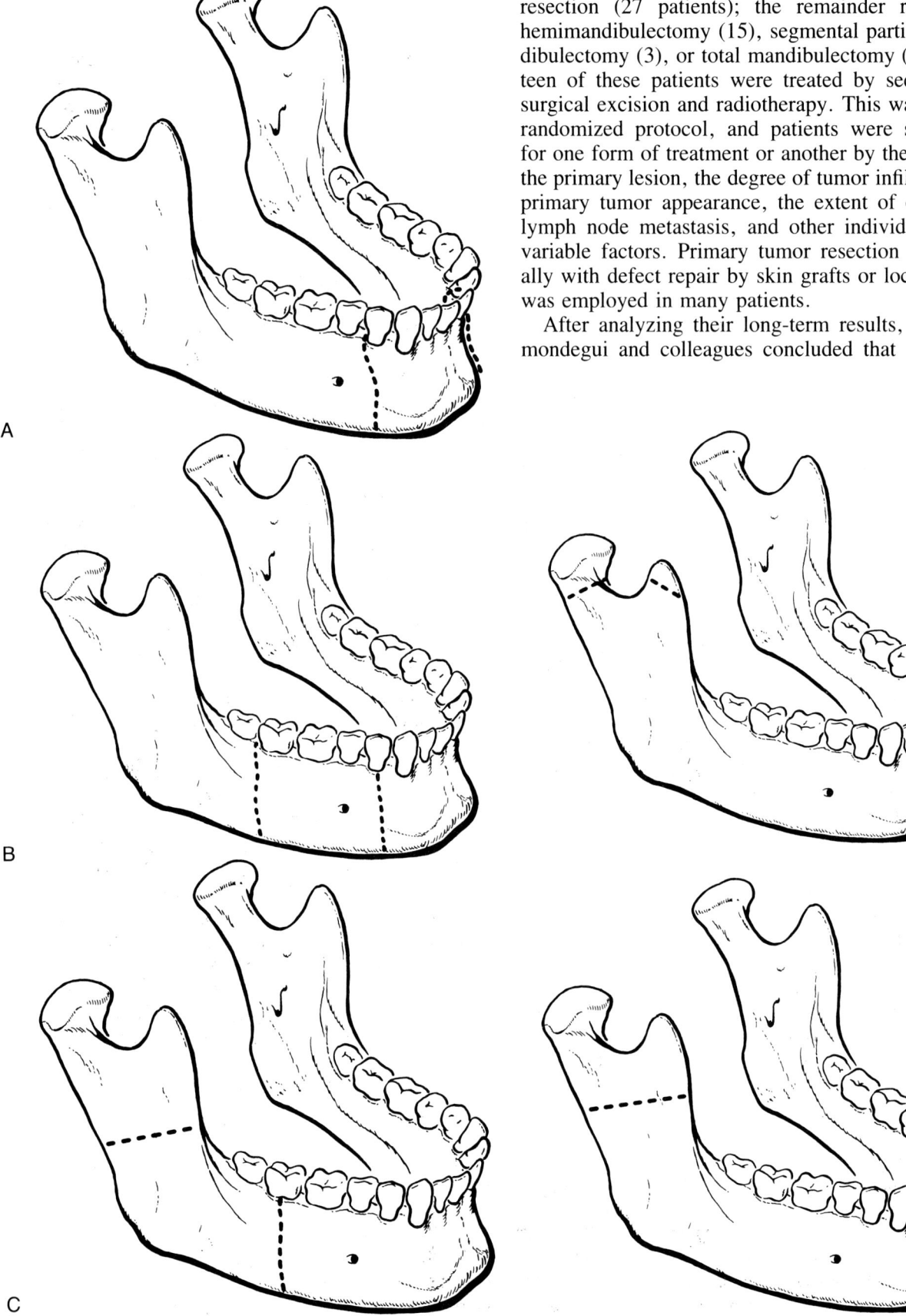

Figure 55. Segmental resection. (A) Anterior (B) Lateral (C) Posterior.

Figure 56. Hemmandibulectomy. (A) Symphysis to condyle. (B) Symphysis to ramus.

resection is extremely effective in controlling T1 and T2-sized tumors and can be accomplished without an unacceptable degree of functional loss. Patients with T1 lesions rarely developed cervical lymph node metastases; when they did, all were salvaged, usually by a neck dissection. This surgical approach was successful in controlling all the primary tumor sites in patients with T2 lesions. Patients with T3 and T4 primaries and clinically negative (N0) necks were controlled effectively by more extensive surgical resection (including neck dissection), but considerable functional loss was seen and surgical reconstruction became more challenging for the larger tumors.

Relatively few variations exist among the resection techniques employed at the present time. These techniques can be classified and illustrated as follows:

I. Marginal resection types.
   A. Anterior arch of mentum—coronal resection or resection of lingual cortical plate for anterior floor of mouth primary (Fig. 58).
   B. Body—resection of lingual cortical one-half of mandible for floor of mouth primary encroaching upon the mandible (Fig. 59).
   C. Body—alveolar (superior) portion resection for early gingival lesion touching the superior oral surface of the mandible (Fig. 60).
   D. Body—resection of submandibular inferior portion for primary tumor or submandibular lymph nodes adjacent or fixed to the periosteum of the inferior margin of the mandible (Fig. 61).

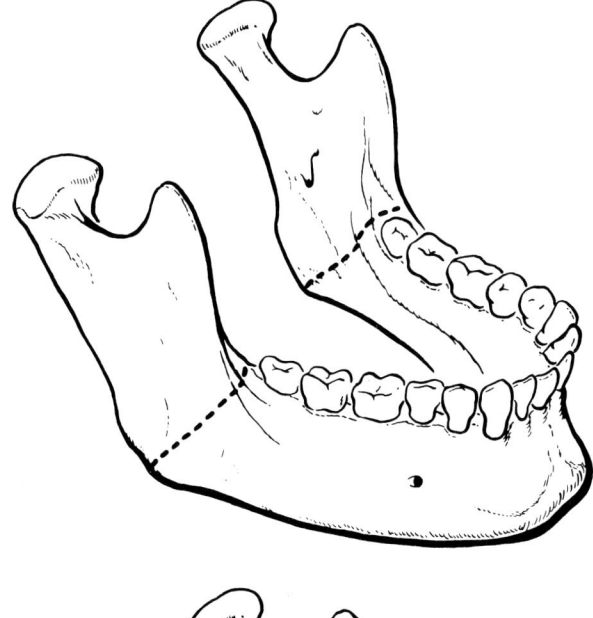
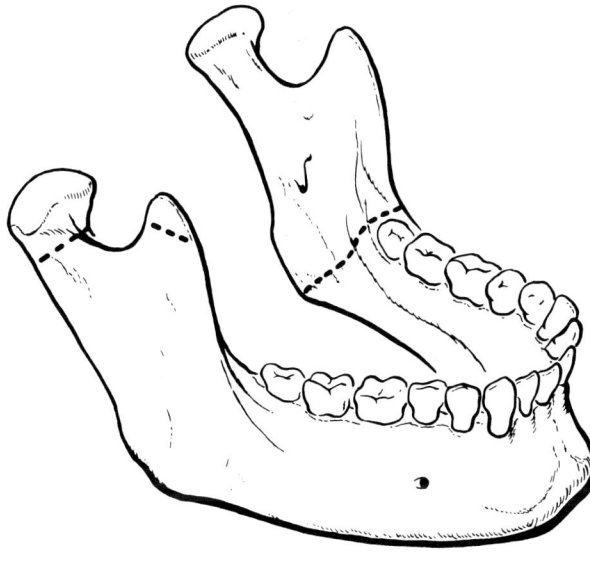
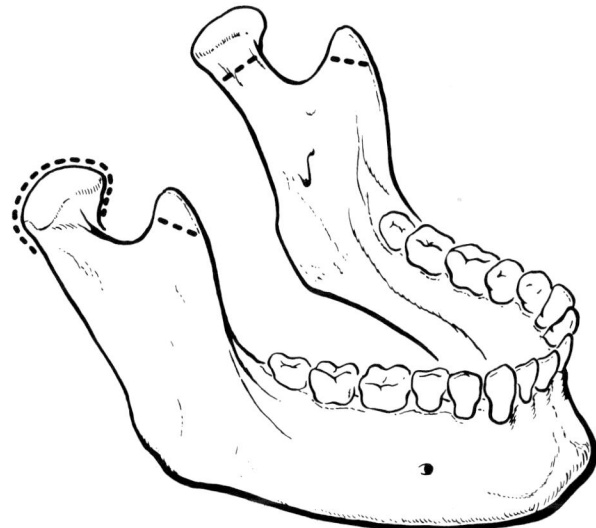

Figure 57. Total mandibulectomy. (A) Angle to angle. (B) Angle to ramus. (C) Ramus to condyle (disarticulation).

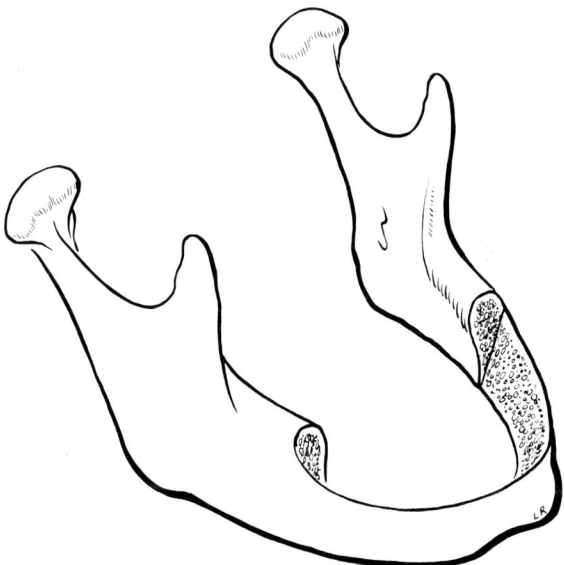

Figure 58. Anterior marginal resection.

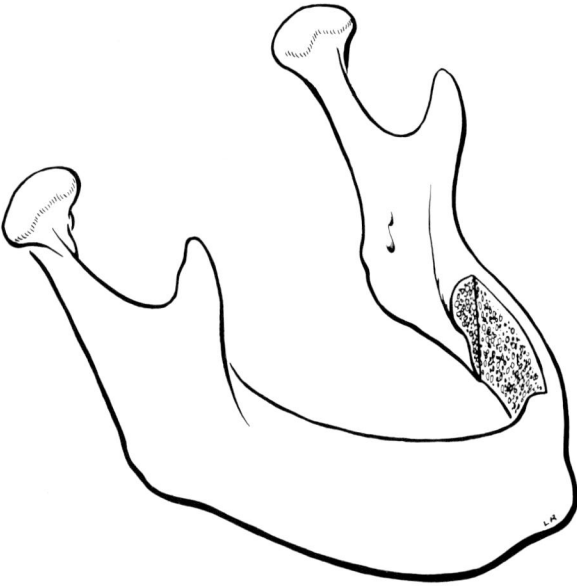

Figure 59. Lingual cortical marginal resection.

II. Segmental resection.
   A. Arch (Figs. 62 to 65).
   B. Body (Fig. 66 to 70.
   C. Angle.
III. Hemimandibulectomy (Figs. 71 to 73).
IV. Total mandibulectomy.

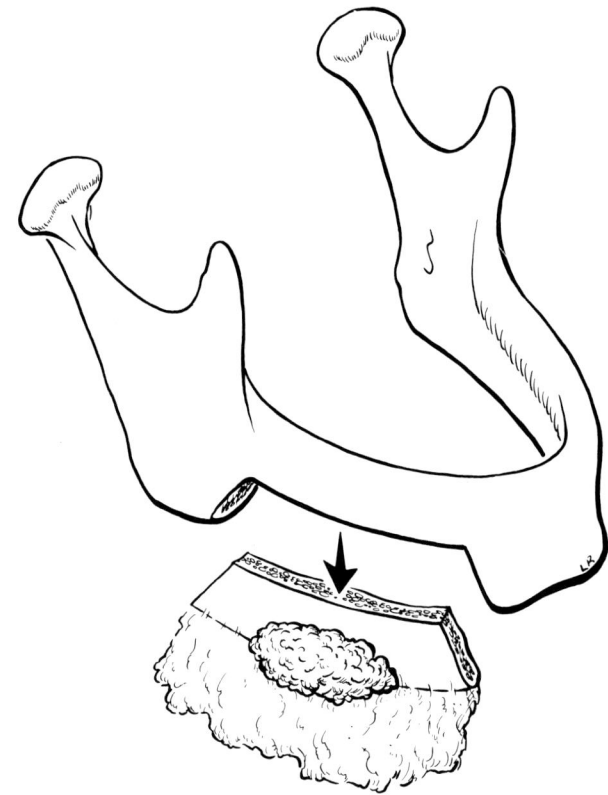

Figure 61. Inferior marginal resection.

Neck dissection should be considered when disease is serious enough to warrant some form of mandibular surgery for an oral cavity or pharyngeal primary. Some form of neck dissection is recommended for all clinically positive (N+ necks and for many N0 necks. Individual surgeons have their own preferences for supraomohyoid neck dissection, modified neck dissection, or radical neck dissection. Numerous reports suggest that approximately one-third of the patients who seem to have an N0 neck will be found to have occult metastatic cancer when resected lymph nodes receive careful

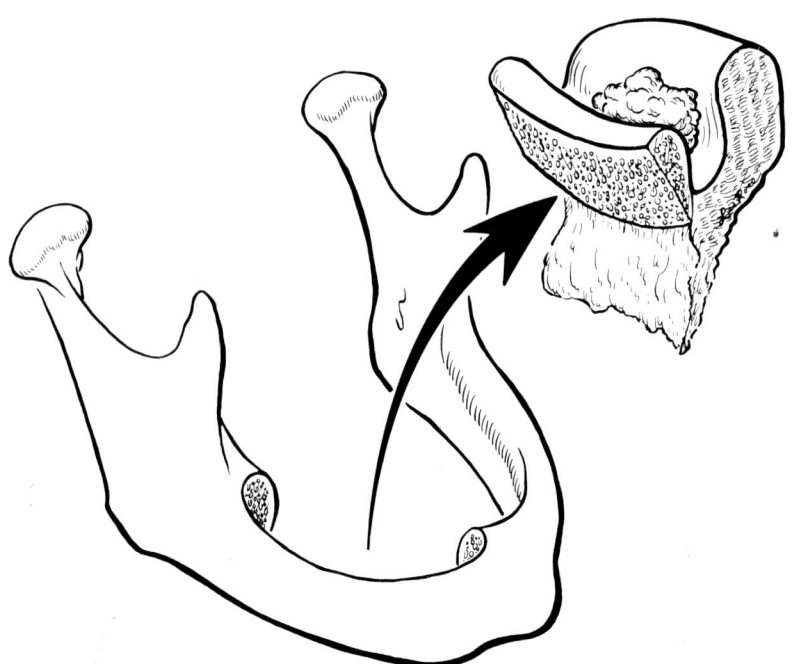

Figure 60. Superior (alveolar) marginal resection.

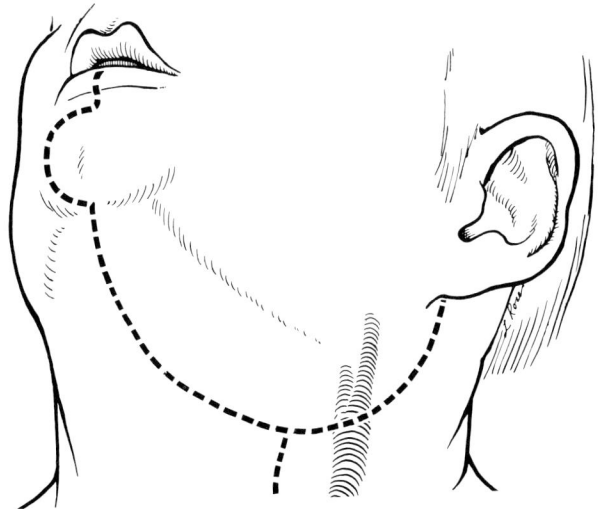

Figure 62. Anterior segmental resection, incision.

histologic study. Of those patients who have cervical lymph node metastases, approximately 20% will have contralateral cervical lymph node involvement.

RATIONAL FOR MANDIBULAR RESECTION

The rationale for including minor or major portions of the mandible in the primary tumor resection

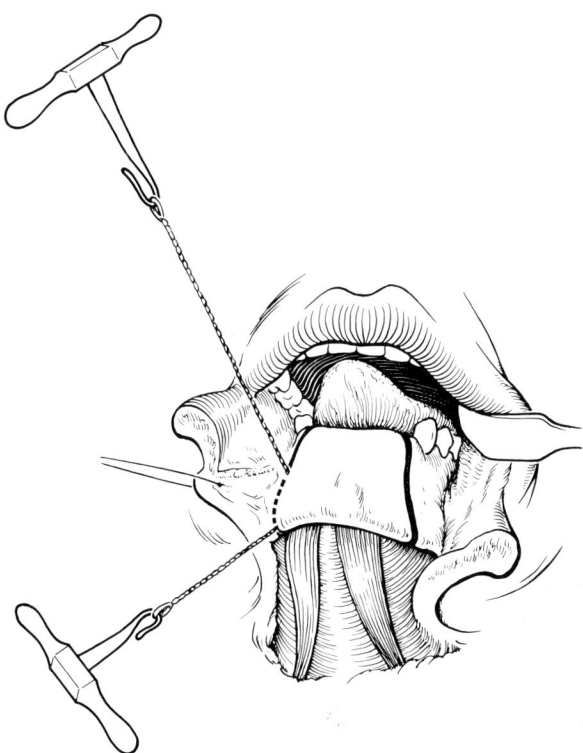

Figure 63. Bilateral anterior mandibular osteotomies.

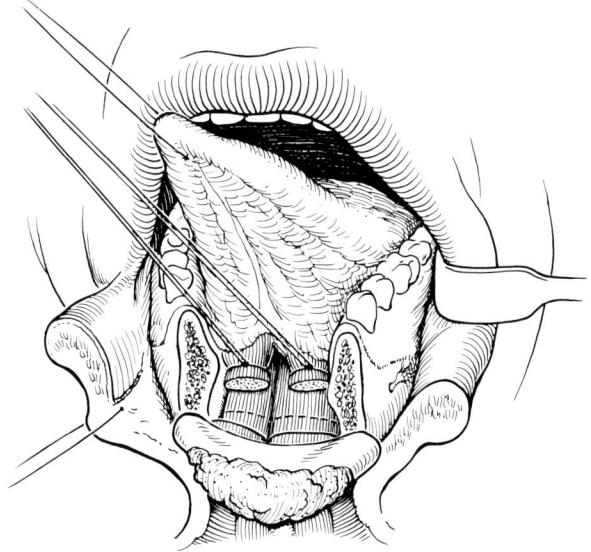

Figure 64. Resection of specimen.

is based upon our observations regarding patterns of treatment that are associated with a high percentage of patient cure and those that are associated with a high percentage of failure. The information that is available can be summarized as follows:

1. Small malignant primaries of the oral cavity can be treated with approximately equal success by radiation therapy or surgery.
2. Patients with mandibular invasion by cancer are unlikely to be cured by radiation therapy and should be managed by resection.
3. Patients with primary carcinoma en-

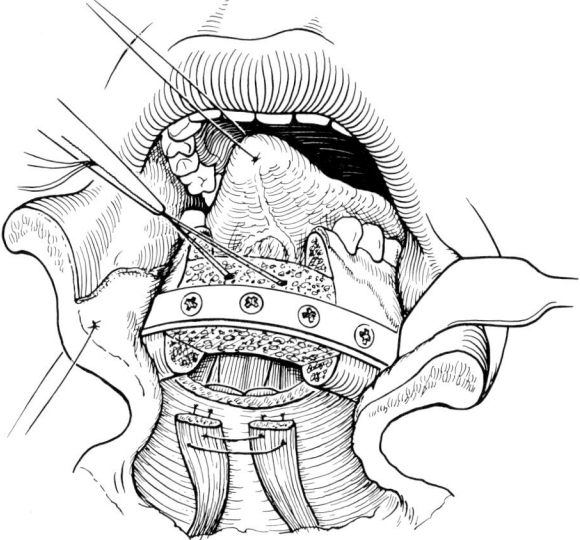

Figure 65. Kirschner wire spacer or dynamic bendable defect bridging (DBDB) plate. (DBDB plate may be used with or without a bone graft.) The two options may be employed sequentailly.

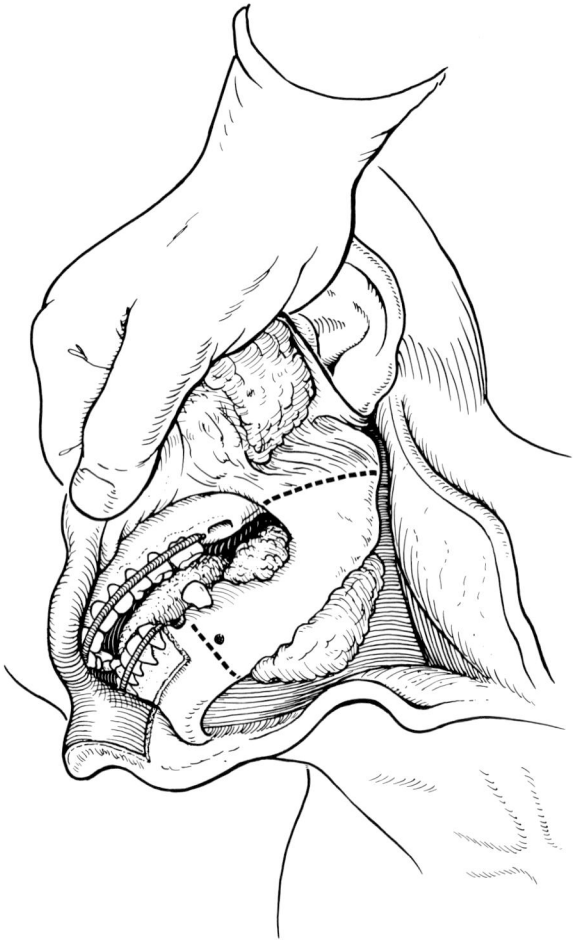

Figure 66. Segmental resection from just anterior to the mental foramen to the ramus, just inferior to the sigmoid notch.

croaching on the mandible and without evidence of cervical lymph node involvement are at risk for occult cervical lymph node metastases, occult invasion of the periosteum or bone, and occult spread of tumor along the inferior alveolar nerve canal.
4. Patients with mandibular invasion by tumor and N0 necks rarely die of distant metastases only.
5. Patients with radiographic evidence of bone invasion usually have more extensive bone involvement than is demonstrated radiographically and should be managed by generous segmental resection or more extensive resection of the mandible.

Taken as a a group, patients with oral cavity carcinoma are usually diagnosed earlier and their cure rates should be in the range of 60 to 75%. Failure to control the primary should seldom occur and most treatment failure will involve residual neck disease. We hope the combination of extensive surgical resection with radiation therapy in a planned sequence will improve the outlook for these patients in future reports. Chemotherapeutic agents such as mitomycin are being investigated for their effectiveness in enhancing radiation therapy. At the present time, the importance of extensive and complete resection at the *initial* operative procedure should be emphasized in view of the low rate of successful salvage by secondary surgery or radiation therapy.

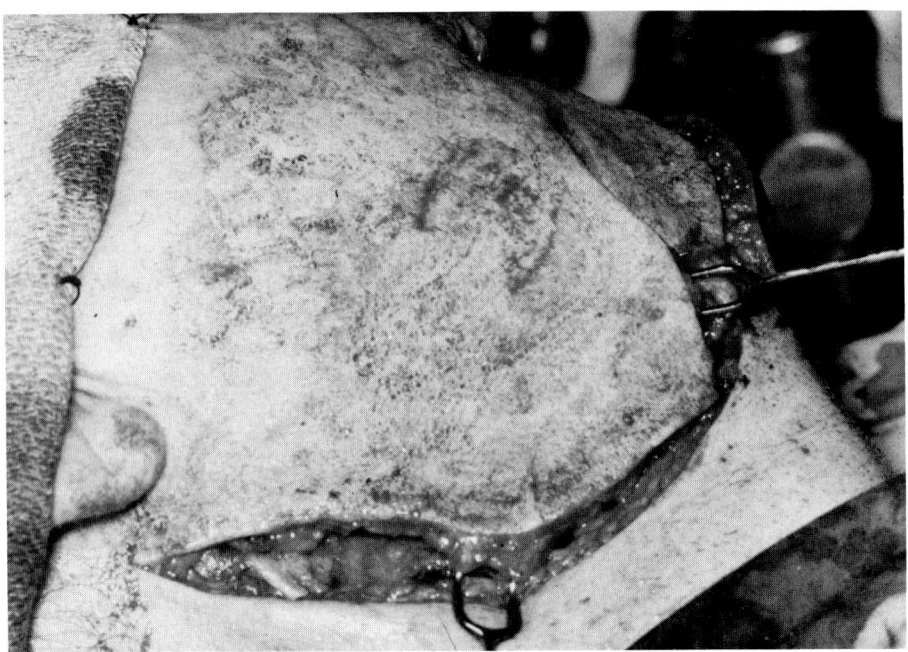

Figure 67. Cervical incision from the mastoid tip to the chin.

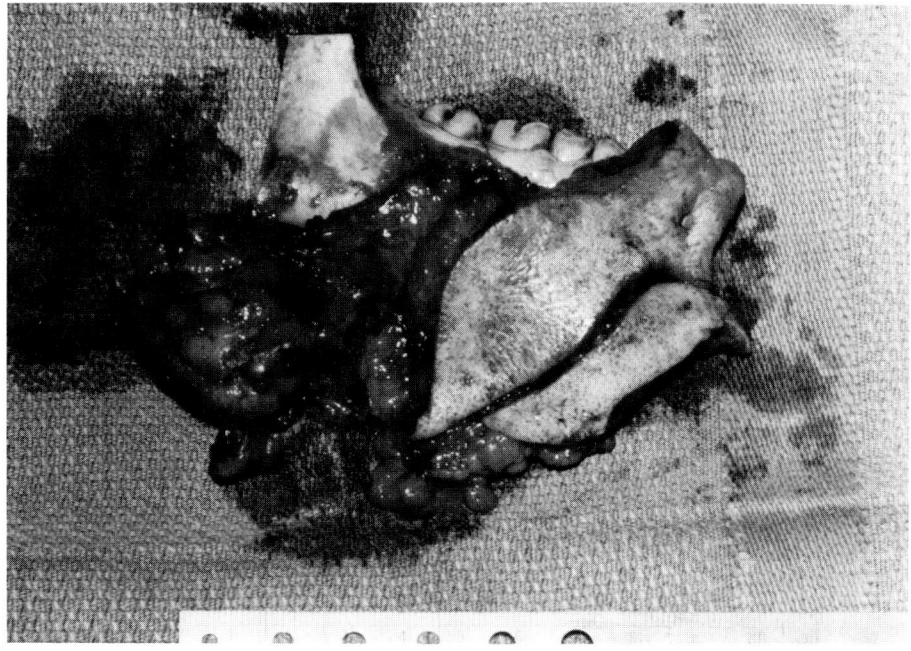

Figure 68. Specimen from laterally. En block resection of lip, skin, suprahyoid neck dissection and hemimandibulectomy.

CONTEMPORARY SURGICAL TRENDS

This section provides brief comments concerning recent trends and new frontiers in an effort to emphasize the dynamic nature of this field. Also, it attempts to place the previous pages into the perspective of recent events.

Some surgeons feel that far too many composite resections of the mandible are being done for reasons that are no longer valid (i.e., to gain access to the primary, to facilitate closure, or just because of tradition). Median or midline mandibulotomy is being proposed as a better way to gain access for tumor resection, including periosteal stripping or marginal mandibulectomy as a means of avoiding

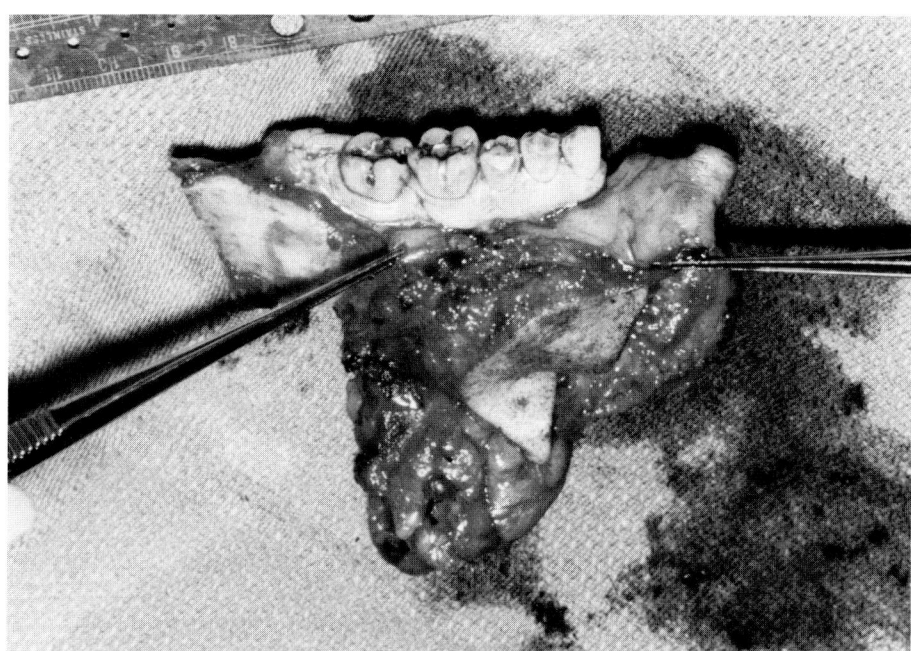

Figure 69. Specimen from superiorly.

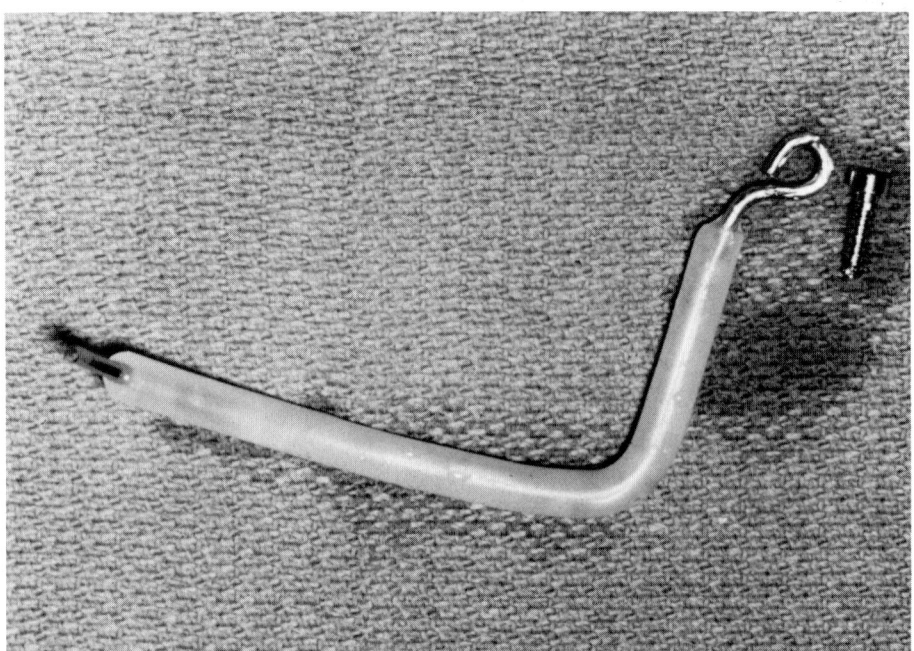

Figure 70. Steinmann pin fashioned as a temporary mandibular replacement. The pin is coated with acrylic, and one end is fashioned for screw attachment to the residual ramus. The other end is inserted into the opposite side of the mandible at the symphysis.

any resection of mandibular segments. Skin grafts, local flaps, and regional flaps offer various opportunities for reconstruction without mandibular resection (Figs. 74 to 76).

Midline mandibulotomy is also being proposed as the surgical approach of choice, even for lesions involving the posterior two-thirds of the cavity. This technique is proposed as an alternative for segmental resection and for posterior or angle mandibulotomy in many instances.

Many surgeons are developing increased confidence in the combination of mandibulotomy with

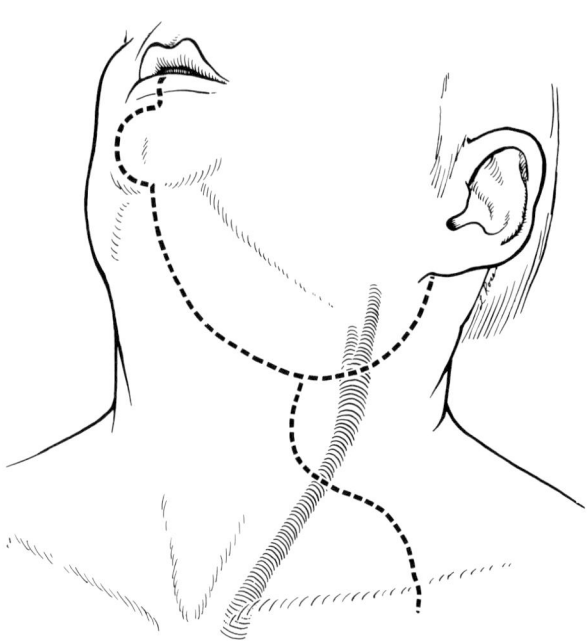

Figure 71. Preferred incision for composite resection of oral cavity primary, adjacent involved mandibular segment, and neck dissection. Lower limb of neck incision is perpendicular to the curved incision (from chin to mastoid tip) and crosses the carotid at only one point.

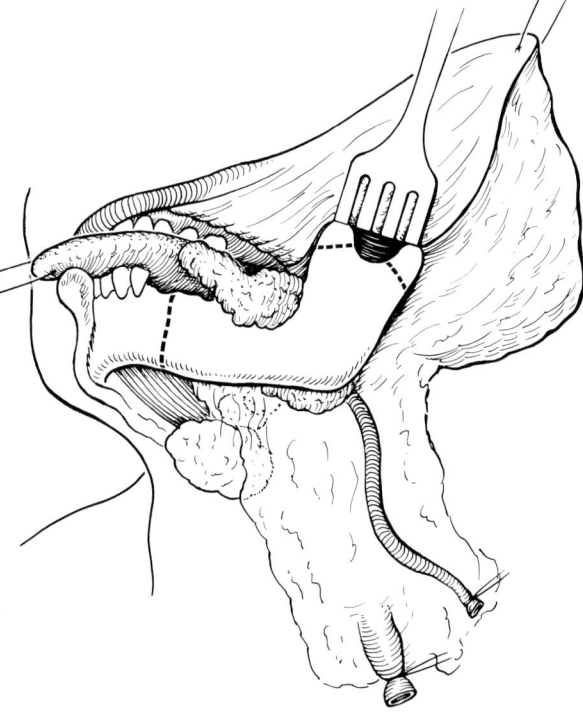

Figure 72. Mandibular osteotomies are performed just anterior to the mental foramen and at the condylar neck.

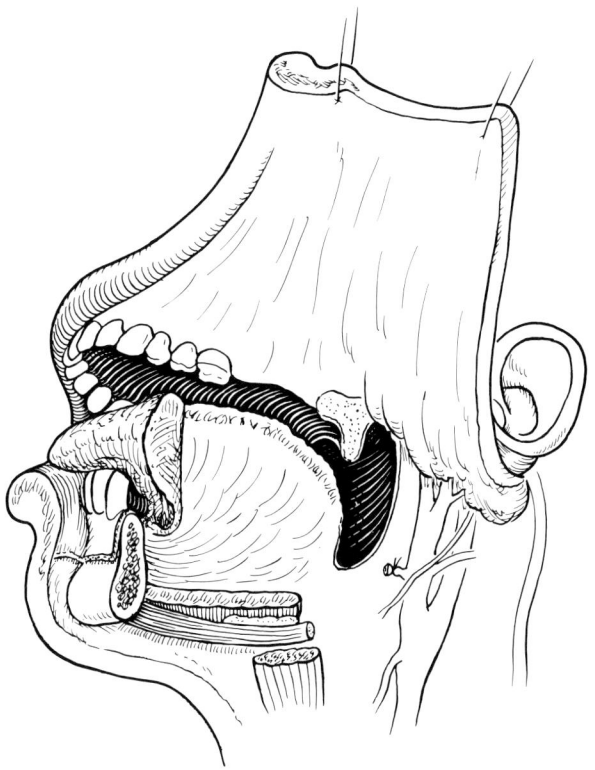

Figure 73. Completion of the composite resection varies according to the location of the primary, and closure may include the use of a tongue flap, deltopectoral flap, or pectoralis major myocutaneous flap.

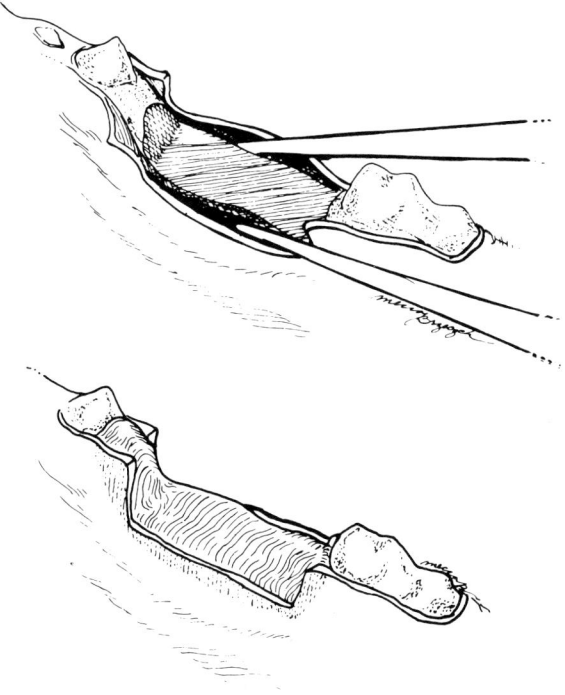

Figure 75. Top. Reflection of the mucoperiosteum to create "pocket" for dermal graft. Bottom. Dermal graft overlying bone and placed into pocket (From Lambert et al., Arch Otolaryngol 110:658, 1984. With permission.)

postoperative radiotherapy. Previously, strong opposition to this combination was based on concerns about the potential problem of postradiation osteoradionecrosis.

Marginal partial mandibulectomy is graining popularity. Routine segmental resection of the mandible is becoming less popular than it was previously.

The "pull-through" operative procedure, in which the primary oral cavity tumor is resected in continuity with a radical neck dissection without mandibulotomy or mandibulectomy, is losing its former popularity.

Findings reported recently have decreased the

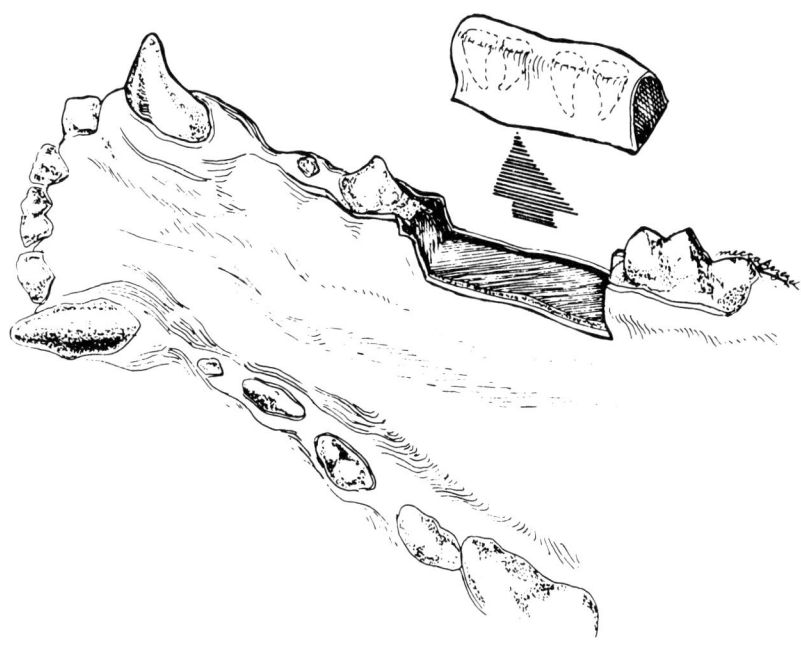

Figure 74. En bloc resection of the mandibular alveolus, including mucosa, bone, and submerged roots. (From Lambert et al.: Arch Otolaryngol 110:658, 1984. With permission.)

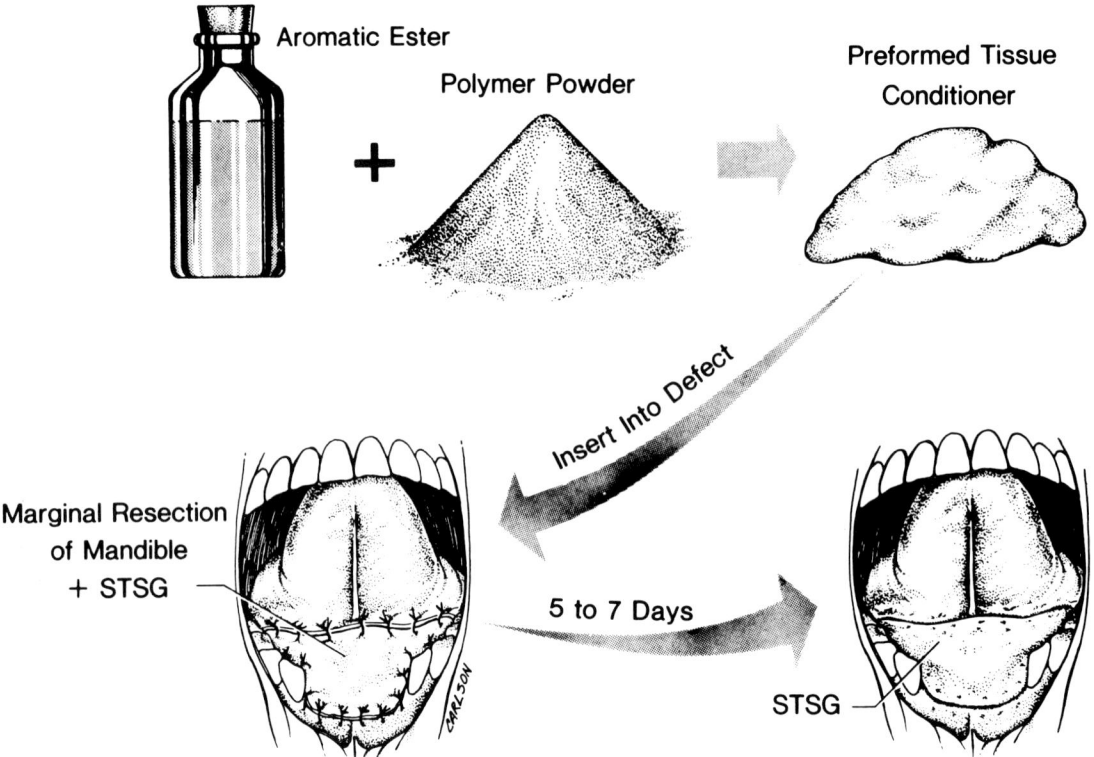

Figure 76. Intraoperative mixing of aromatic ester and polymer powder results in soft, pliable material that conforms to any intraoral defect. (From Teichgraeber Arch Otolaryngol 110:464, 1984. With permission.)

concern regarding cancer involvement of the mandibular periosteum in patients with primary lesions that do not encroach on the mandible.

Some surgeons are suggesting that marginal resection techniques are feasible (in carefully selected patients) even when there is minor cortical bone invasion with tumor.

To preserve the integrity of the mandibular arch has become the object of greater concern and increased effort. This conservative approach appears to be justified, particularly by the lack of evidence that it compromises patients' survival and by the abscense of any routinely reliable, single-stage reconstructive technique for mandibular defects.

Some surgeons are expressing a preference for immediate stabilization of mandibular defects using the simplest techniques (e.g., Steinmann pinbone cement) to obtain spacing and stabilization as an interim management technique. They feel that more complex reconstructive techniques can be performed more appropriately and more successfully at a later time.

The "split-rib" mandibular reconstructive techniques have been adopted by a number of surgeons. Others, however, report difficulty in achieving the level of success reported from Sweden.

Osteo-integrated myocutaneous pectoralis major muscle flaps (and others) along with microvascular composite myoosseous grafts are being investigated intensively. These are highly specialized reconstructive procedures and, at present, the number of patients and even the number of medical centers involved are rather small. If these techniques should become routine, they might alter the patterns of surgical resection in the direction of more radical surgery for this patient group.

Some controversy focuses on the management of recurrent carcinoma in primaries arising near the mandible. As stated previously, dealing effectively with the tumor at the initial procedure must be emphasized. Salvage rates are low with either surgery or radiation therapy. If the tumor recurs at the primary site but a previously N0 neck remains N0, some surgeons would propose that a composite resection be performed. Others feel that if the tumor recurs at the primary site but a previously N0 neck remains N0 and the patient has had prior radiation therapy, a neck dissection is not necessary. Conversely, if there is a primary recurrence and evidence of cervical node metastasis, the prognosis for survival is so poor that even radical surgery offers little.

Laser excision of oral cavity lesions is gaining popularity. Surgeons limited this modality to very small lesions initially, but with growing confidence and good results, we find a trend toward larger laser excision, even for lesions quite near the mandible. Laser therapy for periosteal invasion has been suggested.

Photodynamic therapy may be a particularly applicable modality for patients with oral cavity lesions because the primary lesions are quite accessible. This technique, based on the selective destruction of tumor cells with the preservation of normal cells, holds considerable promise.

Intraoperative radiation therapy may be appropriate for some patients with tumor invasion of the periosteum. The facilities for administering intraoperative radiation therapy are increasing, and this modality may carve out a place in the management of some patients with cancer encroaching upon the mandible.

Because of the unpredictable outcome with all bone grafting techniques, hyperbaric oxygen (HBO) therapy after bone graft reconstructive surgery has attracted considerable interest. The use of HBO is particularly attractive on a theoretical basis when fibrosis following surgery and irradiation compromises the vascular supply at the recipient site in the patient. Daily HBO therapy promotes increased collagen synthesis and induces angiogenesis, the formation of new, additional capillaries. Daily HBO has been reported to improve the success rate of bone graft reconstruction from a range of 20 to 60% to rates higher than 90%.

DENTAL ISSUES

Any surgical procedure involving the mandible can be associated with postoperative infection. When radiotherapy has been used in this region, the vascular supply to the teeth, the mandible, and the soft tissues in the region is decreased. These factors combine to increase the incidence of infection and osteoradionecrosis associated with any mandibular surgical procedure, including dental extraction.

The patient must be permitted to make an informed decision regarding the risks and requirements of retaining the teeth when radiotherapy is given. Patients whose teeth are in good repair and who will comply with postoperative fluoride therapy and other oral hygiene measures may do well. On the other hand, individuals whose teeth are in poor repair, who have significant periodontal disease, who are slated for full-course radiation therapy, and/or who are likely to demonstrate problems of postoperative compliance should receive a strong recommendation for preoperative dental extraction. The more severe the problems appear to be, the greater the risk of postoperative osteoradionecrosis. The decision becomes really a matter of whether they wish to retain their teeth at the risk of ultimately losing their jaw. Despite the advances associated with HBO therapy and other regimens that are available, these patients remain at risk for an extremely debilitating course of events.

Beumer and associates[11,12] reported experience with dental extraction before and after radiation therapy. Preoperative dental extraction followed by radiation therapy resulted in localized bone necrosis at the sites of dental extraction in 17 of 120 patients (14%). Although nearly all of these patients responded promptly to conservative management, we are reminded of the importance of planning the dental extraction long enough before radiation therapy to provide adequate time for the extraction sites to heal. Mandibular molar teeth associated with advanced periodontal disease represent the greatest risk for osteoradionecrosis; their selective removal with preservation of other teeth can be considered. Conversely, dental extraction following radiation therapy poses a more serious problem. When mandibular teeth were extracted, intraoral bone exposure persisted for more than 3 months in 13 of 45 patients (29%). The incidence of bone necrosis increased when the amount of radiation administered exceeded 6,500 rad and when 75% or more of the mandibular body was included within the radiation therapy field. Because of the severity and chronicity of these problems, root canal therapy is recommended rather than dental extraction as the means of resolving dental infectious problems in the irradiated mandible.

UNCOMMON MANDIBULAR TUMORS

Histologically, the diagnosis of squamous cell carcinoma will be made in about 95% of the patients who present with malignant tumors involving or encroaching on the mandible. Other pathologic conditions and problems that may occur are reviewed in this section. *Multiple myeloma* is the most common malignant tumor of bone, but it is rarely seen as a surgical problem involving the mandible.

Osteogenic Sarcoma (Osteosarcoma)

Osteogenic Sarcoma (osteosarcoma) is quite uncommon, occurring in only 1 in 100,000 persons in the United States each year. About 6% of the osteosarcomas reported involve the jaw; these are approximately evenly distributed between the maxilla and the mandible. When the long bones of the extremity are involved, osteogenic sarcoma appears to have a survival rate of approximately 20%. In the mandible, the 5-year survival rate is reported to be higher, ranging from 30 to 40%.[13]

The signs and symptoms of osteogenic sarcoma are localized pain, swelling, and loose teeth involving the mandible. This malignancy appears in patients whose average age is 34 years. Radiographic assessment of the mandible usually reveals a lytic lesin. Radical resection of the mandible accounts for the highest survival rates and radiotherapy does not seem to add to the survival in most of the series that have been reported. Because of the high local recurrence rate and the high incidence of distance metastases when surgical treatment is not successful, some physicians feel that radiation therapy and chemotherapy should be added to the treatment regimen.

Of those patients who die of osteosarcoma, approximately 85% develop local recurrence and 80% develop distant metastases.

Ameloblastoma

A rather rare epithelial neoplastic odontogenic tumor, the ameloblastoma tends to be nontender, slow-growing, and deforming. Palpation of the mandible often reveals dental disruption and a lobulated surface. Ameloblastoma seldom metastasizes, but recurrence rates range from 30 to 40% in the reported series. Management consists of total removal of the tumor via intraoral or extraoral block resection with an adequate margin of normal bone around the tumor. The amount of bony margin usually varies according to the size of the tumor. Curettage does not provide an effective treatment. Neck dissection is performed only in patients who present with obvious cervical lymphadenopathy.

Adenoidcystic and Mucoepidermoid Carcinoma

Malignant tumors of the minor salivary glands may encroach on the mandible from their point of origin in the mouth or may present as primary intraosseous tumors. Primary intraosseous mucoepidermoid carcinoma has been described by Grubka and co-workers[14] as a painless swelling in the region of the third molar, commonly seen in patients in their fifties. Conservative excision of the tumor, sparing the mandibular arch integrity and the inferior alveolar neurovascular structures if possible, is the recommended surgical management.

American Burkitt's Lymphoma

When the mandible becomes involved with American Burkitt's lymphoma, patients present a picture that can be confused with some of the malignant tumors we have discussed. These patients present with toothache, numbness of the lip and gum, loose teeth, and radiographic abnormalities. The diagnostic distinctions are important as Burkitt's lymphoma is treated by chemotherapy rather than surgery. Survival is approximately 30% in the series reported by Seraban and associates.[15]

Metastatic Carcinoma

The mandible may be a metastatic site for tumors originating in the kidney, breast, or lung. It may also become involved in the spread of squamous cell carcinoma or basal cell carcinoma (particularly the aggressive spindle cell variant of basal cell carcinoma).

The physician's index of suspicion should be particularly high when the patient complains of numbness or paresthesia involving the lip or alveolar epithelium, when there is unexplained mandibular discomfort, or when there is radiographic evidence of expansion of the neurovascular canal within the mandible. Tumor cell spread through the perineural lymphatics of the inferior alveolar nerve is considered the most common route of progression. Radiographic changes are often far behind the actual location of tumor involvement, necessitating a radical approach for this group of patients.

REFERENCES

1. Guillamondegui OM, Oliver B, Hayden R: Cancer of the anterior floor of the mouth: Selective choice of treatment and analysis of our failures. Am J Surg 140:560–562, 1980
2. Beahrs OH, Myers MH (eds): Manual for Staging of Cancer, Ed. 2. Philadelphia: JB Lippincott, 1983
3. Gilbert S, Tzadik A, Leonard G: Mandibular involvement by oral squamous cell carcinoma. Laryngoscope 96:96–101, 1986
4. Slaughter ED, Roseser EH, Smejkal WF: Excision of the mandible for neoplastic disease. Surgery 26:507–522, 1949
5. Ward GE, Robben JO: A composite operation for radical neck dissection and removal of cancer of the mouth. Cancer 4:98–108, 1951
6. Marchetta FC, Sako K, Badillo J: Periosteal lymphatics of the mandible and intraoral carcinoma. Am J Surg 108:505–507
7. Marchetta FC, Sako K, Murphy JB: The periosteum of the mandible and intraoral carcinoma. Am J Surg 122:711–713, 1971
8. Baker HL, Woodbury DH, Krause CJ, et al.: Evaluation of bone scan by scintigraphy to detect subclinical invasion of the mandible by squamous cell carcinoma of the oral cavity. Otolaryngol Head Neck Surg 90:327–336, 1982

9. Noyek AM: Bone scanning in otolaryngology. Laryngoscope 89 (Suppl 18):1–87, 1979
10. Weisman RA, Kimmelman CP: Bone scanning in the assessment of mandibular invasion by oral cavity carcinomas. Laryngoscope 92:1–4, 1982
11. Beumer J, Harrison R, Sanders B, et al.: Preradiation dental extractions and the incidence of bone necrosis. Head Neck Surg 5:514–521, 1983
12. Beumer J, Harrison R, Sanders B, et al.: Postradiation dental extractions: A review of the literature and a report of 72 episodes. Head Neck Surg 6:581–586, 1983
13. Clark JL, Unni KK, Dahlin DC, et al.: Osteosarcoma of the jaw. Cancer 51:2311–2316, 1983
14. Grubka JM, Wesley RK, Monaco F: Primary intrasseous mucoepidermoid carcinoma of the anterior part of the mandible (case report). J Oral Maxillofac Surg 41:389–394, 1983
15. Sariban E, Donahue A, Magrath IT: Jaw involvement in American Burkitt's Lymphoma. Cancer 53:1777–1782, 1984

7 Management of Mandibular Fractures

Byron J. Bailey, M.D., F.A.C.S.

Head and neck trauma contributes significantly to mortality and morbidity in the United States. Vehicular accidents account for most of these injuries, but other major etiologic factors include personal assaults, falls, sports injuries, and industrial accidents. Mandibular fractures are responsible for a majority of the patients who require hospitalization for care after sustaining maxillofacial injuries.

The large volume and the complexity of mandibular fractures have created considerable interest among the practitioners of many professional disciplines: emergency room physicians, otolaryngologists-head and neck surgeons, general plastic surgeons, oral surgeons, and dentists, to name several. Each discipline approaches the problem from a slightly different perspective and each has a specific contribution to make in the management of a specific individual; nevertheless, one physician must serve as the "team leader" to facilitate coordination and communication among professionals and with family members.

PATIENT ASSESSMENT

The cardinal principles of assessment follow:

1. Rule out the presence of any potentially lethal injuries before doing anything else.
2. Find all injuries sustained, by conducting an orderly sequential examination.
3. Establish treatment priorities for multiple injuries.
4. Request consultation for those injuries outside your area of expertise.

Mandibular fractures account for the largest number of facial bone fractures except for those involving the nasal and septal area. Fractures of the mandible are multiple (56%) more often than they are single, and they are open into the oral cavity or dental space (64%) more often than they are closed. The body and angle of the mandible are most commonly involved (Fig. 77) and the patients are usually young adult males (Fig. 78).

Physical examination of the mandible usually reveals pain on movement, point tenderness, and crepitus on palpation, along with malocclusion (Figs. 79 to 81). The probable location of mandibular fractures should be apparent to the physician before obtaining roentgenograms.

Severe, multiple mandibular fractures can destroy the integrity of the hyoid mandibular musculoskeletal system, in collapse of the upper airway. When these patients present with a decreased level of consciousness, they must be positioned on their sides and watched carefully for signs of respiratory distress. Before taking any steps to assess or treat mandibular fractures, the physician must rule out the presence of intrathoracic or intraabdominal injuries, occult hemorrhage, or cervical spine instability.

Careful physical examination usually provides an accurate assessment of the fracture sites. Palpation and inspection of the teeth and the occlusion usually reveal a specific type of malocclusion (illustrated in Figs. 82 to 84). Obvious step-off points or loose teeth adjacent to the fracture lines are usually reliable signs of fracture.

Detailed information can be obtained from panoramic roentgenographic films and from traditional lateral oblique views of the mandible. Polytomography in the area of the TM joint may be indicated in certain difficult cases.

More detailed general information is available from the current sources listed in the Bibliography at the end of this chapter. Limitations of space do not permit a more detailed elaboration of the nonsurgical aspects of mandibular fracture assessment.

PLANNING TREATMENT

Treatment goals are the restoration of anatomic alignment of the fragments, restoration of the preinjury occlusion, retention of the full range of temporomandibular (TM) joint motion, and the avoidance of infection, malunion, and nonunion.

Certain common preoperative conditions influence the management and outcome of mandibular

62 Surgery of the Mandible

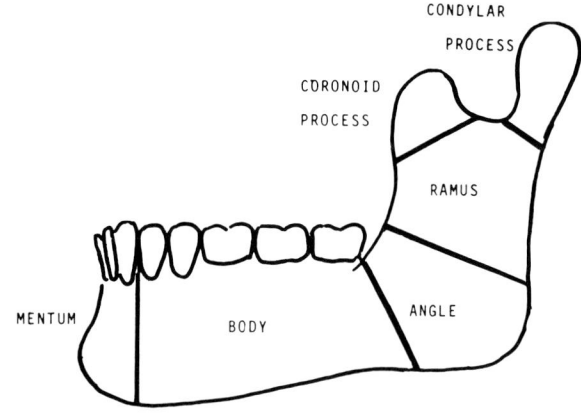

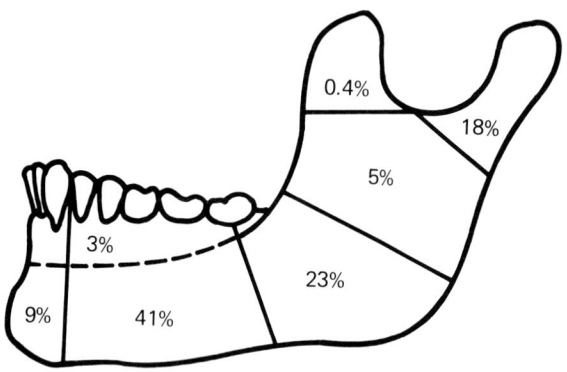

Figure 77. (A) Anatomic regions of the mandible. (B) Frequency of fracture involving each region. (From Bailey BJ and Gaskill JR: Laryngoscope 77: 1137–1154, 1967. With permisison.)

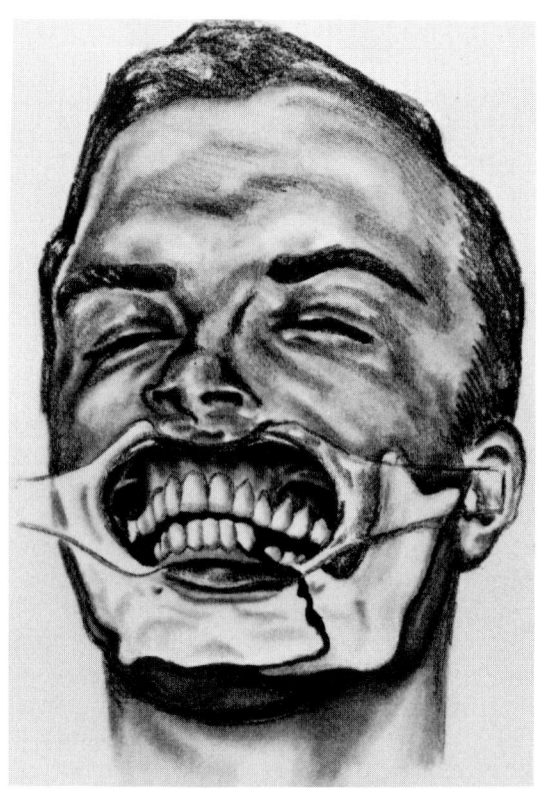

Figure 79. Dental malocclusion with mandibular fracture. (From English G (ed): Otolaryngology. Maryland, Harper & Row, 1972, p. 5. With permission.)

fractures. An unerupted third molar tooth weakens the mandible in the region of the angle, predisposes this area to fracture, and is associated with a higher incidence of postoperative complications, including infection and malunion. Alcohol or narcotic addic-

AGE DISTRIBUTION

```
8-9    ┌── 12
10-19  ├───── 35
20-29  ├─────────────────────── 192
30-39  ├────────── 84
40-49  ├──────── 59
50-59  ├── 18
60-69  └─ 6
```

Figure 78. Age distribution of the patients with mandibular fractures.

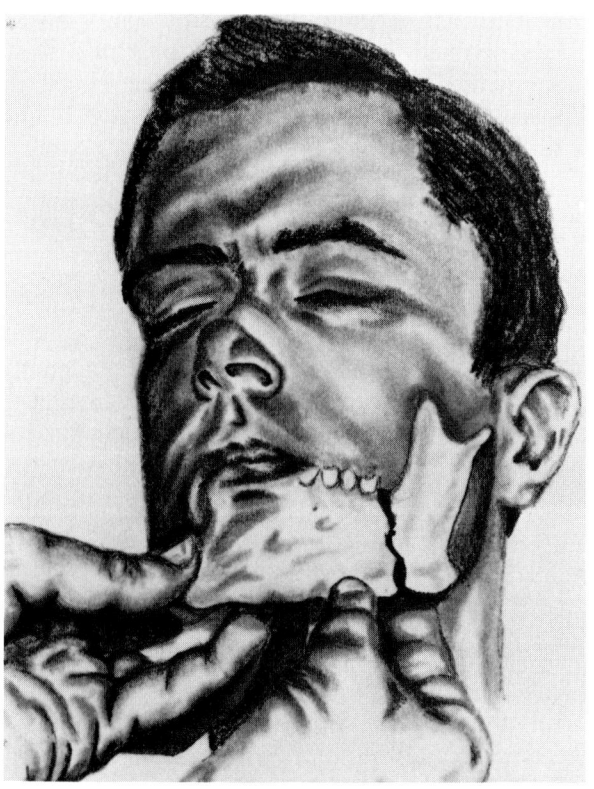

Figure 80. Palpation of the mandible for point tenderness, contour irregularity, or false motion. (From English G (ed): Otolaryngology. Maryland, Harper & Row, 1972, p. 5. With permission.)

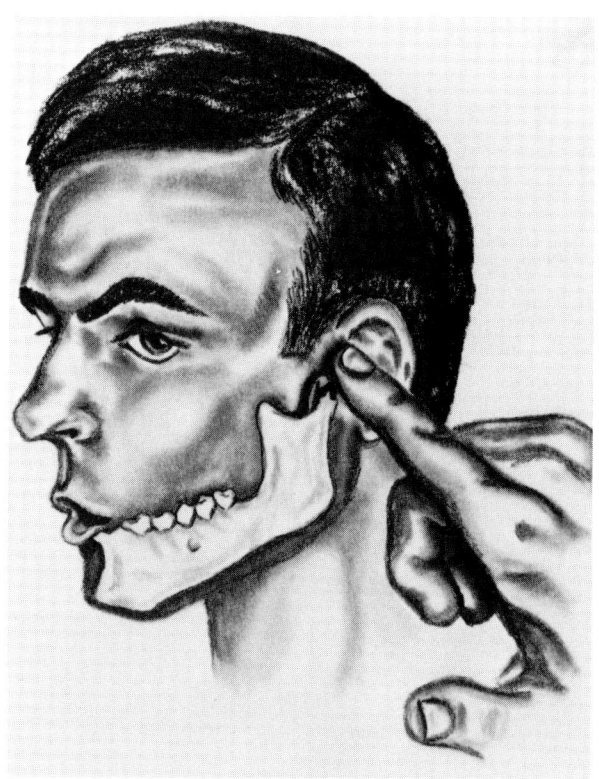

Figure 81. Palpation in the region of the condylar neck. (From English G (ed): Otolaryngology. Maryland, Harper & Row, 1972, p. 5. With permission.)

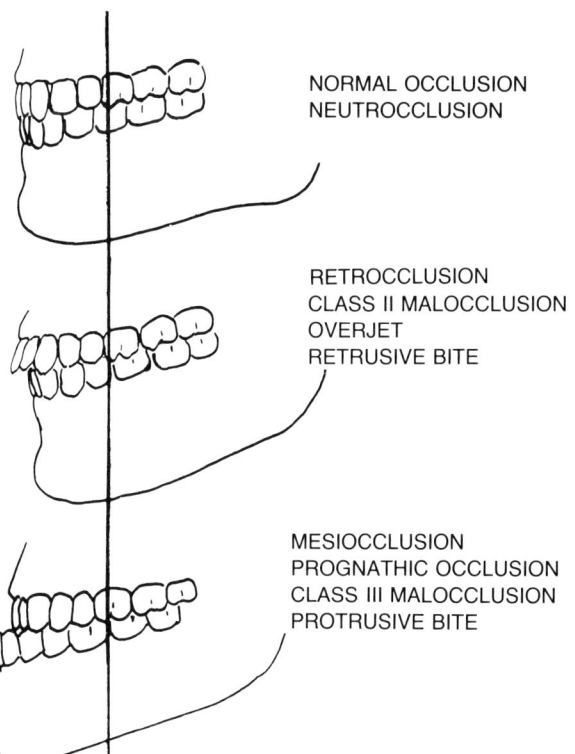

Figure 82. Occlusal relationships with reference to the mesial buccal cusp of the first molar maxillary tooth. It should be aligned with the buccal groove of the first mandibular molar tooth.

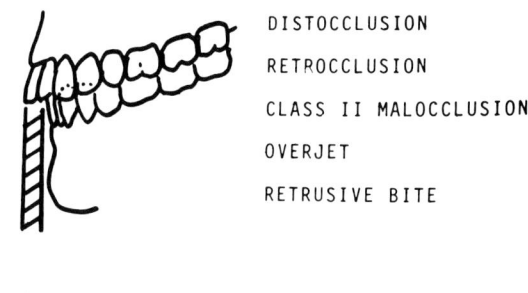

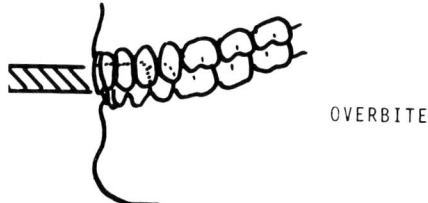

Figure 83. Overbite contrasted with overjet refers to the relationship of the incisor teeth.

tion may hinder the evaluation of a patient and cause difficulty in diagnosing a closed head injury.

Significant associated injuries have been reported in 20 to 40% of patients who are seen with mandibular fractures. Failure to address the associated injury places approximately one-sixth of these patients at risk for a lethal outcome or for significant disability. Cerebral concussion is the most commonly noted associated injury; and if there has been a period of unconsciousness, this diagnosis should be made. Subdural hematoma and related central nervous system injury must be considered in developing the management plan. Other facial bone fractures, facial soft tissue injuries, and eye injuries are significant and must not be overlooked.

In organizing the sequence of management, keep in mind that, whenever possible, all underlying skeletal injuries should be repaired whenever possible prior to the management of soft tissue lacerations that are located adjacent to these fractures.

MANAGEMENT PRINCIPLES

Fortunately, most of the patients who sustain mandibular fractures possess relatively good dentition. Statistically, the most common types of mandibular fractures respond to management by simple, well-standardized techniques. Even so, treatment should always be planned carefully and matched in each case to the needs of the patient and the goals outlined above.

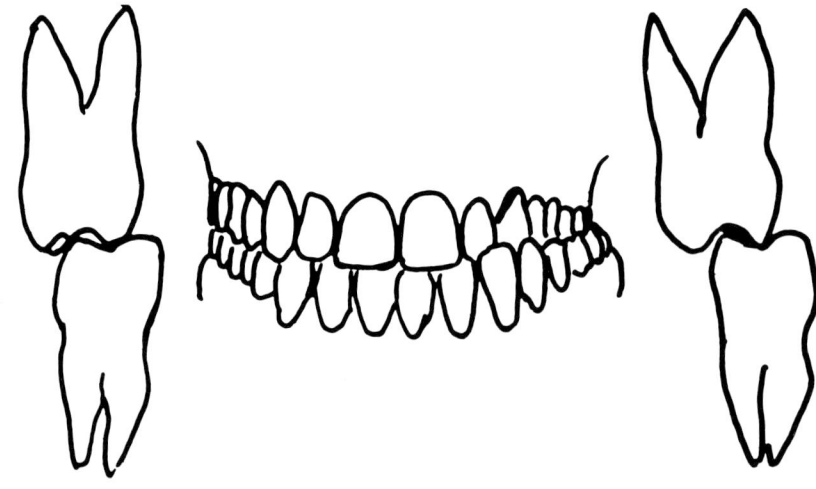

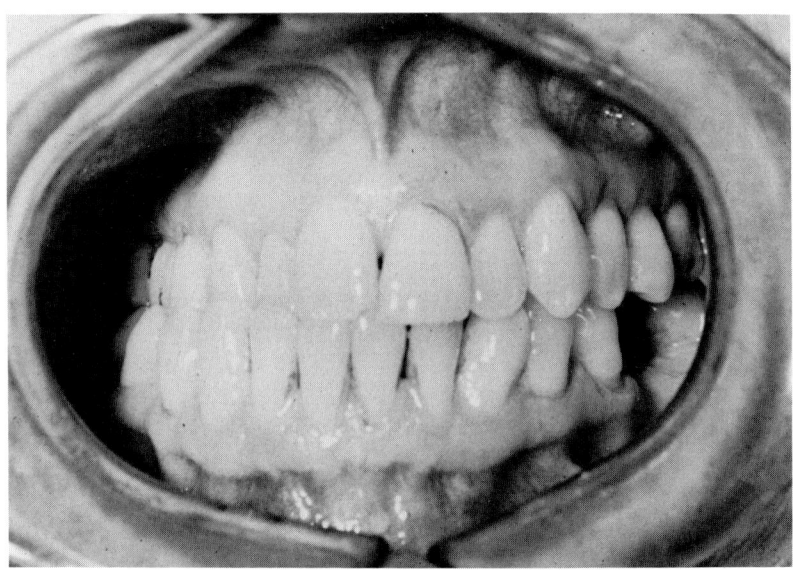

Figure 84. Crossbite is a disturbance of the occlusion of the dental arches when viewed anteriorly. (A) Diagram (B) Patient photograph.

Local anesthesia is adequate for most patients with mandibular fractures, as they will require only closed reduction and immobilization of the fracture site. Local anesthesia has been sufficient for approximately two-thirds of our patients, while general anesthesia is reserved for patients who are excessively apprehensive or uncooperative or who require an open reduction with interosseous wire fixation of their fractures.

Local anesthesia is achieved by preliminary spraying with Cetacaine or 4% Lidocaine application to the gingiva. The inferior alveolar nerve is blocked bilaterally. Greater palatine nerve block anesthetizes the maxilla and palate. Infiltration superiorly and posteriorly in the buccal sulcus and along the alveolar ridge enhances the degree of anesthesia achieved so that wiring techniques can be performed without excessive discomfort.

SURGICAL TECHNIQUE

Variations in the mandibular fractures, the number and condition of teeth, and the patient's general medical condition necessitate some individualization in every case. As a rule, patients with a fracture of the mandibular body (shown in Fig. 85) can be managed successfully by one or another form of dental wiring or by the application of dental arch bars combined with the use of elastic band traction. The management becomes more complex when numerous teeth are missing or when those present are in poor repair. Unfavorable dentition will sometimes necessitate open reduction and interosseous wiring techniques. No effort should be made to correct preexisting malocclusion during the course of fracture management.

Often, teeth will be present in the fracture line

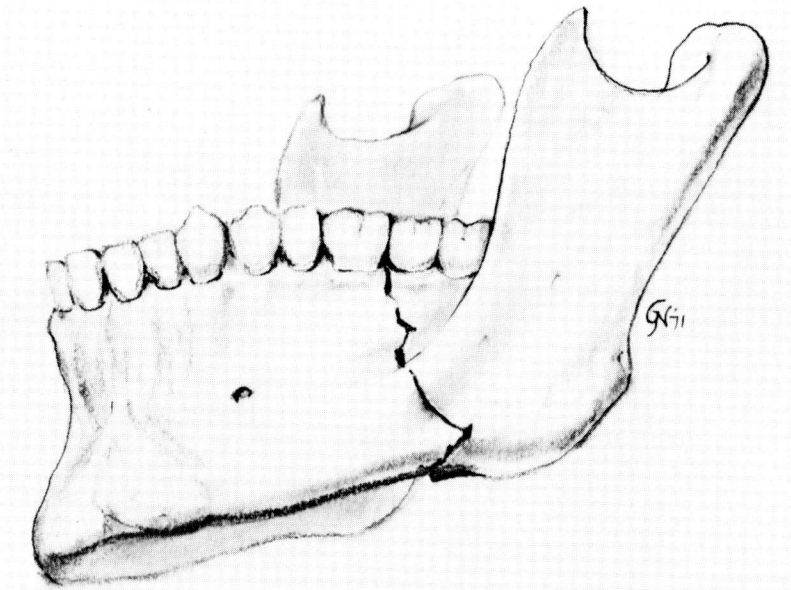

Figure 85. Fracture of the mandibular body with teeth present proximal and distal to the fracture line. (From English G (ed): Otolaryngology. Maryland, Harper & Row, 1972, p. 5. With permission.)

and questions will arise as to the indications for removal. When these teeth are stable and free of obvious fracture involving the root or the pulp of tooth, they are better left in place, as they are likely to survive and are not prone to induce infection. When these teeth are fractured or when they are extremely loose, and thus liable to become dislodged and aspirated, removal is preferable. In general, we have chosen to avoid intraoral incisions to approach mandibular fracture sites and we have limited the use of plating of mandibular fractures to those rare instances when no alternative seemed feasible. We prefer elastic band traction to intermaxillary wiring for intermaxillary fixation.

The instruments used most commonly to repair mandibular fractures are shown in Figure 86.

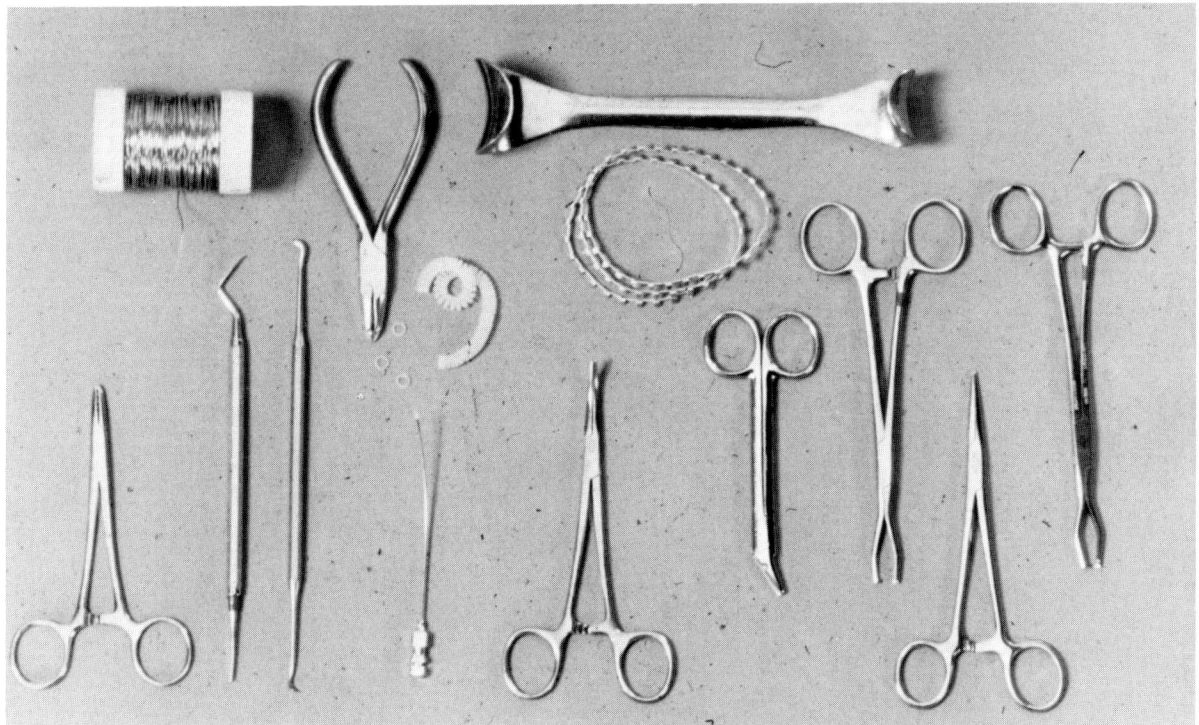

Figure 86. Surgical instrumentation includes (from upper left, clockwise) #25 stainless steel wire, wire cutters, 3/8 inch orthodontic elastic bands, cheek retractor, bone-grasping forceps, wire cutters, curved 18 guage spinal needle, dental gauze packers, and hemostat.

APPLICATION OF DENTAL ARCH BARS—INTERMAXILLARY ELASTIC BAND IMMOBILIZATION

We prefer lightweight, malleable arch bars that have the flexibility to be shaped to the configuration of the dental arch. These arch bars are trimmed to a length that permits their extention from the posterior margin of one dental arch to the same location on the opposite side. We use no. 25 or no. 26 stainless steel wire to ligate the dental arch bars to the teeth. We prefer to ligate the arch bars to the molars posteriorly and then to the canine teeth and finally to as many of the intervening teeth as possible so as to achieve maximum stability for the duration of of immobilization. Incisor teeth are excluded from ligation because their shallow root structure is vulnerable to partial or complete evulsion by the steady pull of the elastic bands.

We use 3/8-in. latex orthodontic elastic bands, to stabilize the mandibular arch bar to the maxillary arch bar because these are particularly suitable for the application of gentle continuous traction. They are superior to wire in that they can be removed easily in the case of an emergency and they can be positioned so that they provide gentle forces in any direction that is desired to achieve correction of the malocclusion produced by the injury.

The technique we employ for ligating the arch bar to the tooth isa simple circumferential ligature (Fig. 87A). The surgeon carefully seats the stainless steel wire around the neck of the tooth on the lingual aspect using a notched dental gauze packer (Fig. 87B). The widest portion of the tooth must

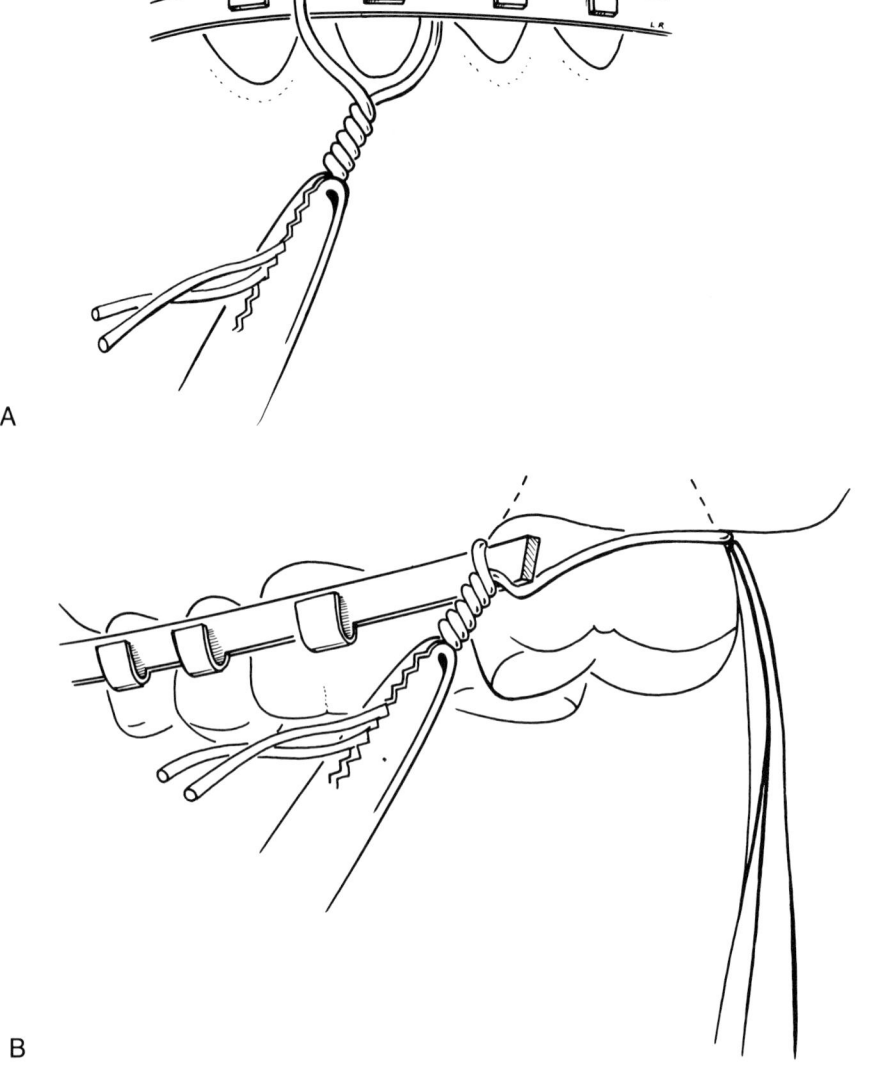

Figure 87. (A) Circumferential ligation of each tooth individually with careful placement of the wire and avoidance of inclusion of soft tissue in the ligature. (B) The wire is "seated" around the neck of the tooth as it is tightened.

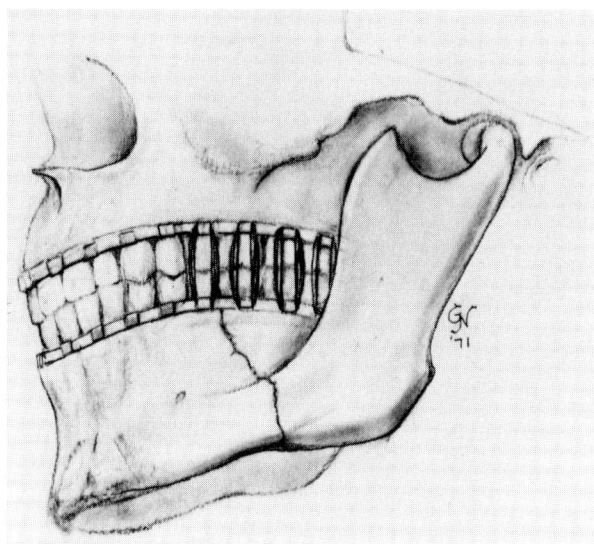

Figure 88. Appearance at the conclusion of the application of arch bars and elastic bands.

be distal to the wire to prevent slipping and consequent loosening of the appliance. Avoid placing any soft tissue in the ligature as its inclusion will produce pressure necrosis and set the stage for infection and loosening of the arch bar.

We prefer to place only two or three elastic bands between the two arch bars at the conclusion of the procedure. This allows the patient to open the mouth in case nausea and vomiting occur. After the patient is awake and alert, the rest of the elastic bands can be applied to achieve the desired degree of immobilization and vectors (Fig. 88).

OPEN REDUCTION AND DIRECT INTEROSSEOUS WIRING

We have found open reduction and interosseous fixation valuable in certain the following situations:

1. Fractures in the region of the angle (Fig. 89).
2. Fractures in the symphysis-parasymphysis region (Fig. 90).
3. Fractures with comminution or fragmentation causing instability.
4. Fractures associated with numerous missing, diseased, or deciduous teeth.
5. Circumstances in which adequate reduction and fragment alignment cannot be accomplished by closed techniques.

In these situations, a favorable result is much more likely when the fracture fragments are exposed and stabilized by direct interosseous wiring so as to achieve the best possible reduction and postoperative stability.

We prefer to apply the arch bars and place a few elastic bands to achieve a rough approximation of good occlusion prior to the open reduction. This permits the dental arches to come into contact and also avoids the unpleasant circumstance in which the interosseous wire breaks during the arch bar application. The lightweight, malleable arch bars can be molded sufficiently to permit their application prior to the fine tuning accomplished by the open reduction.

Except for the rare situations in which an appropriate laceration exists over the fracture line, we prefer to make our skin incisions approximately 2 cm inferior to the margin of the mandible and to approach the mandible from its inferior aspect. Avoid injuring the marginal branch of the facial nerve, which is located just deep to the platysma. This nerve should be identified and carefully retracted out of the operative field to ensure its protection. The mandibular periostium is exposed and incised along the inferior margin of the mandible; evaluation permits the exposure of the frac-

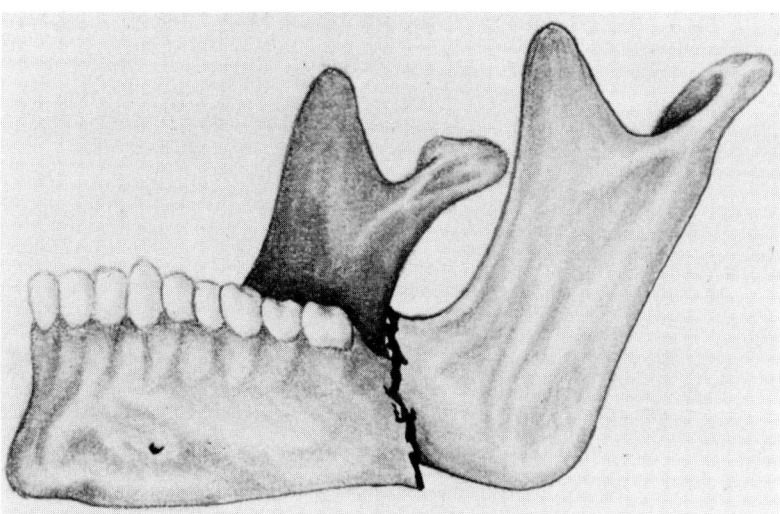

Figure 89. Fracture involving the angle of the mandible.

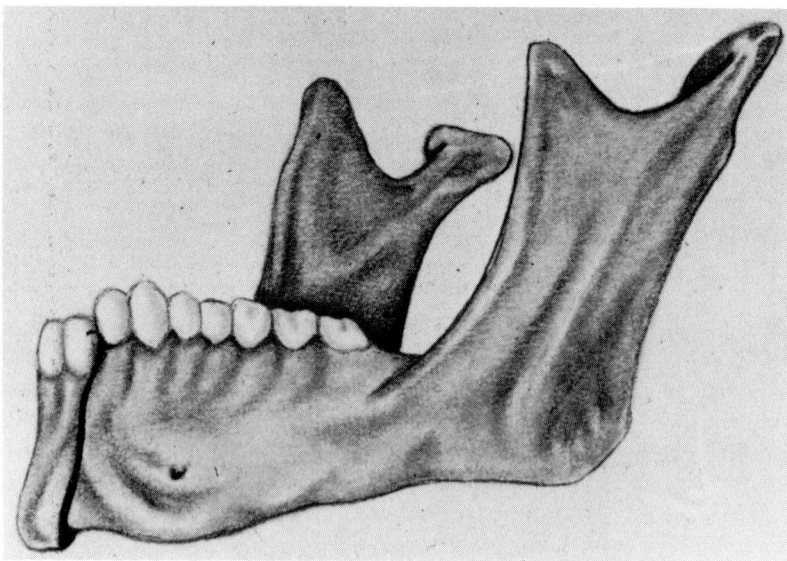

Figure 90. Fracture of the symphysis of the mandible.

ture sites (Fig. 91). Modified Kocher forceps or bone forceps are used to grasp the fracture segments, which are realigned as carefully as possible (Fig. 92). Approximately 7 to 9 mm from the inferior margin and from the fracture line, holes are drilled through which the stabilizing wires will be passed. We prefer the figure-of-eight wiring technique, which permits passage of the ligature from laterally to medially through both drill holes. The wire ends are then twisted together and the twisted end is passed into one of the drill holes (Fig. 93). This provides a stable fixation which is sufficient in most patients (Figs. 94 to 97).

CIRCUMFERENTIAL WIRING— SPLINTS AND DENTURES

When the patient is endentulous (Fig. 98) or has inadequate dentition for the application of arch bars, the surgeon may need to utilize the patient's dentures or to prepare custom dental splints to accomplish immobilization. One of the most common techniques involves preparing the patient's dentures by drilling holes at several locations and ligating the arch bars to the preexisting dentures (Fig. 99). This arch bar-denture combination is then wired into place around the mandible (man-

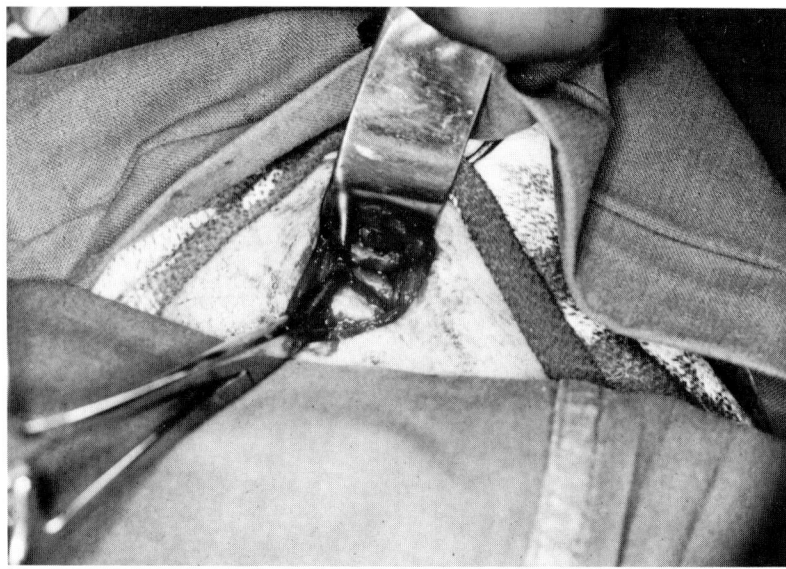

Figure 91. Exposure of the fracture from the inferior aspect.

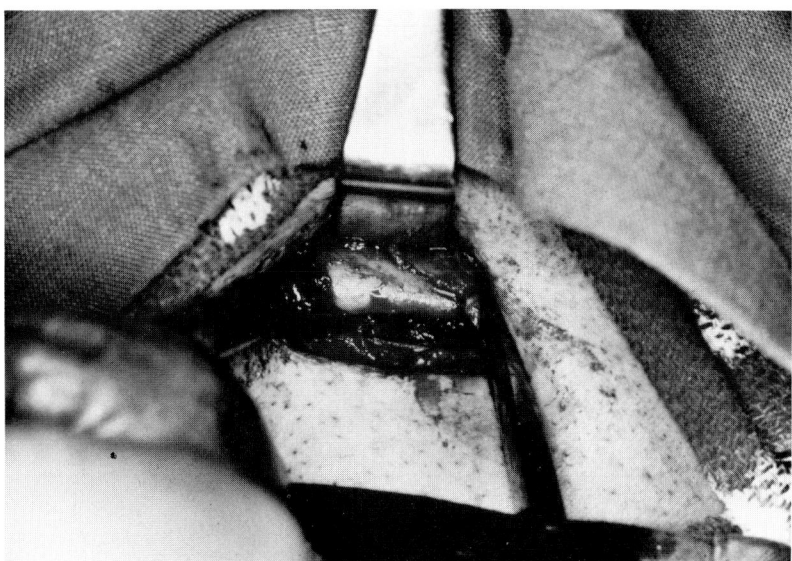

Figure 92. Reduction of the fracture.

dibular denture) or suspended from the zygomatic arch and pyriform aperture (maxillary denture). A curved 18-gauge spinal needle is used to pass the circumferential wire. This technique (as indicated in Fig. 100) avoids the necessity for small incisions in the skin and the need to position the wire against the mandible by sawing it to and fro in a manner that might injure adjacent vascular structures or nerves (Figs. 101 to 104). The same principle applies to passing suspension circumferential wires around the zygomatic arch (Fig. 105). Anterior stability and immobilization are obtained by drilling small holes in the floor of the pyriform aperture and dropping wires from these to small holes made through the denture (Fig. 106). Removal of these suspension wires and circumferential mandibular

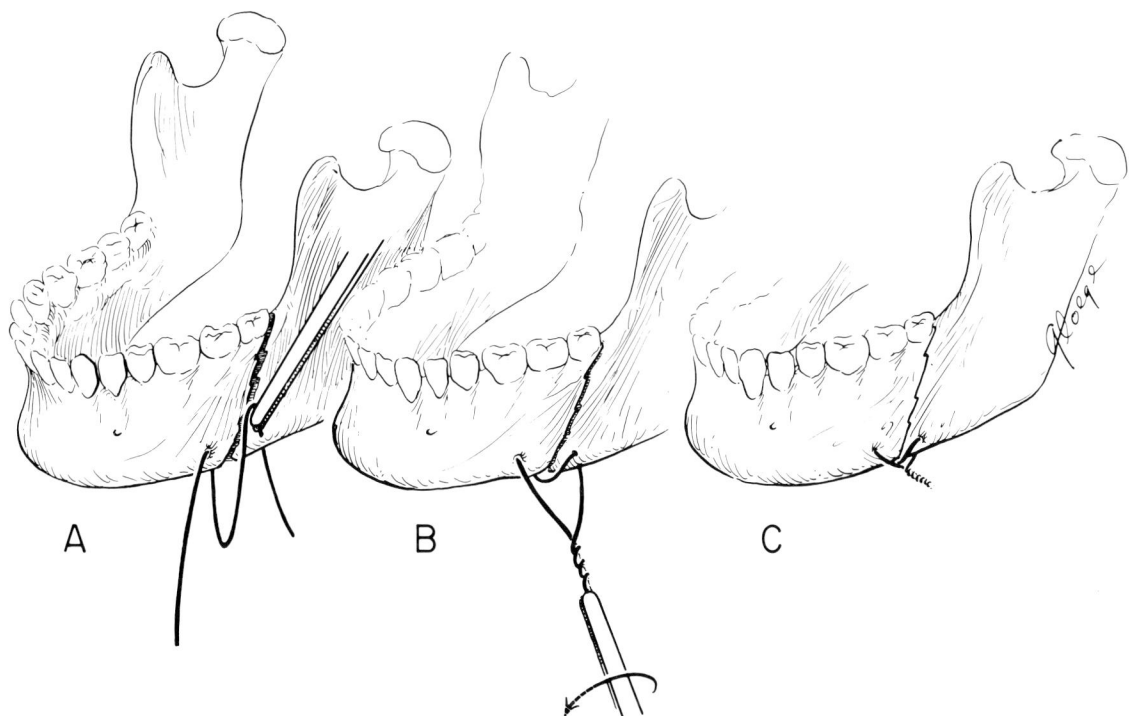

Figure 93. The Figure 8 wiring technique. (From Bailey BJ and Gaskill JR: Laryngoscope 77: 1137–1154, 1967. With permisison.)

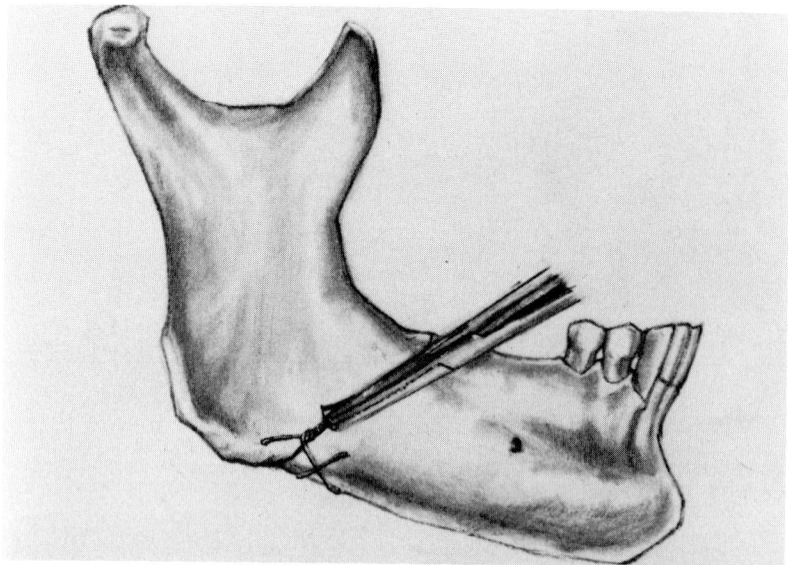

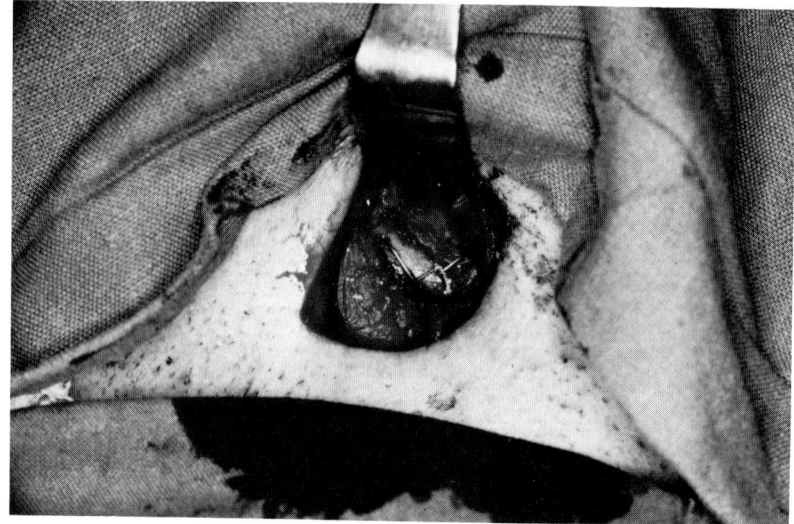

Figure 94. Completion of the wiring at the angle. (A) Diagram (B) Patient photograph. (From Baily BJ and Clark WD: Ear Nose Throat J: 371–378, 1983. With permisison.)

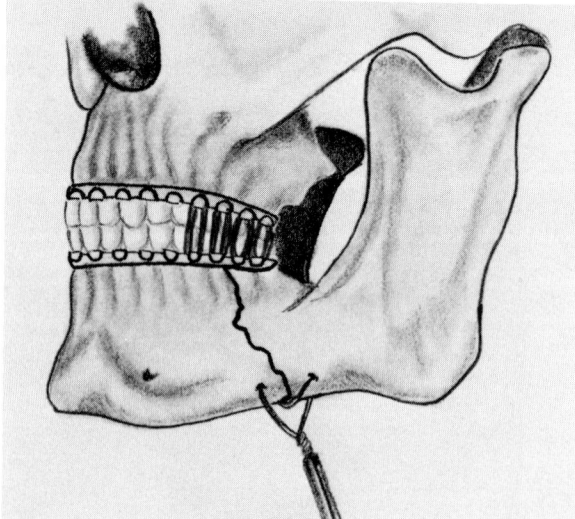

Figure 95. Diagrammatic representation of the open reduction and direct interosseous wire fixation technique for an angle fracture. (From Bailey BJ and Clark WD: Ear Nose Throat J: 371–378, 1983. With permission.)

wires can be accomplished readily under local anesthesia. A light premedication with analgesic and/or barbiturate may be helpful.

PRINCIPLES OF MANAGEMENT FOR SPECIFIC FRACTURES

Mandibular Body

Body fractures are common in young adults, who usually have adequate dentition with teeth proximal and distal to the fracture line. The application of dental arch bars and immobilization using orthodontic elastic bands suffice in most patients to provide the stability for healing in good occlusion.

Some patients have complicating factors such as bone fragments in the fracture line, nonreducible fractures (Figs. 107 and 108), extensive hematoma, unfavorable fracture line (Fig. 109), or problems

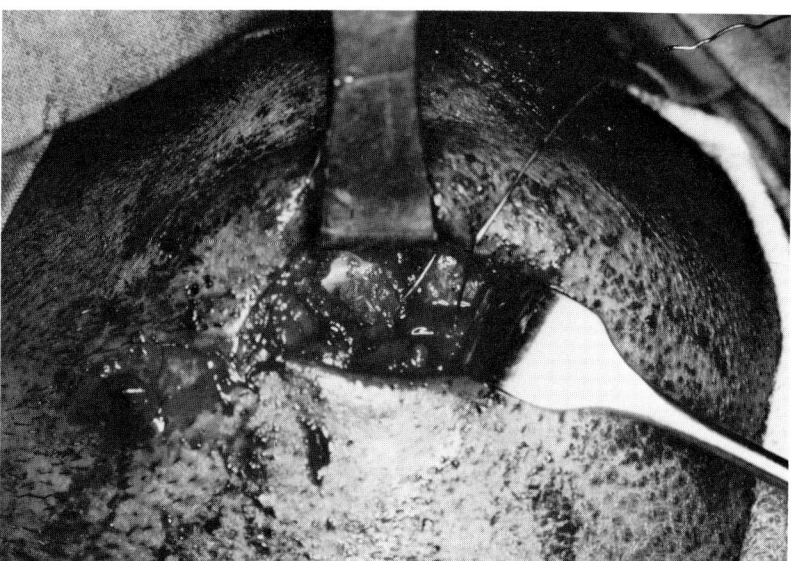

Figure 96. Completion of direct wiring of a fracture at the symphysis.

with patient cooperation. Under these circumstances, open reduction and direct interosseous wiring may increase the probability of a desirable outcome.

Condylar Neck

The history of management patterns for this injury is a chronical of varied approaches. The pendulum has swung recently from frequent recommendations for open reduction and direct interosseous wiring to preference for a much more conservative approach. Surgical exposure and wiring of condyle are generally felt to be unnecessary. As in all surgery, exceptions may be indicated; when the condyle is driven into the temporal bone or is malpositioned so as to interfere with chewing, a

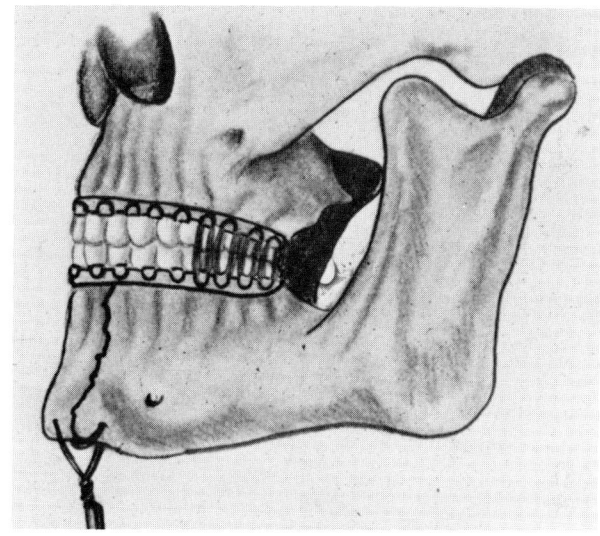

Figure 97. Diagram of open reduction and direct wiring of a fracture at the symphysis.

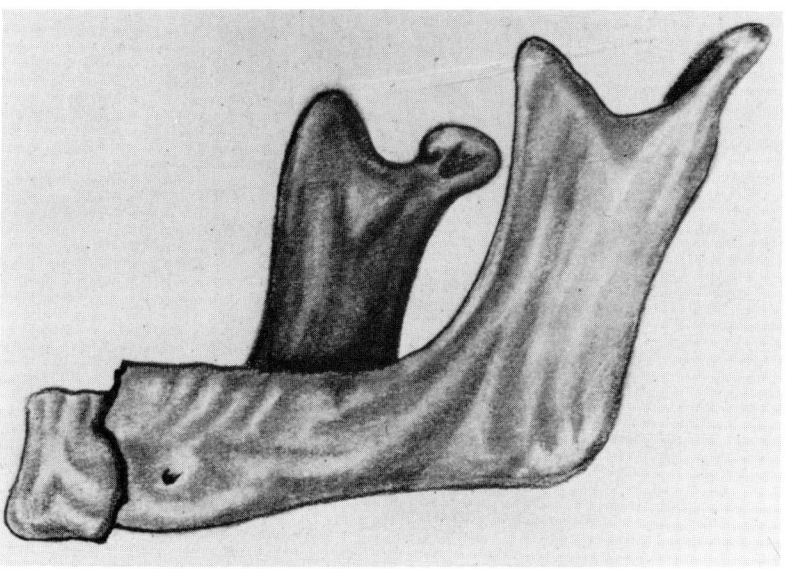

Figure 98. Fracture of an edentulous mandible.

72 Surgery of the Mandible

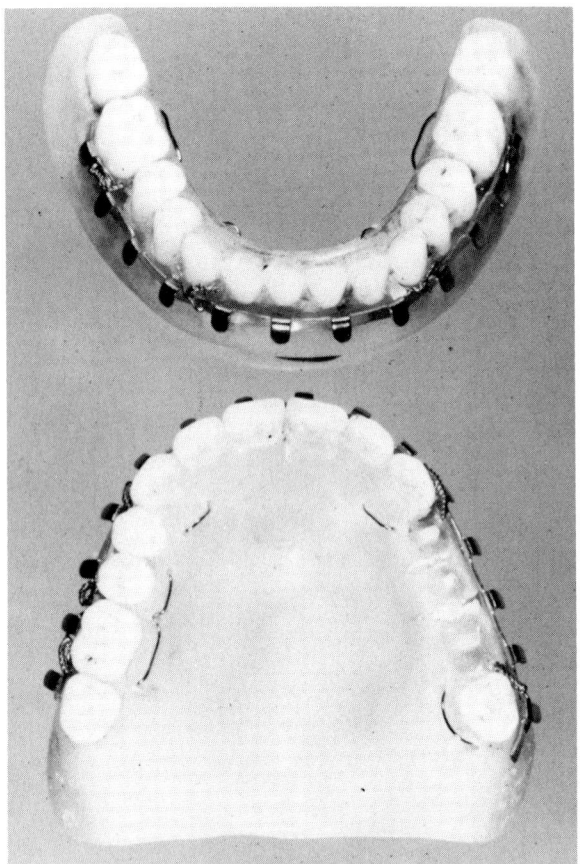

Figure 99. Ligation of arch bars to dentures.

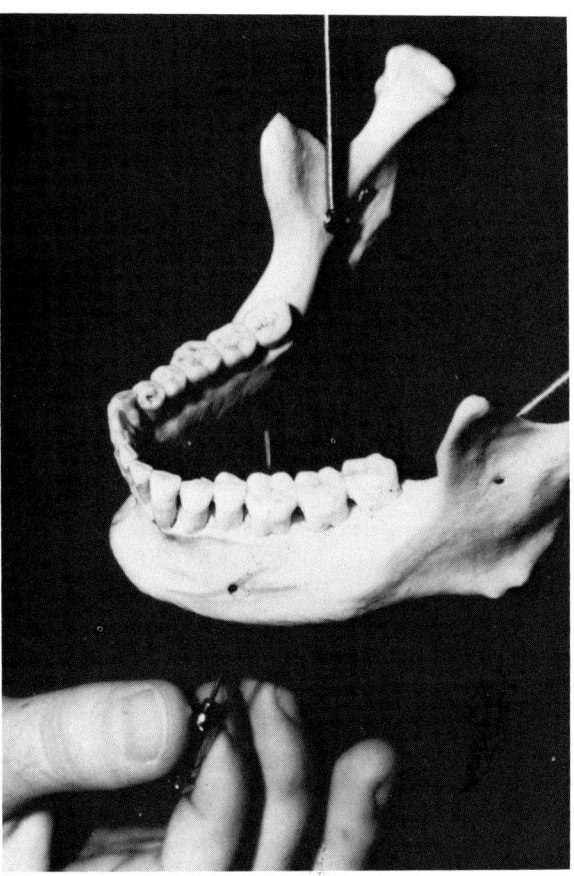

Figure 101. Passing the curved spinal needle (with obturator in place) into the oral cavity.

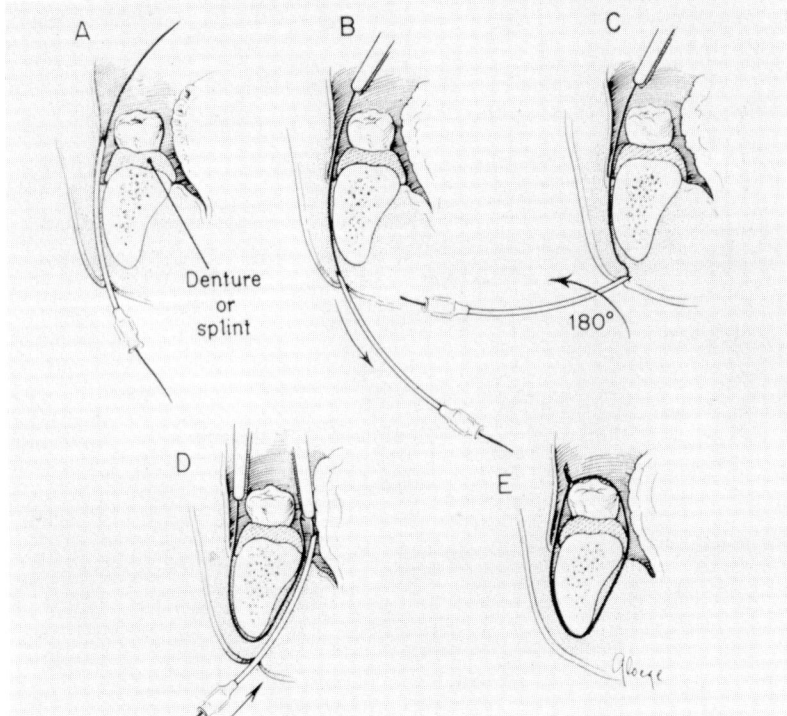

Figure 100. Circumferential wiring technique using an 18 gauge curved spinal needle. (From Bailey BJ and Gaskill JR: Laryngoscope 77: 1137–1154, 1967. With permisison.)

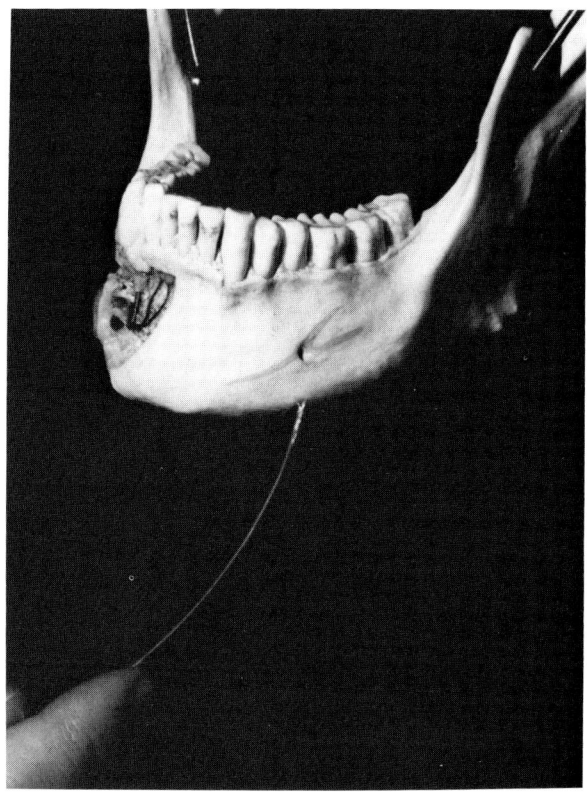

Figure 102. After the obturator is withdrawn, the wire is passed through the needle and grasped with a hemostat. The needle is withdrawn to the level of the inferior mandibular border.

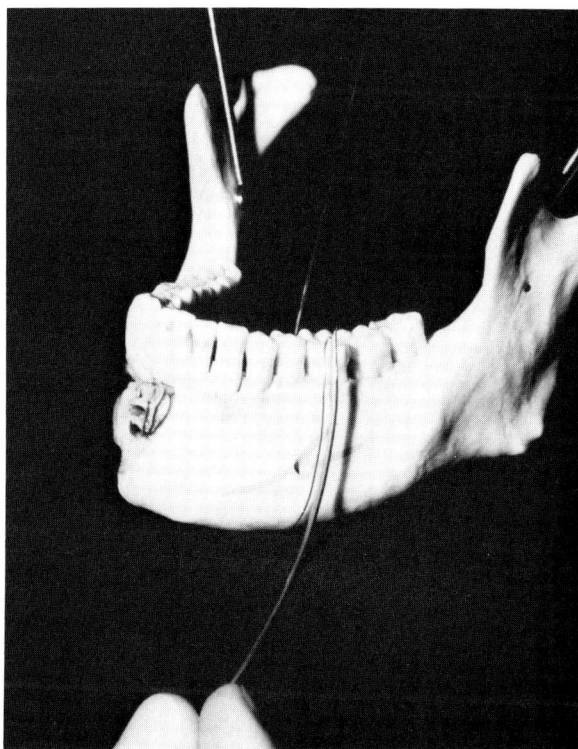

Figure 103. Passing the curved needle upward along the buccal margin of the mandible, dragging the wire ligature along.

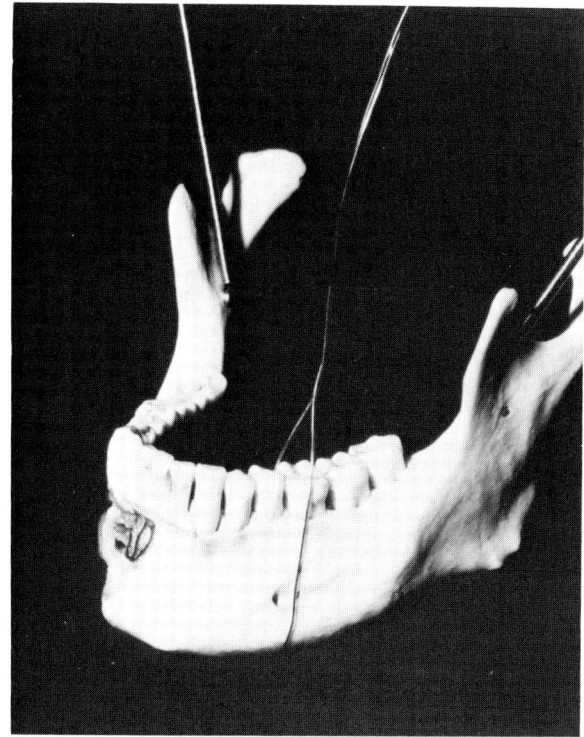

Figure 104. The wire end is grasped and the denture may be ligated securely in place.

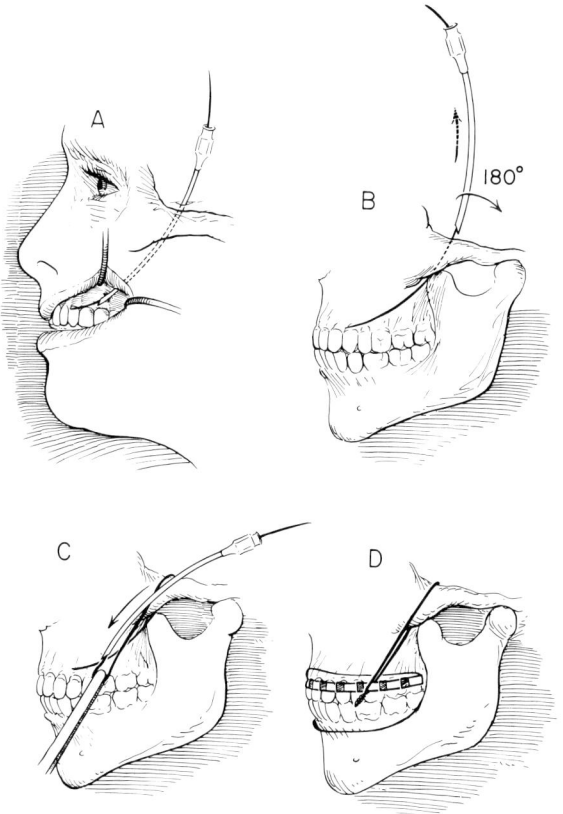

Figure 105. Circumferential wiring around the zygomatic arch to support and stabilize the upper denture. (From Bailey BJ and Gaskill JR: Laryngoscope 77: 1137–1154, 1967. With permisison.)

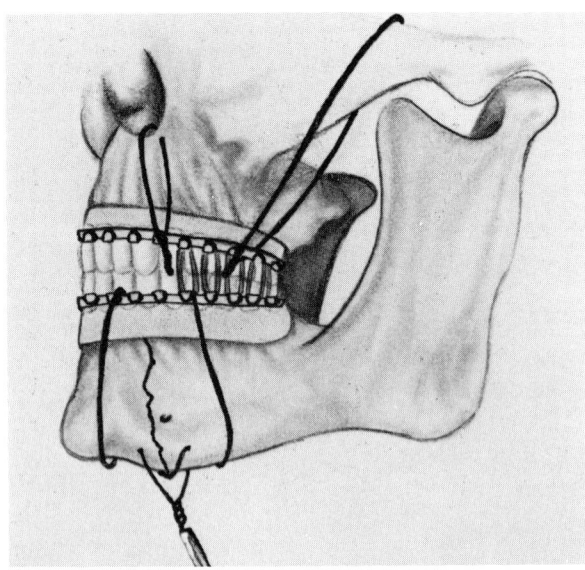

Figure 106. Diagrammatic representation of circumferential wiring and immobilization using patient's dentures and arch bars with intermaxillary stabilization.

more radical approach can be considered. Nevertheless, as a general rule, the application of dental arch bars and elastic band traction is sufficient for those patients who can be brought into good occlusion and maintained in that position for a period of 4 to 6 weeks.

Unilateral fractures of the condylar neck that are relatively asymtomatic and not associated with marked jaw deviation on opening, as well as many unilateral condylar neck fractures in young children, can be managed adequately by placing the patient on a regimen consisting of a soft diet and sequential weekly examinations to observe for adequate healing. Fractures in this area may heal with minor malunion or malocclusion but resolve during the first year following the injury because of extensive bone remodeling and realignment with growth. This phenomenon is said to follow Wolff's law, which deals with the process of bone changes that occur in response to local stress and forces following muscle tension and muscle action.

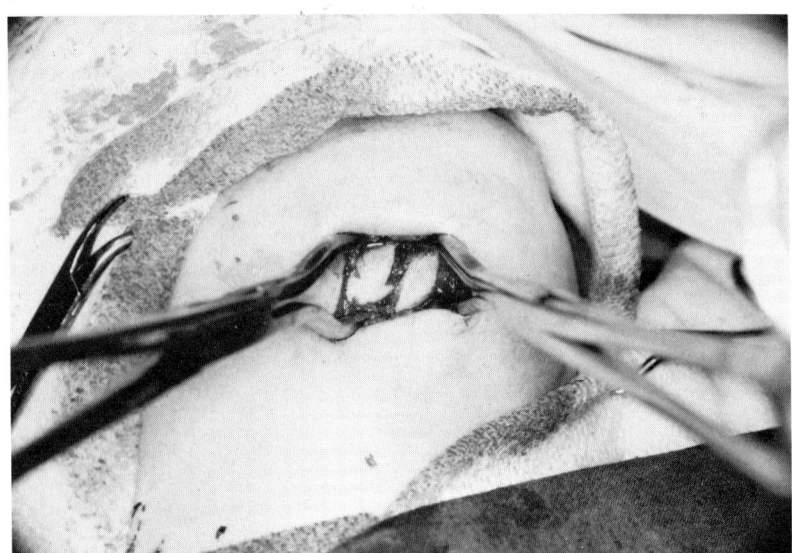

Figure 107. Patient with fracture involving body of mandible; unsuccessful attempt at management by closed reduction. The tongue and groove configuration was not reducible, except by an open approach.

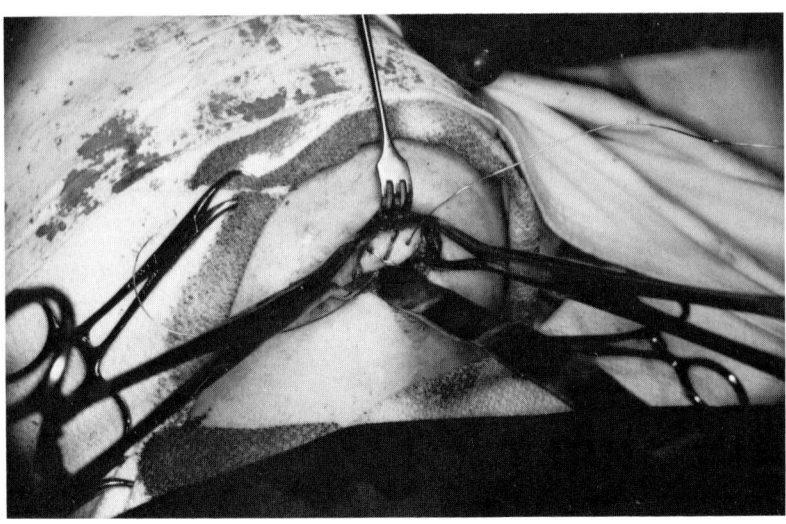

Figure 108. Reduction and direct interosseous wiring of proximal and distal fragments.

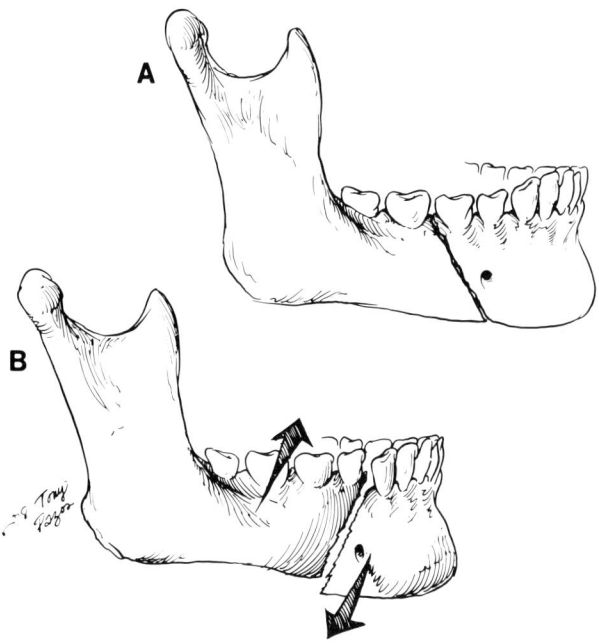

Figure 109. An unfavorable fracture line involving the mandible. The muscles of mastication will oppose the forces of the suprahyoid musculature and will tend to increase the displacement and instability of the fracture. (A) Favorable. (B) Unfavorable. (From Snow JB (ed) Controversy in Otolaryngology. Pennsylvania, W. B. Saunders Co., 1980, p. 484. With permission.)

Mandibular Angle

The mandibular angle is the most frequently fractured anatomic area because of its configuration and the common fracturing force vectors. The mandible is thinner in the region of the angle and the tendency of fracture fragments to override in this location makes precise assessment of the fracture more difficult. Remember that these fracture lines are usually oblique when viewed from laterally and from inferiorly. Precise realignment of fracture fragments at the angle is important to avoid postoperative minor malocclusion. These are unstable fractures and the routine use of open reduction and direct interosseous wiring is wise (Fig. 110).

The proximal and distal bone segments are held securely in the bonegrasping forceps, while drill holes are made. Remember that one of the drill holes is likely to pass through both fragments, while the other drill hole passes through only one fragment. For this reason, as soon as the drill is withdrawn from the hole that passes through both fragments, the wire should immediately be passed through the hole before any slippage occurs. The combination of arch bars with direct interosseous wiring and elastic band intermaxillary fixation is satisfactory treatment for fractures involving the mandibular angle.

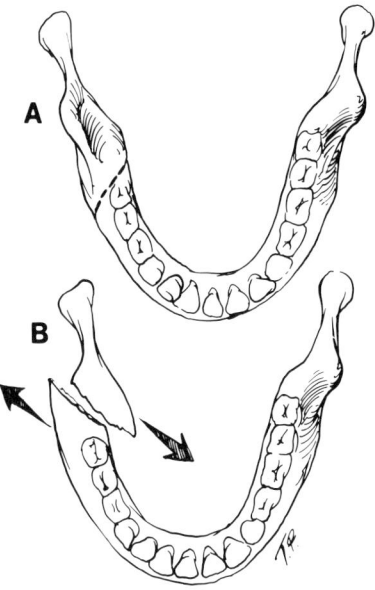

Figure 110. Unstable fracture lines involving the angle of the mandible. (A) Stable. (B) Unstable. (From Snow JB (ed) Controversy in Otolaryngology. Pennsylvania, W. B. Saunders Co., 1980, p. 484. With permission.)

Mandibular Symphysis and Parasymphyseal Region

Whether direct interosseous wiring is necessary for fractures in this region, is a controversial question. In our opinion, while this wiring may sometimes exceed what is minimally required, these fractures should be considered generally unstable. Healing in poor alignment occurs frequently, but because this is such a serious complication, we routinely employ open reduction and direct interosseous wiring. The inferior margin of the mandible is easily accessible in this location and only minimal morbidity is associated with the addition of direct interosseous wiring. Analysis of a large series of patients frequently shows that this approach to be cost effective and associated with a lower percentage of postoperative malocclusion than is seen when direct interosseous wiring is not utilized.

SPECIAL CONSIDERATIONS

This section supplements the discussion of general principles presented above. Here we will report the management of six patients who exemplify our application of the general principles to particular clinical situations. We do not intend to imply that this is the only satisfactory treatment or that it is the best plan for management. These patients were chosen because the surgical management was simple, cost effective, and readily available to most practitioners, and because the outcome was satisfactory in every case.

1. *Gunshot wound of the mandible.* The patient is a 78-year-old male who sustained a gunshot wound from a 38-caliber pistol. The bullet entered the region of the right submandibular gland, passed through the body of the mandible on the right and into the oral cavity, and then continued through the hard palate, lodging in the right maxillary sinus. The patient neither lost consciousness nor suffered any neurologic deficits other than numbness of the right chin and lower lip secondary to the severing of the inferior alveolar nerve. He sustained no other injuries and his general health was satisfactory.

Radiographic studies demonstrated the loss of approximately 1 cm of the body of the mandible on the right. Some small bony fragments were dispersed through the surrounding soft tissue along the path of the bullet.

The patient was managed by closed reduction and realignment of the proximal and distal mandibular segments with the application of an external biphase fixation appliance (Figs. 111 and 112). After 10 weeks of external fixation, the appliance was removed and the patient was placed on a soft diet for another 10 weeks. Subsequently, the patient was able to wear dentures, and he has enjoyed an essentially normal mandibular function.

Follow-up films, obtained 8 years after the original injury, demonstrated the complete bony bridging of the defect. Our impression is that defects up to 1.0 to 1.5 cm can be successfully managed in this manner.

2. *Severely comminuted fracture of the mandible.* A 52-year-old black male sustained multiple injuries in a serious automobile accident. He sustained

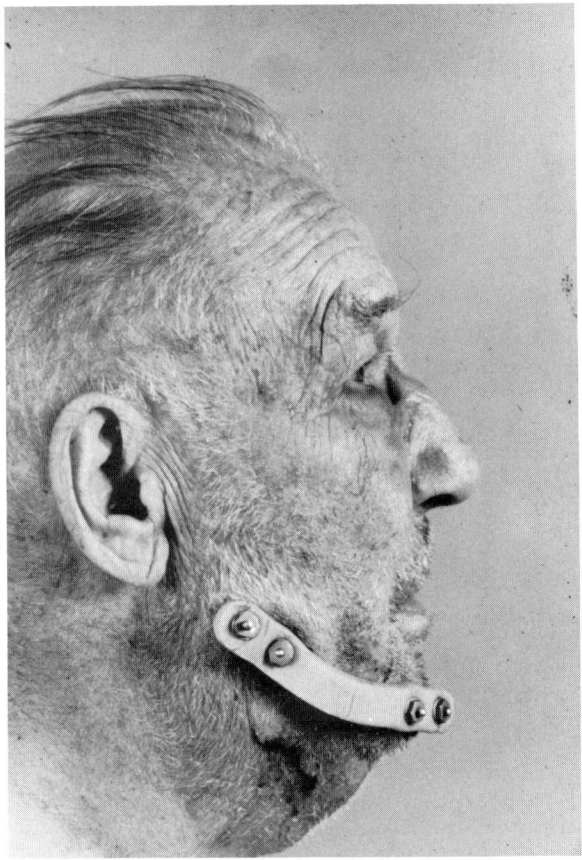

Figure 111. External fixation using a biphase acrylic splint.

a right pneumothorax, a closed head injury with subdural hematoma, and a severely comminuted mandibular fracture involving the region of the right mandibular body and parasymphyseal area.

Satisfactory management of the pneumothorax and evacuation of the subdural hematoma were

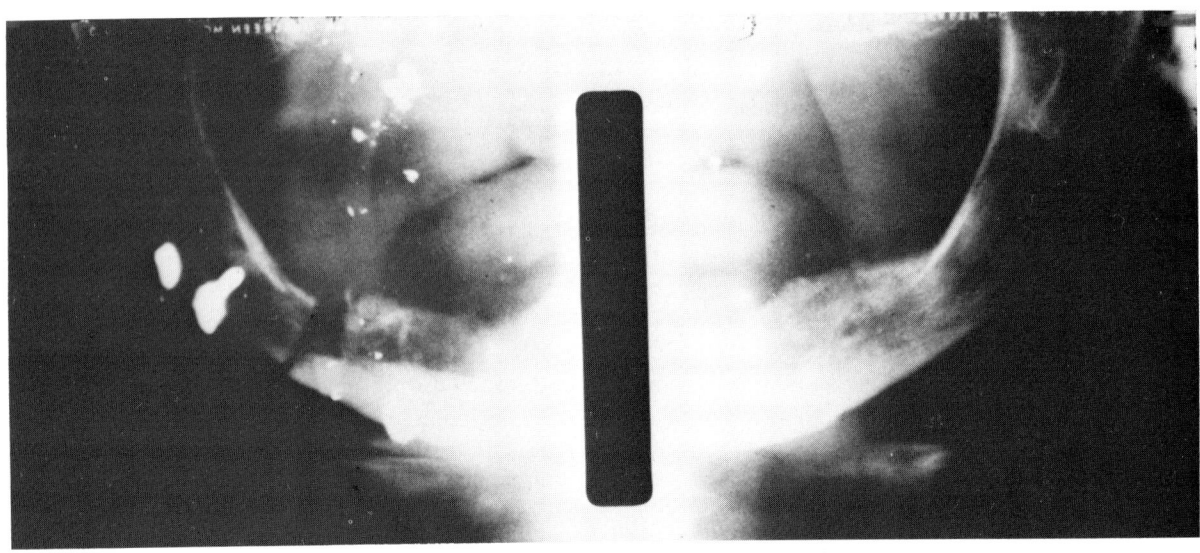

Figure 112. Panoramic radiographic view of a gunshot wound of the mandible. Defect is approximately 1.0 cm.

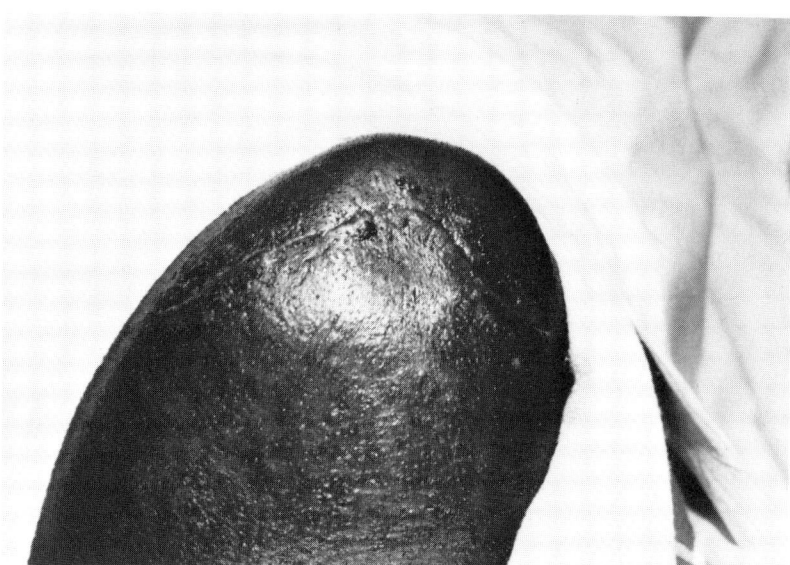

Figure 113. Curved laceration over severely comminuted fracture fragments attached by lingual periosteum.

accomplished, and the patient regained consciousness approximately 6 days after his initial injury. At that point, we were consulted regarding the comminuted mandibular fracture.

A long, curved laceration over the area of the mandibular fracture had been closed in the Emergency Room. This laceration was reopened for exposure of the area of mandibular fracture. Five major fragments were involved. The periosteum had been torn away from the external surface of these mandibular fragments, but they were still attached on their lingual surface (Figs 113 and 114). The widely displaced fragments were brought into their preinjury relationship with each other and wired together. (Fig. 115). Arch bars were applied, excluding ligation of the teeth in the region of the comminuted fractures. This permitted the restoration of normal occlusion for healing during an 8-week period. This patient illustrates the viability of major bony fragments, even when the remaining periosteal attachment involves less than 50% of the fragment.

3. *Inadequate dentition with mandibular fractures.* This 24-year-old white male sustained a comminuted, unstable fracture in the region of the mental symphysis. Numerous mandibular teeth were missing and those remaining were inadequate for the application of a mandibular archbar. A lingual splint was fashioned from acrylic; this functioned to splint the mandibular fragments in good alignment as well as to provide a point for attachment for the arch bar in the spaces where teeth were missing. A maxillary arch bar was also applied and the patient was placed in elastic band intermaxillary fixation (Fig. 116).

The appliance was removed at 6 weeks and the

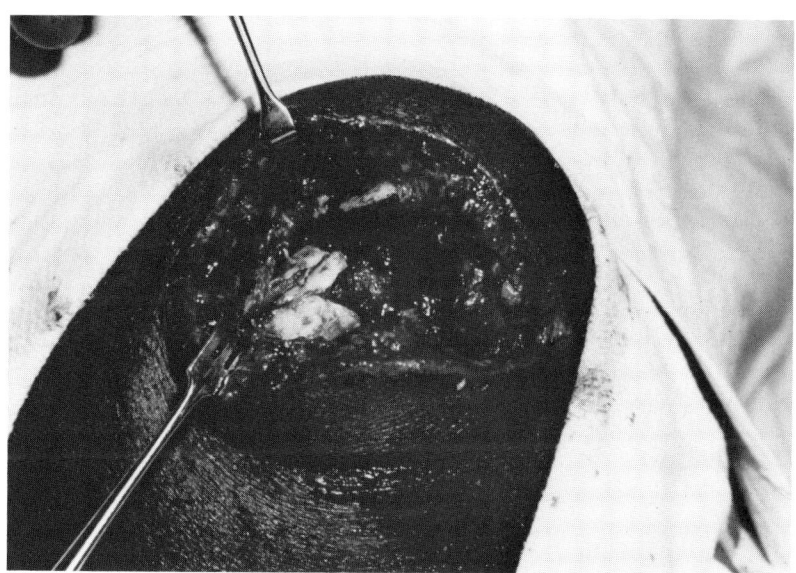

Figure 114. Multiple major fracture fragments attached by lingual periosteum.

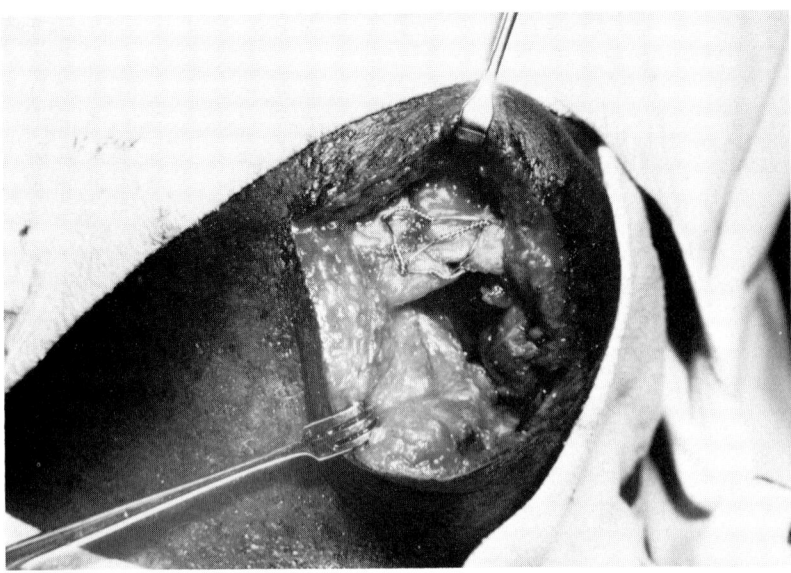

Figure 115. Direct wiring of multiple fragments.

patient enjoyed a satisfactory postoperative result. An excellent review of the various options available for custom acrylic splints to be used in the treatment of mandibular fractures is presented in the article by Jackson and Wetmore (see Bibliography). Examples of this technique that we have employed in our practice are shown in Figures 117 and 118.

4. *Fracture of the atrophic-edentulous mandible.* A 68-year-old white female fell in her home and sustained a fracture in the region of the right mandibular body and the left condylar neck. The fracture of the body was displaced approximately 1 cm and was unstable. The mandible was atrophic, having a height of approximately 19 mm displaced approximately 1 cm, and was unstable.

Open reduction and direct interosseous wiring were chosen to manage the region of the right mandibular body. The fracture line was approached from inferiorly, and minimal periosteal elevation was performed (Fig. 119). Drill holes were created and a figure-of-eight wiring was accomplished. Further stabilization and immobilization were achieved by applying arch bars to the patient's dentures and fixing them in position by circumferential wiring techniques (Figs. 120 and 121).

Our routine recheck of the original fracture site when we finished positioning the dentures revealed that the reduction had not been maintained (Fig. 122). Therefore, we reestablished the precise anatomic reduction and repeated the original wire fixation (Fig. 123). At this point, the desired stability had been achieved, and we closed the wound. The patient enjoyed a benign postoperative recovery and a good long-term result.

The vertical height of the mandible is a critical factor in the management of edentulous patients

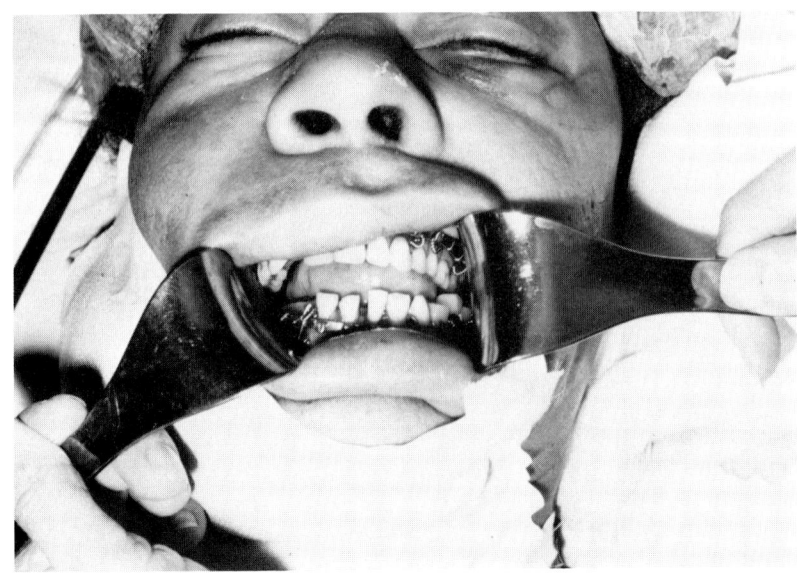

Figure 116. Custom acrylic lingual splint for stabilization of a comminuted fracture involving the symphysis.

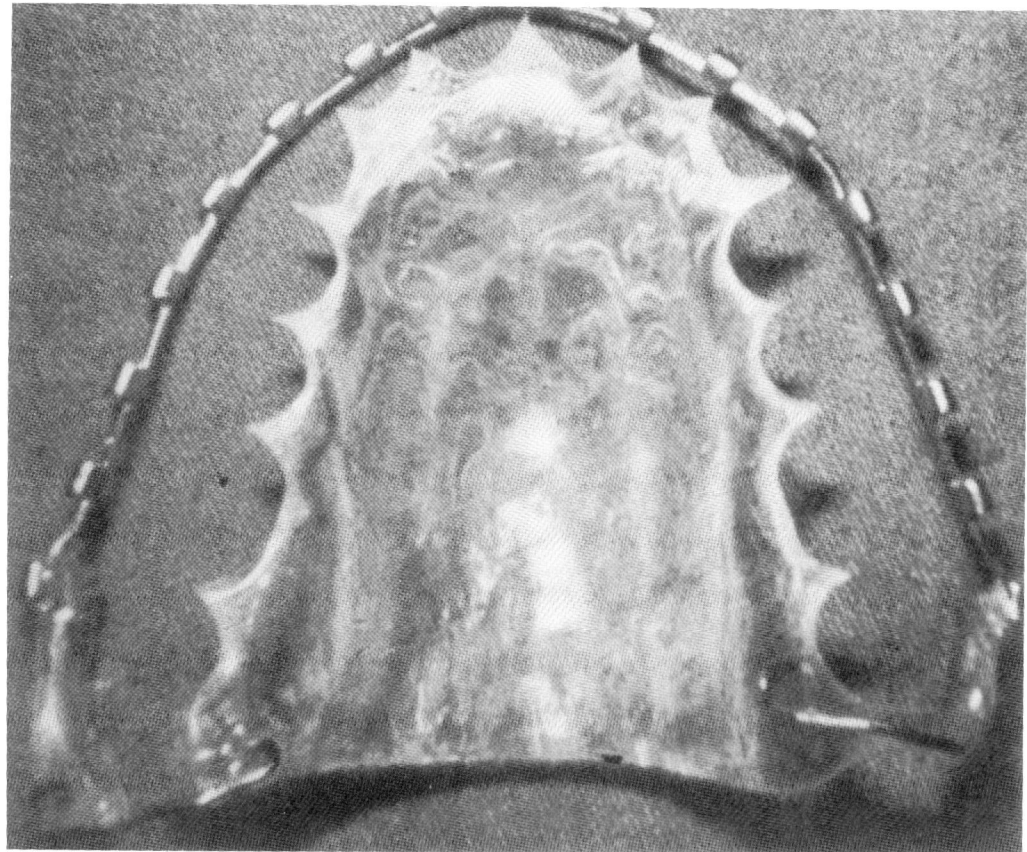

Figure 117. Maxillary acrylic palatal splint incorporating arch bar. (From Jackson MJ and Westmore SJ: Arch Otolaryngol 106:25–30, 1980. With permisison.)

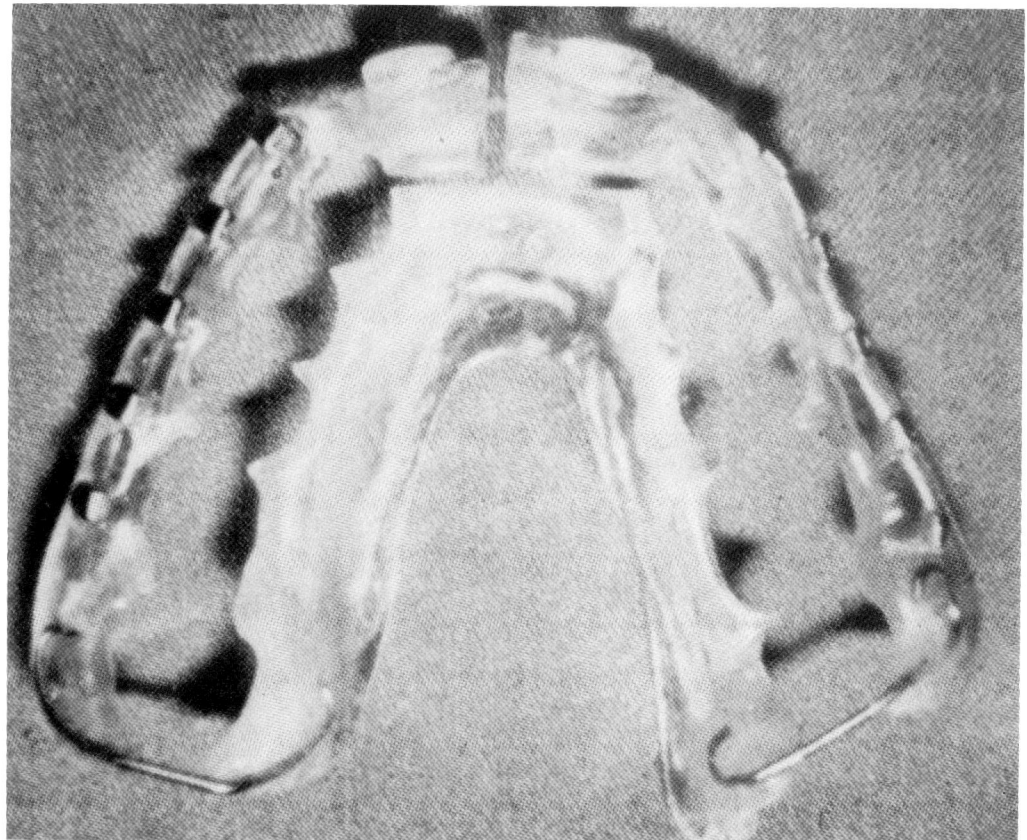

Figure 118. Mandibular labial-lingual splint constructed to corrected alignment of mandible. Note malleable wires hinging lingual section to labial-buccal section and acrylic buttons on each side of symphysis. (From Jackson MJ and Westmore SJ: Arch Otolaryngol 106:25–30, 1980. With permisison.)

80 Surgery of the Mandible

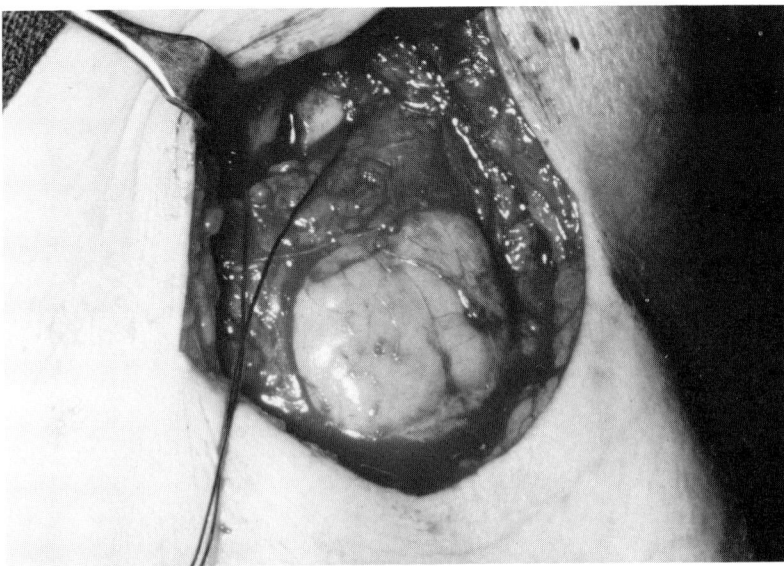

Figure 119. Exposure of displaced fracture of atrophic, endentalous mandible.

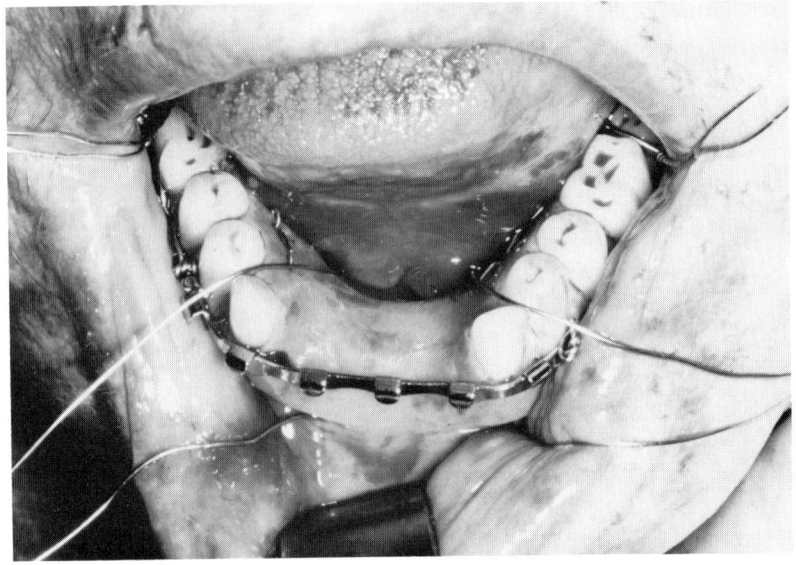

Figure 120. Circumferential wiring of mandibular denture.

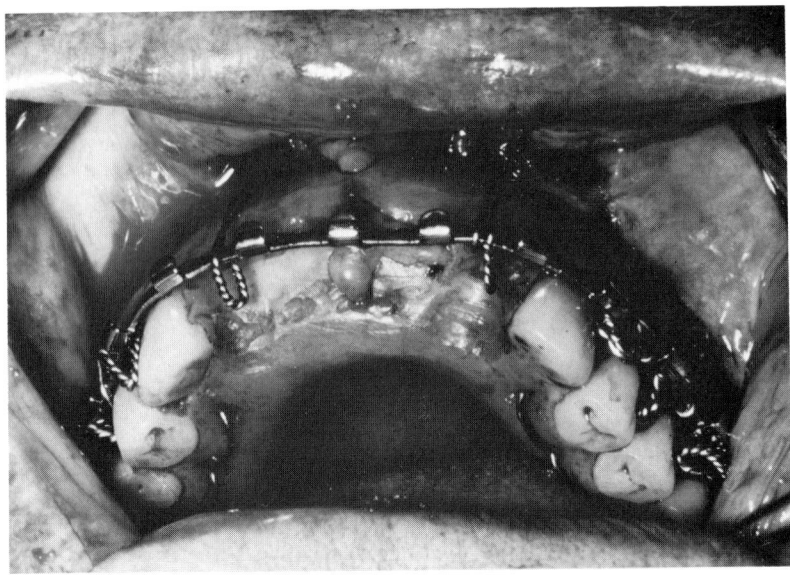

Figure 121. Circumferential wiring of maxillary denture.

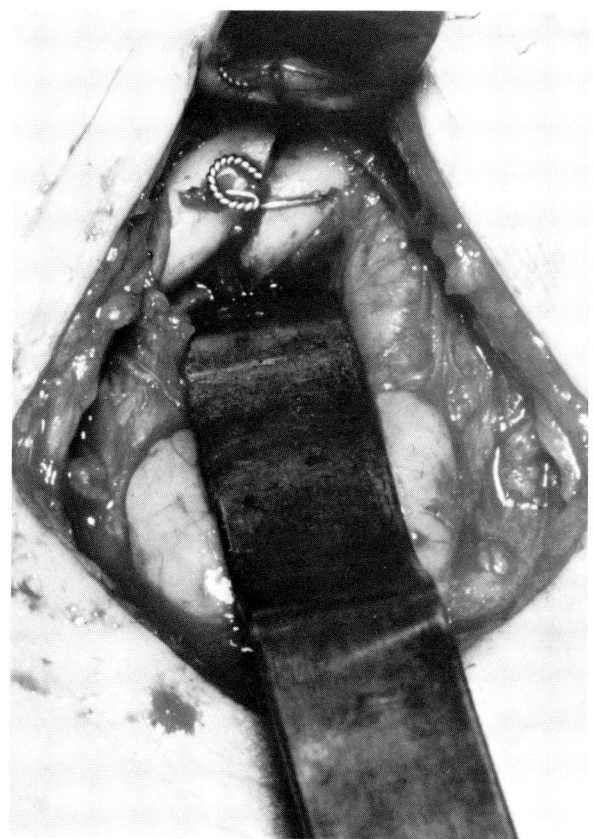

Figure 122. Displaced direct wiring site, prior to correction.

with mandibular fractures. The atrophic nature of the mandible (when its height is 2 cm or less) affects the outcome by causing instability and reducing the size of the area of bony contact between the fragments as well as being associated with a reduced blood supply.

When a denture or splint is used to reinforce the immobilization, it must cover the fracture line and extend beyond the fracture line at least 1 cm. The other options available for these patients include closed reduction, external fixation devices, and internal fixation devices such as a compression plate. The disadvantage of the compression plate technique in the presence of an atrophic mandible is that the extensive periosteal elevation required results in further loss of an already compromised blood supply. The introduction of a substantial foreign body is a further disadvantage.

Generally, when the fracture has more stability than was the case with the patient described here, closed reduction techniques are far more effective. Review of the literature indicates that no matter what technique is used, a fracture involving an atrophic edentulous mandible will be complicated by nonunion of the fracture in about 20% of patients. Therefore, wisdom dictates keeping treatment to the minimum extent possible. Naturally, when inadequate stability results from the conservative approach, more radical intervention is indicated.

5. *Mandibular fractures in children.* The patient is a 4-year-ole white male who sustained a mandibular fracture in a fall from a bicycle. He suffered fractures involving the right mandibular angle and the left body of the mandible. Displacement of approximately 1 cm resulted at the right mandibular angle. The patient was treated by open reduction and direct interosseous wiring of the right angle and by the application of arch bars and elastic band traction. The mandibular arch bars were reinforced by circumferential wires to relieve some of the tension on the deciduous teeth during the healing period. Only three elastic bands were used on each side (Fig. 124). The two drill holes were placed

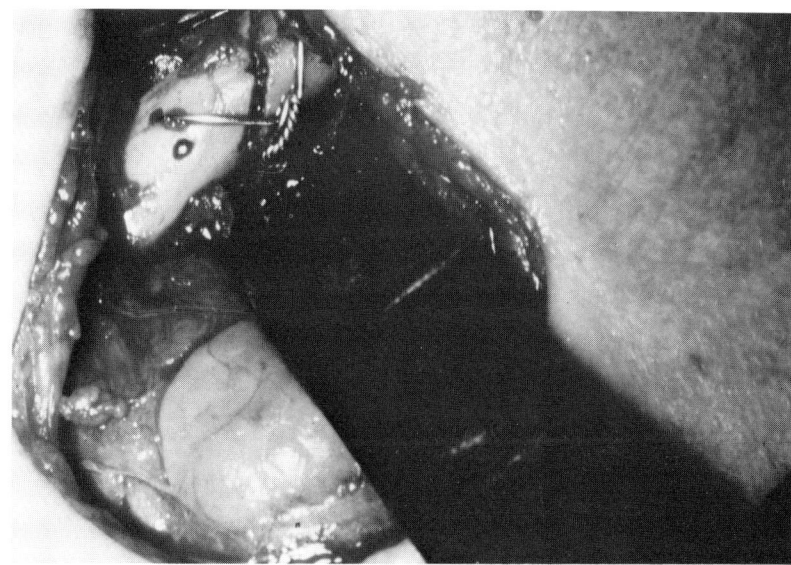

Figure 123. Displaced direct wiring site, after correction.

82 Surgery of the Mandible

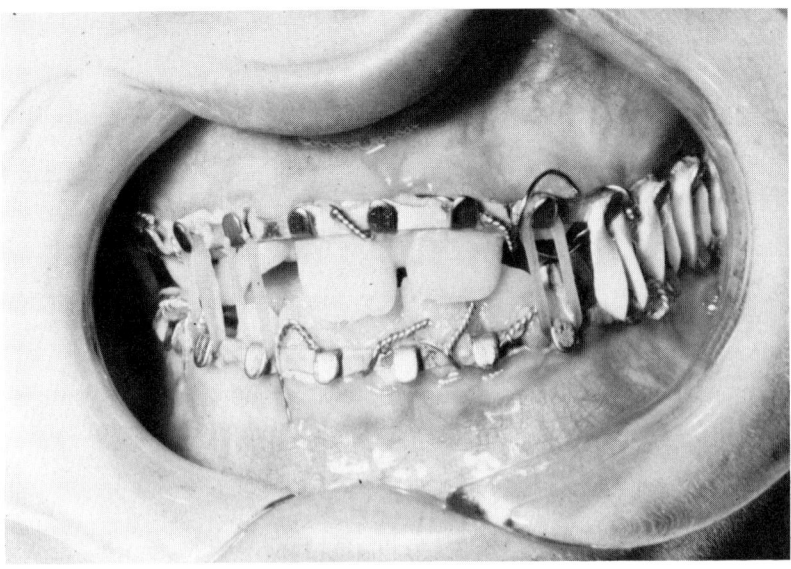

Figure 124. Arch bars and elastic band traction.

approximately 4 mm from the inferior margin of the mandible to avoid an adjacent tooth bud (Fig. 125). Iatrogenic injury to a tooth bud may prevent tooth eruption or cause abnormal dental development and eruption.

Fractures occurring in children account for approximately 5% of all mandibular fractures. About 1% of all mandibular fractures occur in children up to the age of 5 years, while another 4 to 5% occur in children 5 to 15 years of age, with the incidence increasing with advancing age.

Because of the instability of the deciduous teeth, arch bars usually cannot be used in patients younger than 3 years and in those between 5 and 9 years of age. In the older group, custom-made splints and circumferential wiring techniques must be used to achieve adequate stabilization and immobilization. For children between the ages of 3 and 5 and those 9 or 10 years of age and older, arch bars and elastic band traction, as used in this patient, may produce an adequate outcome. Open reduction is not employed unless the fracture is significantly displaced or quite unstable.

The parents of these patients must be given counseling preoperatively so they will understand that abnormalities of mandibular or dental development may arise in the future. Failure to inform the parents that these problems may result from the fracture could cause them to conclude erroneously that the problems result instead from the surgical intervention. The medical/legal implications of this misinterpretation are obvious and worth avoiding.

6. *Late repair of malunion.* A 23-year-old white female sustained a fracture involving the right mandibular angle and the left condylar neck. Because these fractures were minimally displaced and appeared to be stable, the initial treatment consisted of the application of dental arch bars with intermaxillary fixation. The patient did not return for any follow-up care for 4 months, at which time she presented with malocclusion as noted in Figure 126. Solid bony union was noted to be present bilaterally, and no symptoms of jaw pain or trismus were present.

The patient was managed by employing bilateral vertical osteotomy of the ramus, accomplished by an inferior approach to the mandibular angle with elevation of the periosteum from the ramus bilaterally. A sagittal bone saw was employed to create the osteotomies as shown in Figures 127–134.

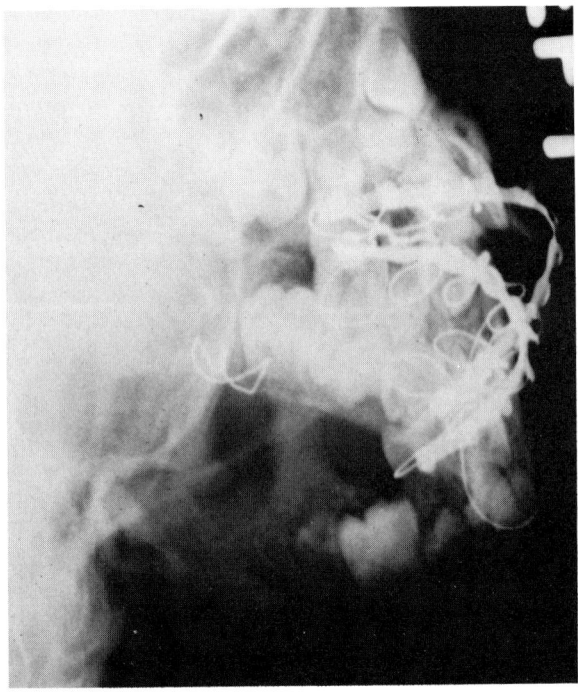

Figure 125. Radiographic view of repair.

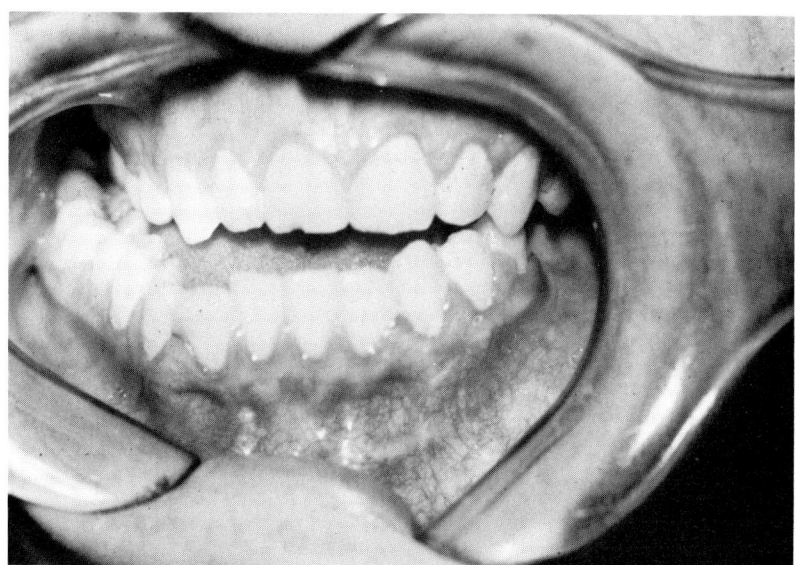

Figure 126. Malocclusion following initial treatment.

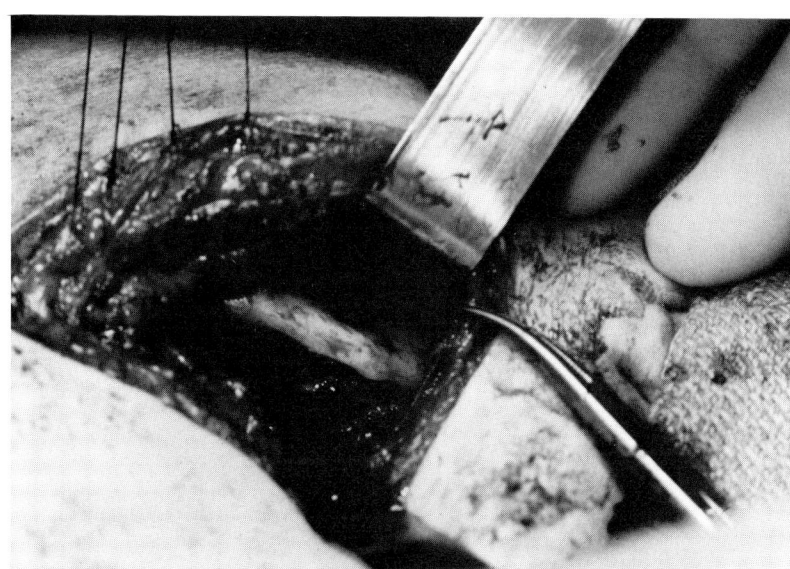

Figure 127. Exposure of ramus and elevation of periosteum.

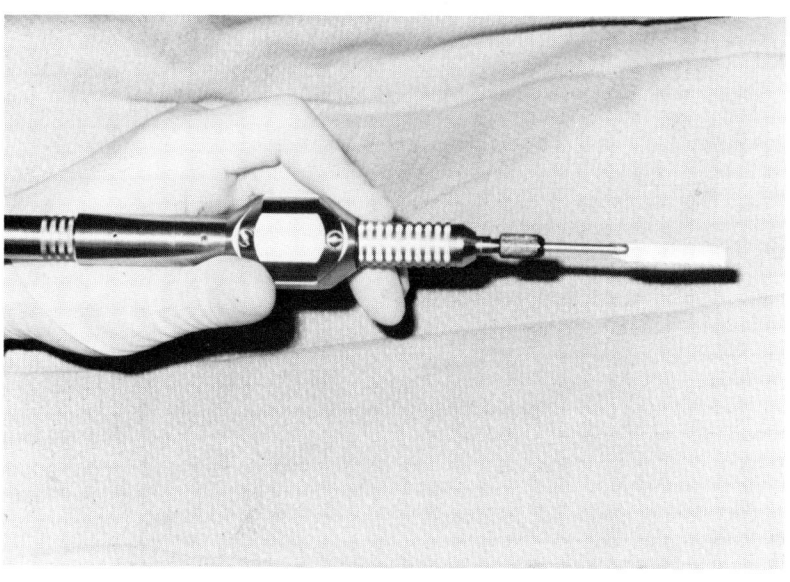

Figure 128. Power sagittal saw for vertical osteotomy.

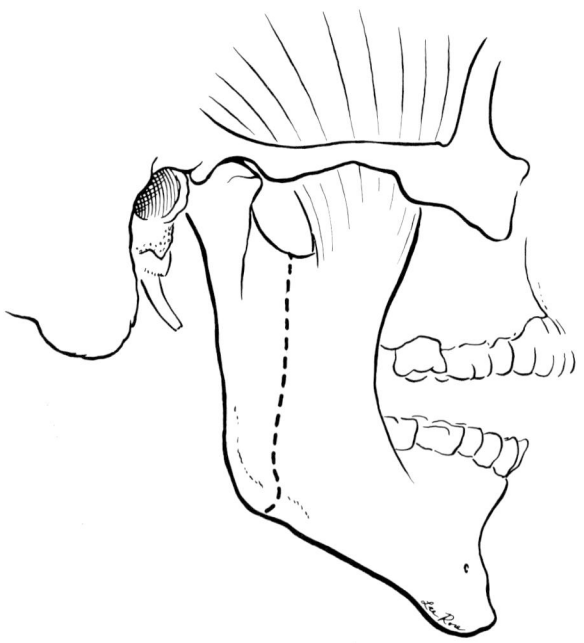

Figure 129. Vertical sagittal osteotomy of ramus.

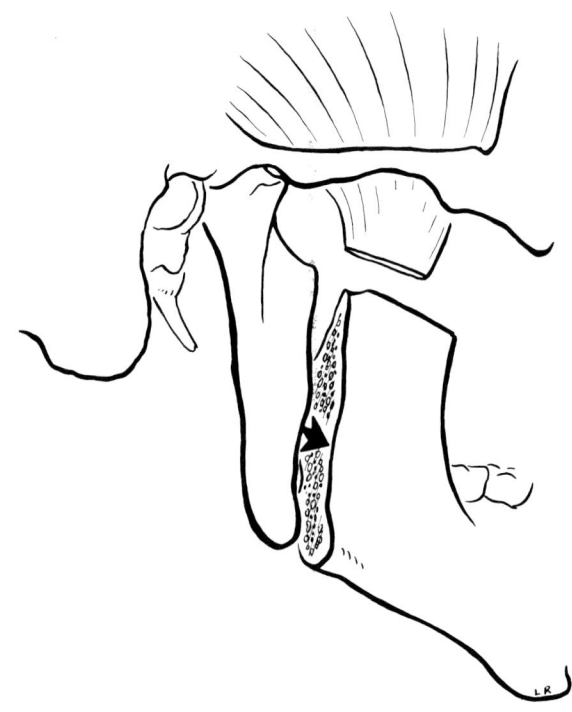

Figure 131. Option for advancement of mandibular arch.

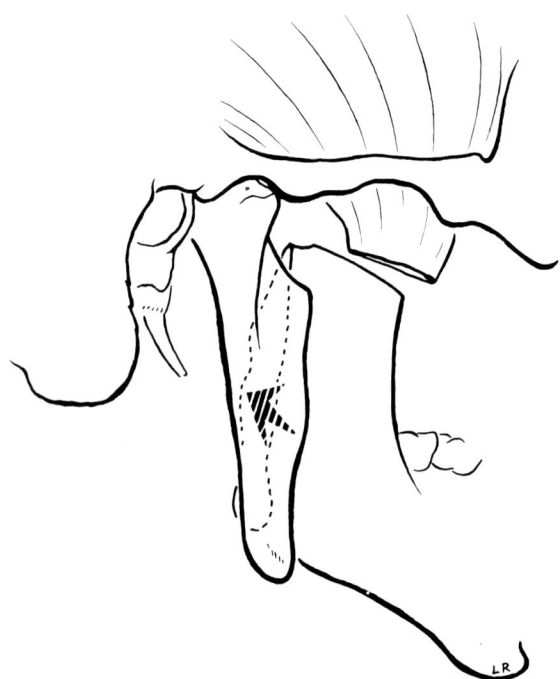

Figure 130. Option for retro-positioning of mandibular arch.

Next, the mandibular arch was repositioned in good alignment with the maxillary dental arch; this relationship was maintained by the application of dental arch bars and elastic band traction. The osteotomy sites were then wired for stabilization. The patient has enjoyed an excellent postoperative result.

Malunion of mandibular fractures can be managed by direct manipulation of the fracture sites for as long as 2 weeks. Beyond this length of time, osteotomy must often be considered to deal with this problem. In some circumstances, osteotomy at the site of the original fracture will be more practical and easily accomplished, while in other patients, such as this individual, vertical osteotomy of the ramus is preferable. The latter technique is useful when the contour of the mandibular arch has not been adversely affected by the malunion process.

These comments are offered as a practical review of the principles of mandibular fracture assessment and treatment. Readers who wish more detailed information should peruse the Bibliography.

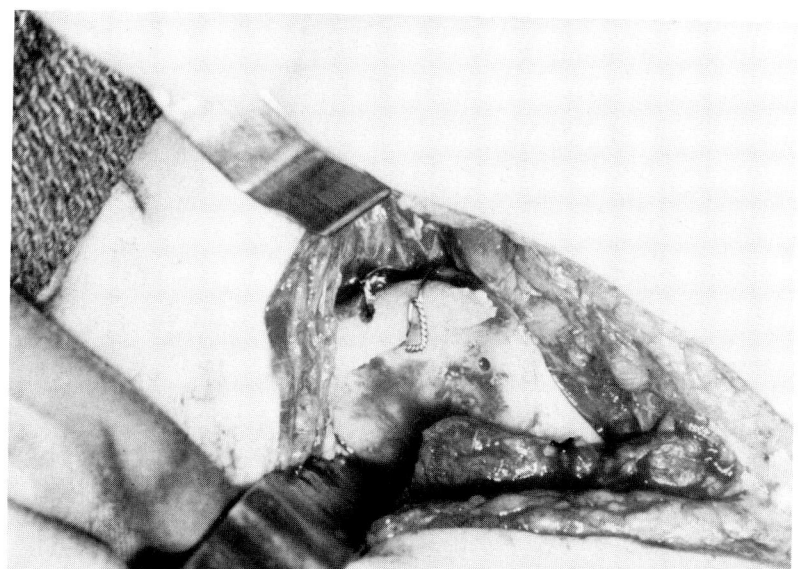

Figure 132. Wire stabilization of osteotomy after restoration of occlusion.

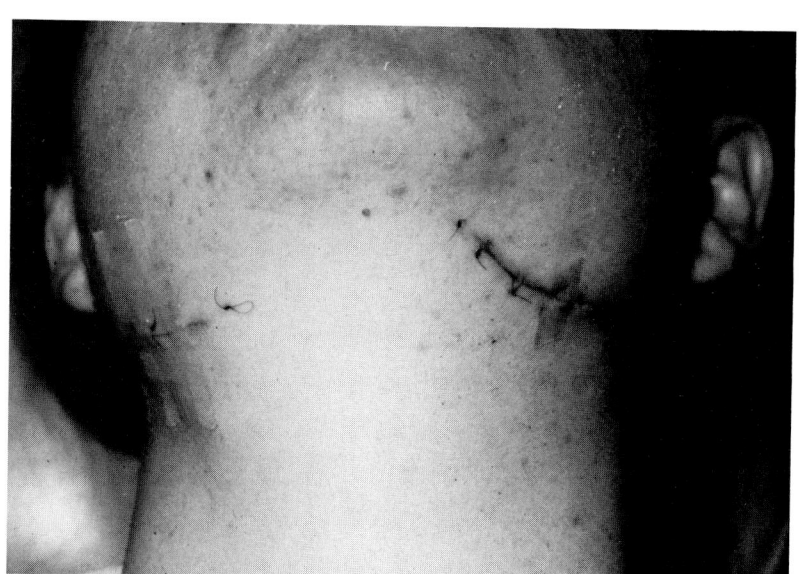

Figure 133. Skin incisions for approach.

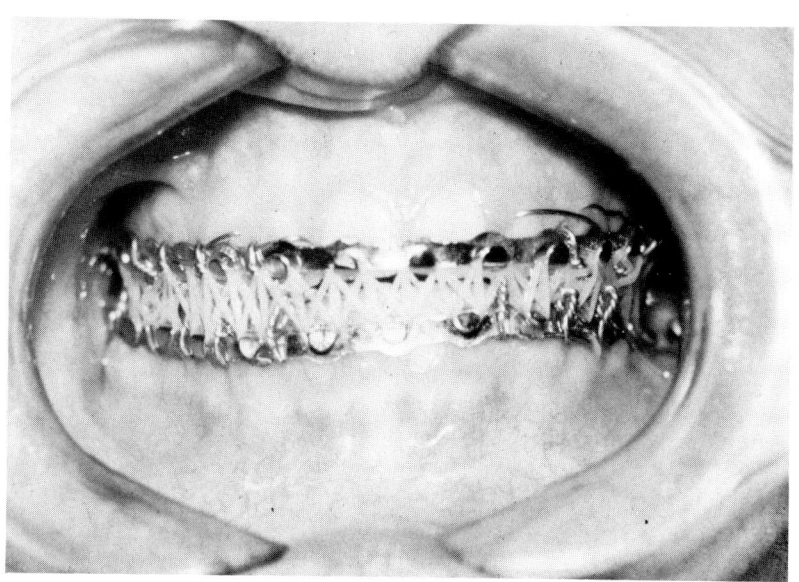

Figure 134. Postoperative occlusion following revision by ramus osteotomies.

BIBLIOGRAPHY

Adams G, Nelms CR: Complicated mandibular fractures. Otolaryngol Clin N Am 9:453–464, 1976

Bailey BJ, Gaskill JR: Fractures of the mandible. Laryngoscope 77:1137–1154, 1967

Converse JM (ed): Kazanjian and Convere's Surgical Treatment of Facial Injuries, Ed. 3. Baltimore: Williams & Wilkins, 1974, pp 145–146, 217–219

Dingman RO, Natvig P: Surgery of Facial Fractures. Philadelphia: WB Saunders, 1964, p 119

Eby JD: Principles of orthodontia in the treatment of maxillofacial injuries. Int J Orthod 6:273–310, 1920

Eid K, Lynch OJ, Whitaker LA: Mandibular fractures: The problem patient. J Trauma 16:658–661, 1976

Fractures of the edentulous mandible: Chalmers J Lyons Academy Study. J Oral Surg 34(11):973–979, 1976

Freidhofer HPM Jr, Salier HF: Experiences with interosseous wiring of mandibular fractures. J Maxillofac Surg 1:248–252, 1973

Gilmer TL: Fractures of the inferior maxilla. Illinois St Dent Soc Trans 67:104, 1881

Gunning RB: The treatment of fractures of the lower jaw by interdental splints. NY State J Med 3:433–448, 4:11–29, 4:274–277, 1861–1862

Ivy RH: Practical method of fixation in fractures of the mandible. Surg Gynecol Obstet 22:670–673, 1934

Jackson MJ, Wetmore SJ: Surgical prosthetic splints as an adjunct in treating facial fractures. Arch Otolaryngol 106:25–30, 1980

James RB, Fredericks C, Kent JM: Prospective study of mandibular fractures. J Oral Surg 39:275–281, 1981

Kazanjian VH: Immobilization of wartime, compound, comminuted fractures of the mandible. Am J Orthod Oral Surg 28:551–560, 1942

Klein JC: Intraoral open reduction. Arch Otolaryngol 103:645–647, 1977

Loesche WJ: Indigenous human flora and bactermia. In Kaplan El, Taranta AV (eds): Infective Endocarditis: An American Heart Association Symposium. Dallas: American Heart Association, 1977, p 40

Obwegeser H: Uber eine Methode der friedhandisen Drahtschienung von Kierferbruchen. Osterreichinschen Z Stomat 49:652, 1952

Risdon F: The treatment of fractures of the jaw. Can Med Assoc J 20:260–262, 1929

Rowe NL, Killey HC: Fractures of the facial skeleton, Ed. 2. Edinburgh and London: E & S Livingston, 1970

Schneider SS: Teeth in the line of mandibular fractures. J Oral Surg 29:107–109, 1971

Siegel LG, Meyerhoff WL: Reduction of mandibular fractures. Otolaryngol Clin N Am 9:439–451, 1976

Soujris F, Lamarche JP, Mirfakhrai AM: Treatment of mandibular fractures by interoral placement of bone plates. J Oral Surg 38:33–35, 1980

Stout R: Manual of Standard Practice of Plastic and Maxillofacial Surgery. Philadelphia: WB Saunders, 1943

Thoma KH: Oral Surgery, Vol. 1, Ed. 5. St. Louis: CV Mosby, 1969, pp 534–538

Wolvjewicz MA: Fractures of the mandible involving the impacted third molars. Br J Oral Surg 18(2):125–131, 1980

8 Bone Plate Osteosynthesis in the Treatment of Mandibular Fractures

Victor V. Strelzow, M.D., F.R.C.S.(C), F.A.C.S.

DYNAMICS OF BONE PLATE COMPRESSION

All modern self-compressing bone plates developed for maxillofacial surgery are based on a similar principle.[1,2] During application, the dynamic interaction between the head of the screw and the shape of the hole in the bone plate occurs due to the *spherical gliding principle* described by the Association for the Study of Internal Fixation. The concept is likened to a sphere rolling down a cylinder: as the screw advances into the bone, the hemispherical undersurface of its head is forced by contact with the incline-shaped hole in the bone plate, and thus glides down the incline-shaped ramp in the bone plate. Further tightening of the screw produces progressively more horizontal movement relative to the plate.

The force vector produced by this movement is parallel to the screw and perpendicular to the bone plate when the screw first engages the ramp built into the plate. As the screw is tightened down, however, the oblique shape of the screw hole forces the initial vector to develop a horizontal component that parallels the plate. Since the geometry of the screw's head and the incline ramp in the bone plate allows movement in only one direction, this axial force vector is expressed as horizontal movement of the screw and bone relative to the plate. By using two such opposing *screw-plate units* on either side of a fracture line, the result will be horizontal movement of the bone segments toward each other, resulting finally in fragment approximation. At that time, this force vector can no longer produce horizontal movement but will be translated into compression across the fracture line. This will continue until the screw has traveled the full length of the oblique ramp in the bone plate or until the breaking point of the metal components are reached or the inherent modiolus of elasticity of the bone is surpassed by the purchase of the screw's threads.

Osteosynthesis refers to the treatment of bone fractures by implantable metal appliances (Fig. 135A to F). *Dynamic compression plates* (DC plates) autonomously generate horizontal movement followed by interfragmentary compression across the fracture line from one or both ends of the plate. *Static fixation plates* (SF plates) have no incline ramps built into their screw holes and achieve no relative movement or axial forces across the fracture line. *Eccentric dynamic compression plates* (EDC plates) are specially modified DC plates with the outside screw holes having incline ramps set obliquely at 45 to 90 degrees to the long axis of the plate so that the forces of movement and compression generated are orientated in these same directions. These plates were developed to help counteract the unwanted splaying open effect inherent with the use of axially compressing dynamic plates. This splaying open effect occurs because the basilar margin of the mandible is used for most plate applications; when its axially orientated screws are tightened, relative movement and subsequent fracture compression primarily occurs at the lower aspect of the fracture interface. This produces a relative splaying open or fanning out of the fracture fragments at their alveolar margin. To help passively counteract this tendency when a DC plate is chosen, a *traction bar* of arch bar material, reinforced with cold-cured acrylic around its circumdental wires, needs to be applied first in mandibles having stable teeth. Then, by choosing an EDC plate which has eccentrically orientated screw holes, a force vector can generate significant compression through to the alveolar margin as well. In the edentulous or poorly dentured mandible where no traction bar can be used, the choice of this plate type is therefore mandatory. Due to its versatility, the EDC plate has now almost completely replaced the DC plate in most routine mandible fracture applications, even in patients with adequate dentition.

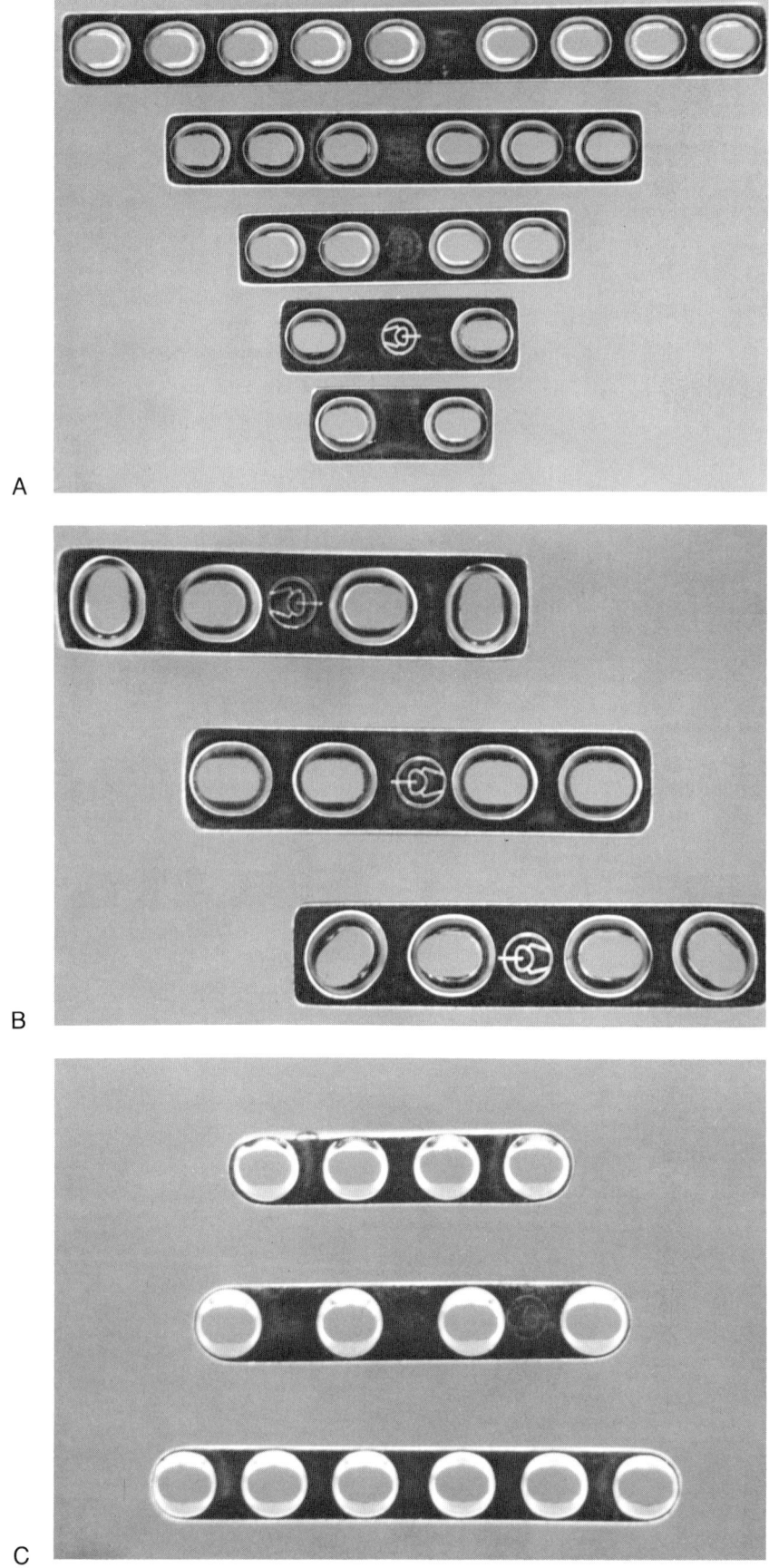

Figure 135. (A) Various sizes of dynamic compression (DC) plates. (B) Top, 90 degree eccentric dynamic compression (EDC) plate; middle, DC plate for comparison; bottom, 45 degree EDC plate. (C) Static fixation (SF) plates.

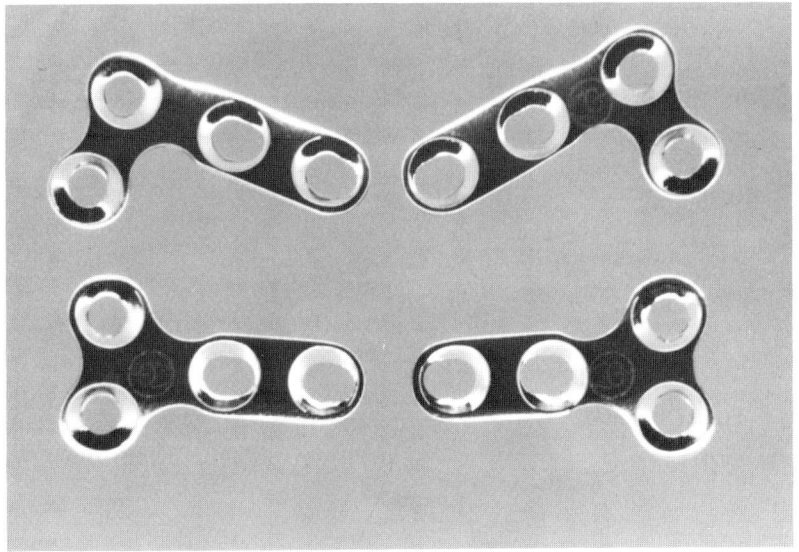

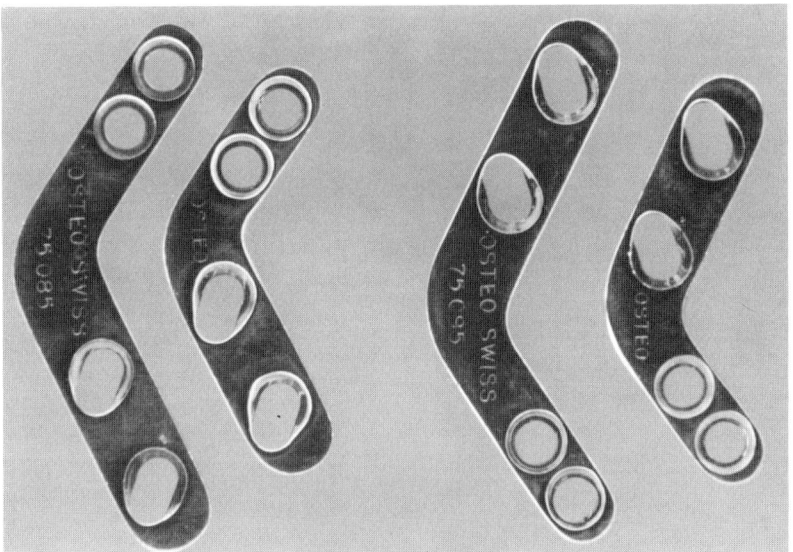

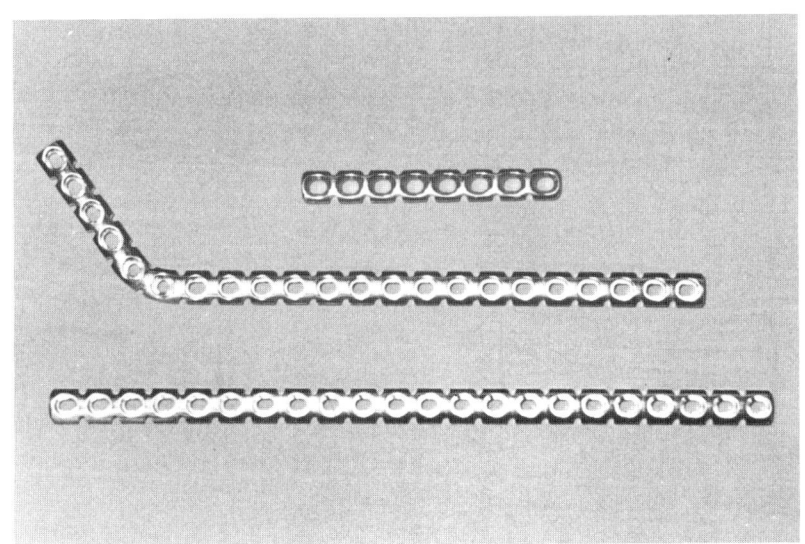

Figure 135. (D) Small "mini-plates" of different shapes. (E) Left and right, small and large angled DC plates. (F) Straight and angled reconstructive plates.

Because the compression plate is usually applied on the outer surface of the mandible, a similar disproportionate compression occurs at the buccal cortex of the fracture with some resultant splaying open of the lingual cortex. This effect is accentuated further because they are applied on the outside of a mandible, which is itself a rounded anatomic structure. Practically, this lingual splaying effect is overcome by slightly overbending the plate in relation to the corresponding curve of the mandible.[3]

EFFECTS ON BONE HEALING

Traditionally, uncomplicated bone healing has usually been studied in long bones held in relative immobilization. This histologic sequence, termed *secondary bone healing,* begins with the development of a fracture hematoma and, depending on the severity of the trauma, a variable degree of bony necrosis especially in the cortical layers. This is followed by a localized inflammatory response and the production of granulation tissue consisting of young fibroblasts and capillary buds which grow into and begin to replace the fracture hematoma. Cellular differentiation occurs with the newly formed chondroblasts laying down matrix and maturing into chondrocytes which in turn further proliferate and fill in the fracture gap with cartilage. A fracture callus derived primarily from the periosteum results in the deposition of structural bone adjacent to its inner surface. Continuing wound maturation produces spicules of calcified cartilage which are then replaced by osteoblasts with osteoid, immature woven bone, and finally by mature lamellar bone which undergoes remodeling in response to the surrounding functional stresses.

With the advent of successful rigid fixation techniques has come the concept of *absolute stability*[4] which describes an ideal situation in which during healing the bone fragments would be held in complete immobilization. Although not attainable in practice, the marked improvement in stability afforded by presently available osteosynthesis does result in a different sequence of bone healing which has been termed *primary bone healing.*[5] At the time of trauma a fracture hematoma still forms, but the bone fragments are so closely coapted and compressed that any potential space for it effectively disappears. Death of the osteoblasts involved at the fracture site still occurs, but the main elements of bone healing originate from cellular ingrowths occurring directly through the patent canals of the adjacent and still viable haversian systems. First surrounding osteoclasts resorb the necrotic bone edges back to healthy osteons, which proceed to tunnel in from both sides and across the coapted fracture line in a growing rootlike fashion. This is immediately followed by buds of neovascularization and by proliferating osteoblasts which subsequently lay down new bone in an already mature lamellar pattern.

Although the initial process of bone healing appears to be more rapid and direct with osteosynthesis, the final strength after removal of the plate is the same in both cases. Dynamic osteosynthesis therefore appears to modify the basic temporal sequence of bone healing by skipping the earlier emphasis on resorption and repair, and proceeding more directly to the latter stages of remodeling seen in the traditional secondary bone healing model. In fact, if after bone plate application there still exists appreciable fragment instability, primary bone healing will change into a process resembling secondary bone healing. This is probably due to the movement disrupting neovascularization during the important early steps of healing and the maturation of the initial fibrous tissue into cartilage and finally bone. In the presence of lesser instability, secondary bone healing will still progress but its individual stages will be prolonged, resulting in delayed union. This is evidenced radiographically by the development of excessive fracture callus, presumably due to a compensatory attempt to stabilize the fragments and complete the healing process. On exploring such a wound a predominantly fibrocartilaginous scar interspersed with islands of immature woven bone is found. In a wound with relatively more fragment instability, the usual sequence of secondary bone healing will not even proceed this far. No significant callus is formed but rather widespread resorption is seen, accompanied by blunting of the fragment ends with histologically nonossified fibrous connective tissue filling in the fracture gap.

In orthopedic applications where the mechanical stresses on bone are often much larger, the use of internal compression plates has been followed by stress fractures and regional osteoporosis. This is due to *stress shielding,* which is the weakening of bone due to interference by the rigid plate with the translation of the surrounding functional loads into compensatory biomechanical bone changes. Described in bioelectrical terms, Wolff's law of bone remodeling results from generation of positive and negative piezoelectric forces resulting from compression (electronegative charges) and tension (electropositive charges) forces on bone.[6] New bone and fracture callus have been shown to form in areas of increased electronegative charges; therefore, by artificially splinting the bone with a metal plate, the translation of the surrounding mechanical forces into local bone remodeling is disrupted.

Also, because of the nonphysiologic compression generated by the bone plate application itself, local compensatory bone resorption and rarefraction may occur. As a consequence, when the plate is removed it will expose the previously shielded bone to a mechanical stress which it may not be able to withstand, thus resulting in a pathologic fracture. It is for this reason that in orthopedics most bone plates are removed as soon as healing is complete in order that the remodeling forces can restore the necessary strength to the newly repaired bone.

In the area of the mandible, however, the removal of compression plates has not generally been necessary in our experience with over 150 platings. This is due to the gradual drop-off in magnitude of the axial compression that occurs over time as a result of this same bone remodeling occurring at the screw sites. By the time primary bone healing is completed, for example, 4 to 6 weeks after plate removal, the effect of any initial "stress shielding" is not clinically significant. Practically this has shown itself to be true because patients in whom plates were not removed have not subsequently gone on to the postoperative sequellae of bone atrophy or pathologic fracture when followed for at least a 5-year period.

INSTRUMENTATION

A comprehensive set of instruments have been developed for every step of the plating process. *Hohmann retractors* (Fig. 136A) provide atraumatic retraction of the soft tissues resulting in less trauma, postoperative edema, and cases of neuropaxia while allowing maximum exposure through minimal skin incisions. The *bone-holding clamp* (Fig. 136A) functions like a hefty towel clip, and the bone-plate holding clamp, which has one sharp and one flat tine, allows hands-free stable fixation of the plate to the bone during screw application (Fig. 136A). *Reduction-compression pliers* (Fig. 136B) have detachable tips through which short screws can be driven into the lower margin of the jaw to manipulate the fragments into accurate anatomic reduction. Closing and locking the plier handles results in more accurate reduction as well as the production of axial precompression across the basilar portion of the fracture plane. The lateral compression rollers, when advanced, rotate the bone fragments about the plier tips to cause reduction and then interfragment compression at the alveolar margin of the fracture site. *Malleable templates* (Fig. 136C) can translate the surface curvature of the jaw to a more convenient working area where *bending irons* and *bending pliers* can correspondingly shape the selected plate. A *drill guide* (Fig. 136D) with a rotatable headpiece directs the accurate drilling of centric holes (neutral or "nonloaded" position for passive fixation), or eccentric holes (active or "loaded" position for dynamic compression) through the plate holes. When the arrow on the head points to zero (i.e., $\rightarrow 0$), the drilled screw hole will be situated at the bottom of the oblique hole in the plate, which results in no significant horizontal or axial compression. When the arrow is rotated toward the figure (i.e., $\rightarrow 8$), however, the screw hole is drilled 0.8 mm up the oblique screw hole ramp, producing roughly this amount of added horizontal movement and therefore potential axial compression. The *depth gauge* (Fig. 136E), graduated in millimeters to measure the depth of the screw holes, is always used after drilling and before tapping, to insure choosing of the proper screw length which will be able to engage both cortices. A *bone tap* is used to enlarge the hole and remove the bone spicules so that the screw will not splinter the brittle cortical plates.

The surgical stainless steel 2.7-mm plates generally used start with two-hole (20-mm) DC plates and proceed up the six-hole (952-mm) sizes, with larger lengths also available (see Fig. 135A). Eccentric dynamic compression plates have fracture-near axially arranged and fracture-far eccentrically arranged screw holes, beginning with four-hole (20-mm) sizes (see Fig. 135B). These are made with 45 degree and 90 degree orientated outer screw holes relative to the long axis of the plate. These plates are generally used with 6- to 18-mm-long, 2.7-mm-wide cortical bone screws which have threads throughout their length, or with medullary (lag) bone screws which are differentiated by only having threads over the distal one-third to one-half of their shafts.

Smaller 2-mm "mini-compression plates" have been added more recently and are thinner and less wide but still provide axially orientated compression. Yet smaller and thinner "mini-plates," which were originally developed for use in the fixation of the small bones of the hand and foot, are produced in various *T, J, L, Y,* and so forth shapes and sizes (see Fig. 135C and D). These mini-plates are quite malleable and often are very useful in areas of thin bone or when fixation only is required between smaller fragments. These are most frequently utilized with 1.5-mm cortical screws.

Angled DC plates are available in two sizes each in left and right configurations, and utilize 2.7-mm cortical or lag screws (see Fig. 135E). One end provides static fixation while the other, which is angled at 120 degrees to the long axis of the first, results in eccentric dynamic compression across the intervening fracture line.

Several other specially designed and shaped plates

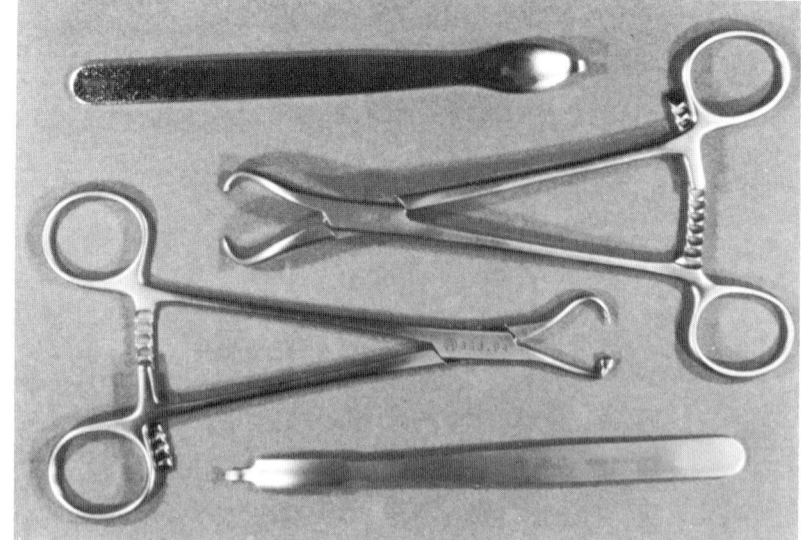

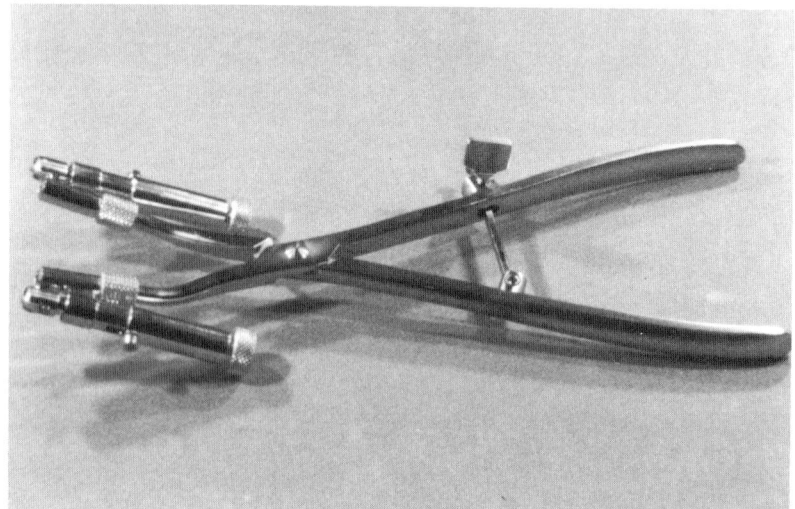

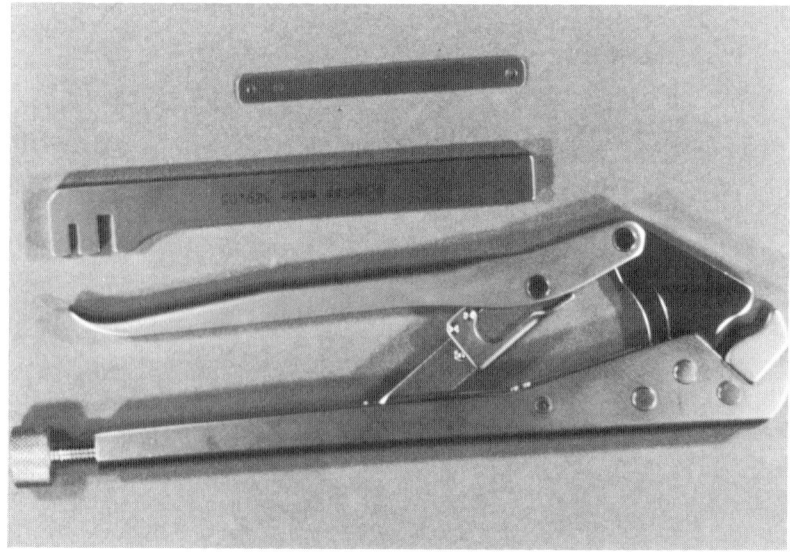

Figure 136. (A) Top and bottom, large Hohmann retractor, bone plate-holding clamp, bone-plate-holding forceps, small Hohmann retractor. (B) Reduction-compression pliers. (C) Top to bottom, malleable template, bending iron, bending pliers.

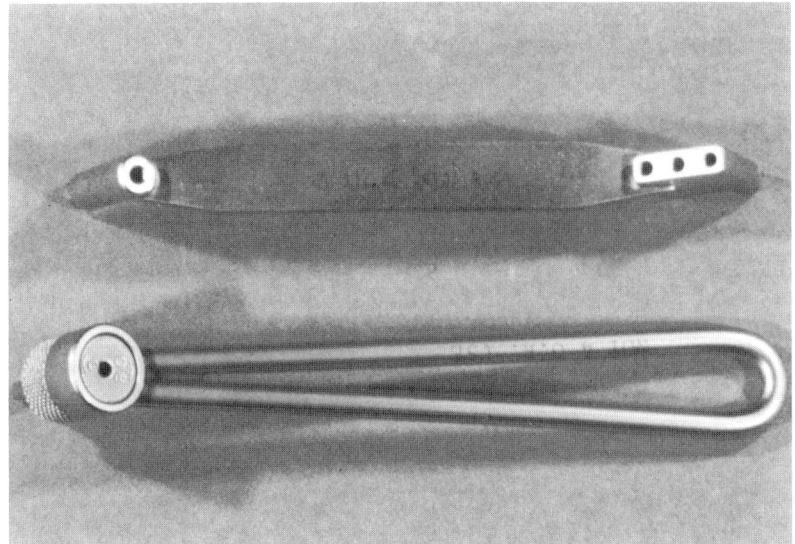

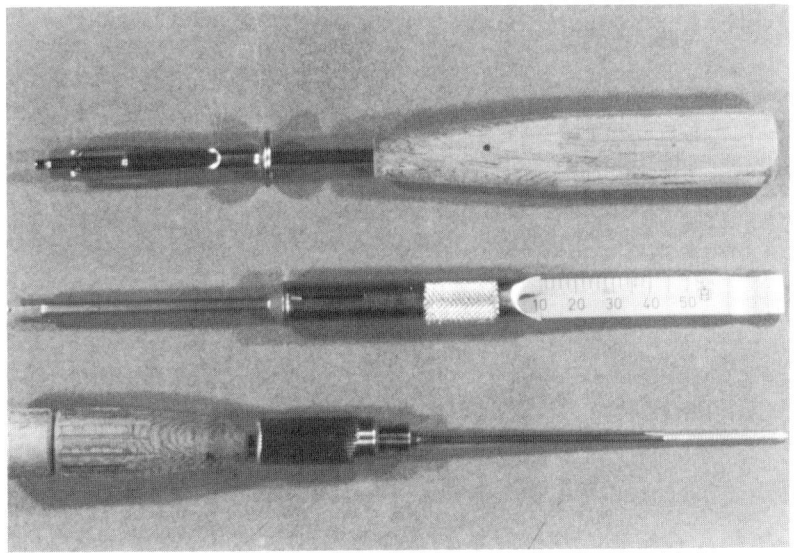

Figure 136. (D) Top, drill guide; bottom, load guide. (E) Top to bottom, screwdriver, depth gauge, bone tap.

with inlays, attached condylar prostheses, and so on, are all basically modifications of the above-described plates. The newest advancement is the development of reconstruction plates with centrically positioned screw holes that provide only fixation (see Fig. 135F). These are available straight, angled, and with and without condylar heads, in 5-hole (58-mm) to 24-hole (192-mm) lengths. Because of V-shaped notches along the side of these plates between the holes, the plates may be bent, by using appropriate bending pliers, in three dimensions to fit almost any complex reconstructive need.

PLATE APPLICATION TECHNIQUE

Preoperatively an accurate dental assessment and consultation with a dental professional in regard to questionably viable teeth, fractured crowns, prosthetic work, etc. that may be involved in the fracture management, should be carried out. After general anesthesia has been induced via nasotracheal tube and the throat packed with 2-in. gauze packing, all of the teeth are inspected and palpated for signs of crown damage, loosening, and the like, and permanently documented. The oral cavity is copiously irrigated with an antibiotic-containing solution and the teeth cleaned with a fluoride-containing dental paste. If clinically or radiographically an unerupted or exposed tooth involved in the fracture line needs to be removed, it is extracted, after which the root socket is curretted. Following this, a water-tight gingival closure with mucoperiosteal buccal or gingival advancement flaps, if necessary, is carried out. Bimanual attempts are then carried out to successfully reduce the fracture and reconstruct the preoperative occlusion.

Arch bar material of sufficient length to bridge at least two to three stable teeth on either side of the fracture line is applied with no. 25 stainless steel circumdental wires. This acts as a tension band to help counteract the alveolar margin splaying that occurs when a DC plate or the axially acting screws of an EDC plate are applied to the basilar margin of the mandible. The nonsterile portion of this procedure is completed by applying two Ernst ligatures (modified Ivy loops) of no. 24 wire, one on either side of the fracture, to both jaws which are then wired together with the teeth stabilized into habitual occlusion.

The decision to use an extraoral approach would be influenced by posteriorly located fractures, the presence of multiple bone fragments, an adequate preexisting external laceration, or the suspicion of missing bone segments. The position of the incision is choosen to complement, if possible, the natural crease lines in the region. A scapel incision is carried down through skin, subcutaneous tissue, and platysma and from there dissection is continued using traumatic forceps and scissors in a layer-by-layer fashion so that the mandibular branch of the facial nerve, if exposed, will not be inadvertently injured. The periosteum is incised along the inferiormost edge of the mandible and the dissection continued in a subperiosteal plane to expose only sufficient bone to allow placement of the plate. With the aid of bone-holding forceps the fragments are distracted, and the fracture site copiously irrigated and examined to insure that no soft tissues, blood clot, or foreign body is present between the bone fragments. The tips of the reduction-compression pliers are applied to either side of the fracture line with 10-mm-long, 2.7-mm-wide cortical screws, and the body of the pliers attached. This allows easy manipulation and accurate reduction followed by the production of interfragmentary precompression. With the advancement of the lateral compression rollers, these forces are translated to the alveolar margin as well. A malleable template is made to slightly overconform to the surface of the mandible and an appropriately-sized EDC plate is shaped accordingly with bending irons and pliers.

The plate is temporarily fixed in the proper position with bone-plate-holding forceps, and a drill guide in the neutral or nonloaded position is used to make the first *fracture-near* screw hole. After measurement with the depth gauge, the screw hole is tapped and the appropriately-sized cortical screw is put in. The opposite fracture-near screw hole is now drilled with the drill guide in the loaded position, that is, with the arrow on its head pointing the 0.8 position toward the fracture line. After measurement and tapping, this screw is inserted and tightened. The eccentric screw holes are always drilled in the loaded position and the alternating sides screws are put in and tightened down in turn. In simple fractures all the rest of the *fracture-far* axially orientated screw holes in the plate are drilled in the centric or neutral position and the screws placed in the same alternating fashion. If the fracture line is oblique, a lag screw technique may be necessary in which the size of the axially orientated screw holes drilled in the proximal bone fragment is the same as the diameter of the screw. The hole in the distal fragment, however, corresponds to the usually smaller drill size. When the medullary or lag screw is then inserted, it will therefore not purchase the proximal cortical bone fragment but successfully engages only the distal fragment. This results in a sandwichlike stable compression of the distal cortical fragment via the screws to the proximal cortical layer and the bone plate.

The choice of an intraoral route is made primarily on the basis of how anteriorly the fracture is positioned. Usually lateral retraction of the cheek will allow the intraoral placement of a plate back to the level of the second premolar and often even further back in older patients. After mucosal injection of 1:100,000 epinephrine solution, a scapel incision is made through the mucosa and periosteum medial to the buccogingival sulcus taking care to avoid the area overlying the branching of the mental nerve. Subperiosteal dissection exposes the lower 2.0 cm of the mandibular margin. The reduction-compression pliers are applied if possible, and a shaped template is transferred to an appropriately-sized EDC plate. Drilling the screw holes is usually not a problem in the symphysis/parasymphysis region but further back a 5-mm percutaneous stab incision may be necessary to accurately use a drill guide and to introduce the screwdriver during plate application.

With either approach, after removal of the pliers and copious irrigation, the wound is closed in multiple layers beginning with the periosteum and immediate soft tissue overlying it. A second fascial layer, if possible, is attempted followed by the platysma muscle and then the deep dermis and epidermis. Hemostasis must be meticulous and all potential dead space must be obliterated. The intermaxillary wires are then taken down and the occlusion rechecked to be sure of having obtained the desired result. Perioperatively, cortical steroids and broad-spectrum antibiotics are employed routinely and without complications. Postoperatively a liquid diet followed by a soft diet and finally a normal diet are progressively introduced and the patient followed at routine intervals until the tension bar is removed at approximately 8 to 12 weeks.

INDICATIONS FOR USE

Bone plate osteosynthesis is an attempt to produce maximally successful fracture healing along with the minimal degree of patient morbidity and inconvenience.[7] Indications for its use in mandibular fractures can be divided into those that help improve surgical technique, and those that attempt to decrease patient morbidity[8] (Fig. 137 to 140).

One of the main technical advantages provided by bone plating is found in patients with poor or inadequate dentition.[9] Arch bars and intermaxillary fixation, long the mainstay of traditional maxillofacial techniques, may be inadequate or impossible in these patients because of the lack of suitably stable teeth. With EDC plates it is unnecessary to modify the patient's own dentures, frequently damaging them in the process, in an attempt to effect fracture immobilization. The commonly available prefabricated splints (i.e., Gunning splints) provide less stability and are often uncomfortable because of individual alveolar differences. This often requires the time-consuming and costly fabrication of customized acrylic splints. In these situations the use of an external fixator or immobilizing appliance—both of which provide less stable fixation—can be avoided. In fractures containing functionally important fragments that need to be accurately reduced and immobilized, for example, to reconstitute the strength or dimension of the alveolar arch, a rigid fixation plate while acting as an internal structural buttress can also help provide the optimum conditions necessary for primary bone healing. When using muliple figure-of-eight wire fixation, individual fragments can be stripped of their remaining periosteal blood supply, especially if they are small, obliquely shaped, involve the alveolar rim, or are found in atrophic mandibles. Absent bone in severe compound comminuted fractures or gunshot wounds can be optionally grafted immediately with the use of fixation plates, providing that sufficient soft tissue coverage can be assured.[10] In revision surgery for nonunion or malunion, the missing or removed bone segment, even if 3 to 4 cm, can be bridged with bone marrow punch grafts or iliac crest grafts held in immobilization by osteosynthesis with little patient morbidity and an excellent chance of success.[11] In patients with mixed dentition, extensive restorative dental work, or active or extensive gingival disease, bone plating can add much-needed interfragmentary stability where circumdental or mandibular wiring may be insufficient or contraindicated.

Choosing bone plate osteosynthesis in an attempt to further decrease unnecessary patient morbidity is particularly applicable in the elderly who often have preexisting medical conditions with specific therapeutic requirements. The distinct advantages of omitting intermaxillary fixation include the avoidance of debilitating weight loss due to restrictions in diet, the maintenance of an oral route for essential medications, and noninterference with speech. For insulin-dependent diabetics, for example, this allows unrestricted exposure to a wider range of equivalent food groups that make up an important aspect of their blood glucose control. For patients with active seizure disorders, uncontrolled alcoholism, or significant illicit drug use, the assurance by rigid fixation of a unrestricted oral airway during healing may be crucial. Maxillofacial patients frequently have other associated cervical or thoracic spine injuries that require long-term regional immobilization in spica casts or halo appliances. These, along with concurrent head injuries which often result in variable periods of altered levels of consciousness, may necessitate nasogastric tube feedings, prophylactic tracheostomy to avoid upper airway problems, and an increased intensity of postoperative nursing care if intermaxillary fixation is used. Simultaneous unrecognized injuries to the temporomandibular joint structures occur with many fractures of the mandible, resulting in various degrees of long-term dysfunction long after the bone fragments have healed. Refraining from immobilizing these joints for 4 to 8 weeks due to intermaxillary fixation may minimize, due to the early return to active mastication afforded by plating, the production of excessive synarthrosis or articular fibrosis. By providing internal fixation, athletes can maintain noncontact physical conditioning, patients may return to employment demanding high physical mobility, students can participate more fully in their vocational training, and businesspeople whose financial success often depends on person-to-person communication can return earlier and with more effectiveness to their jobs without the social and functional limitations associated with an external fixation device. Not the least important patient-related indication is the use

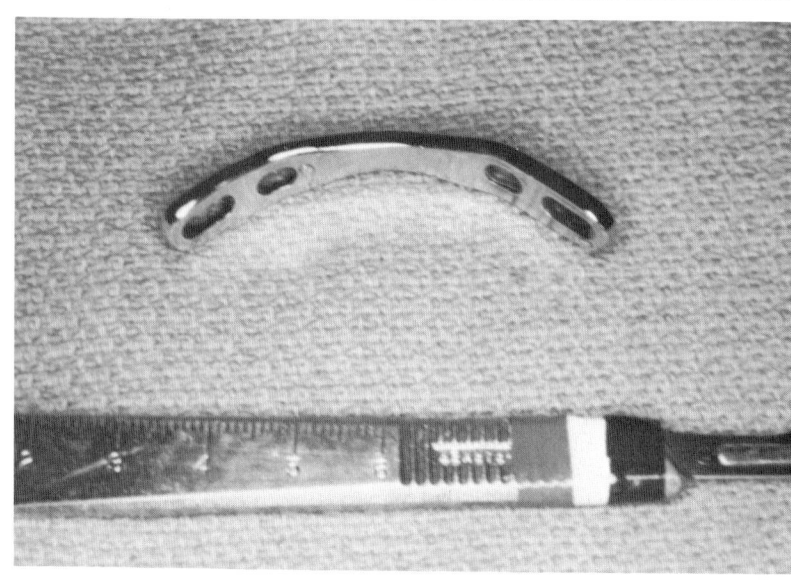
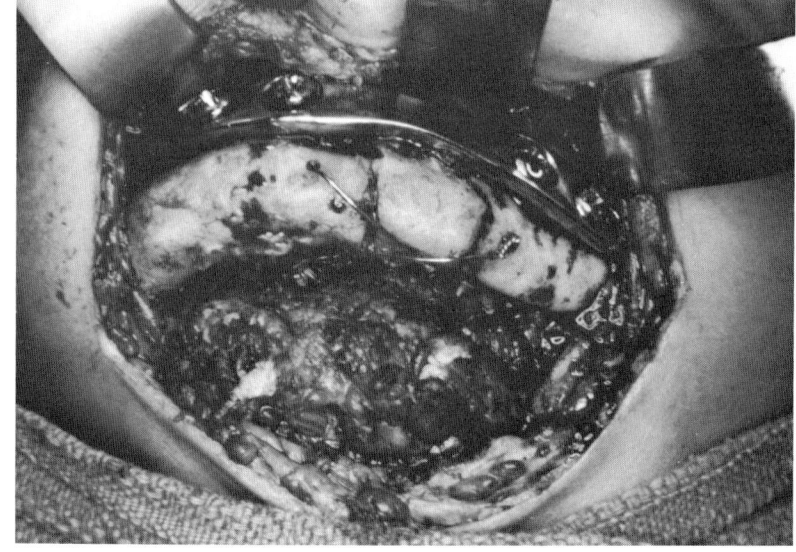

Figure 137. Teenage male with closed head injury and compound comminuted parasymphyseal fracture which failed two efforts at intermaxillary fixation due to noncompliance. (A) Intraoral view of fracture site. (B) Four-hole DC plate appropriately bent. (C) Triangular bone segment wired in place and plate applied through submental approach.

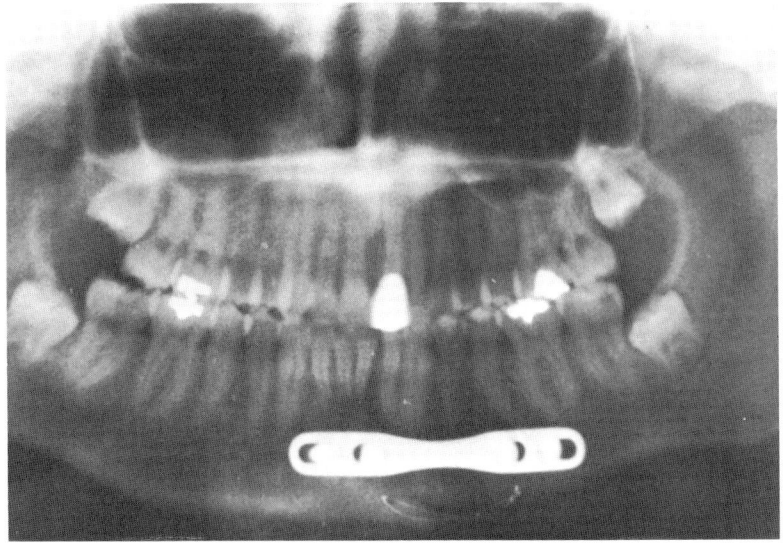
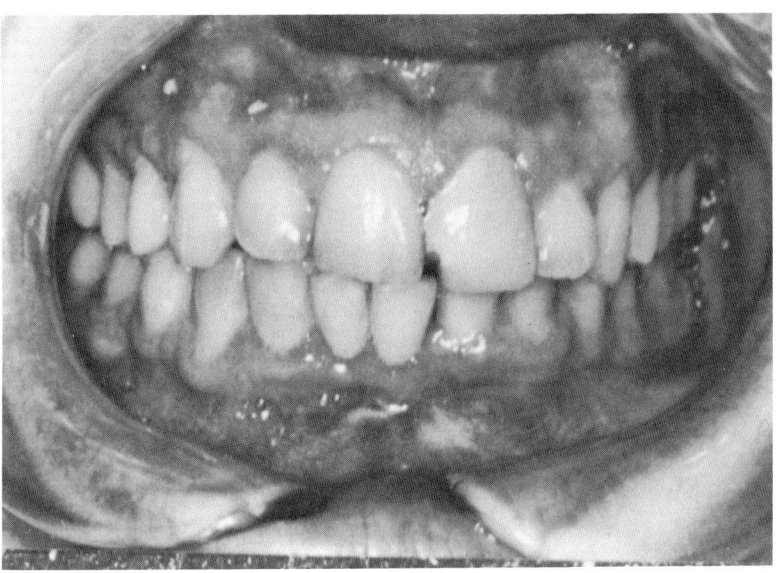

Figure 137. (D) Panoramic radiograph, 12 months postoperatively. (E) Restored habitual occlusion, 12 months postoperatively.

of osteosynthesis in those who, because of social, psychological, or personal reasons, are not willing to have their teeth wired together, especially as a therapeutic alternative is available.

POTENTIAL COMPLICATIONS—AVOIDANCE AND TREATMENT

The technical aspects of applying bone plate osteosynthesis in mandibular fractures have been highly refined and extensively tested through basic research and clinical experience involving thousands of patients. The appropriate plate correctly applied in the right clinical circumstance should result in a complication rate approaching zero. Realistically, however, the surgery of trauma frequently involves uncontrollable variables and hence some complications do occur.[12]

Soft tissue infection is the most common concern when dealing with implantable foreign bodies such as plates. Its occurrence is not related to the use of plating per se but rather to the degree of soft tissue trauma and contamination at the time of surgery. A conscientious regime of mouth hygiene including preoperative dental consultation if indicated, and in compound fractures with extensive soft tissue trauma the use of broad-spectrum antibiotics, can help to minimize soft tissue infection. Intraoperatively before plating, the oral cavity must be copiously irrigated with an antibiotic-containing solution and the teeth brushed with a fluoride-containing toothpaste. Similar repeat irrigations during the plate application decrease the potential contagion

98 Surgery of the Mandible

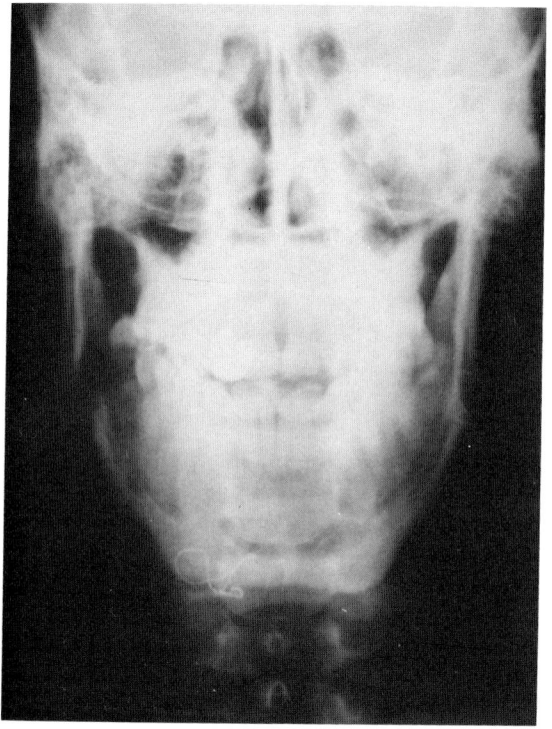

Figure 138. Young male with acute right-angle fracture but also evidence of old healed right parasymphyseal and left-angle fractures (figure-of-eight wires seen on x-ray). (A) Mandible film showing right angle fracture. (B) Preoperative occlusal imbalance due to the patient's previous failure to maintain intermaxillary fixation.

at the implant site as well. Atraumatic soft tissue handling, conservative trimming of potentially devitalized soft tissue, and a multiple-layered closure to obliterate any potential dead space for hematoma or seroma formation are essential. Only rarely is it necessary to use a small-diameter soft Silastic suction drain left beneath the platysmal layer and irrigated out before attachment to the suction bulb. If evidence of wound infection occurs, the initial treatment plan includes conservative debridement and wound care, provision of adequate drainage, and intravenous broad-spectrum antibiotic coverage.

Osteitis or osteomyelitis is most often seen with the loss of soft tissue coverage leading to failure of fixation, and when teeth have been inappropriately left in the fracture line. Preoperative dental evaluation and treatment is often omitted from treatment plans because of interspecialty rivalry, but is often most helpful, especially in view of the

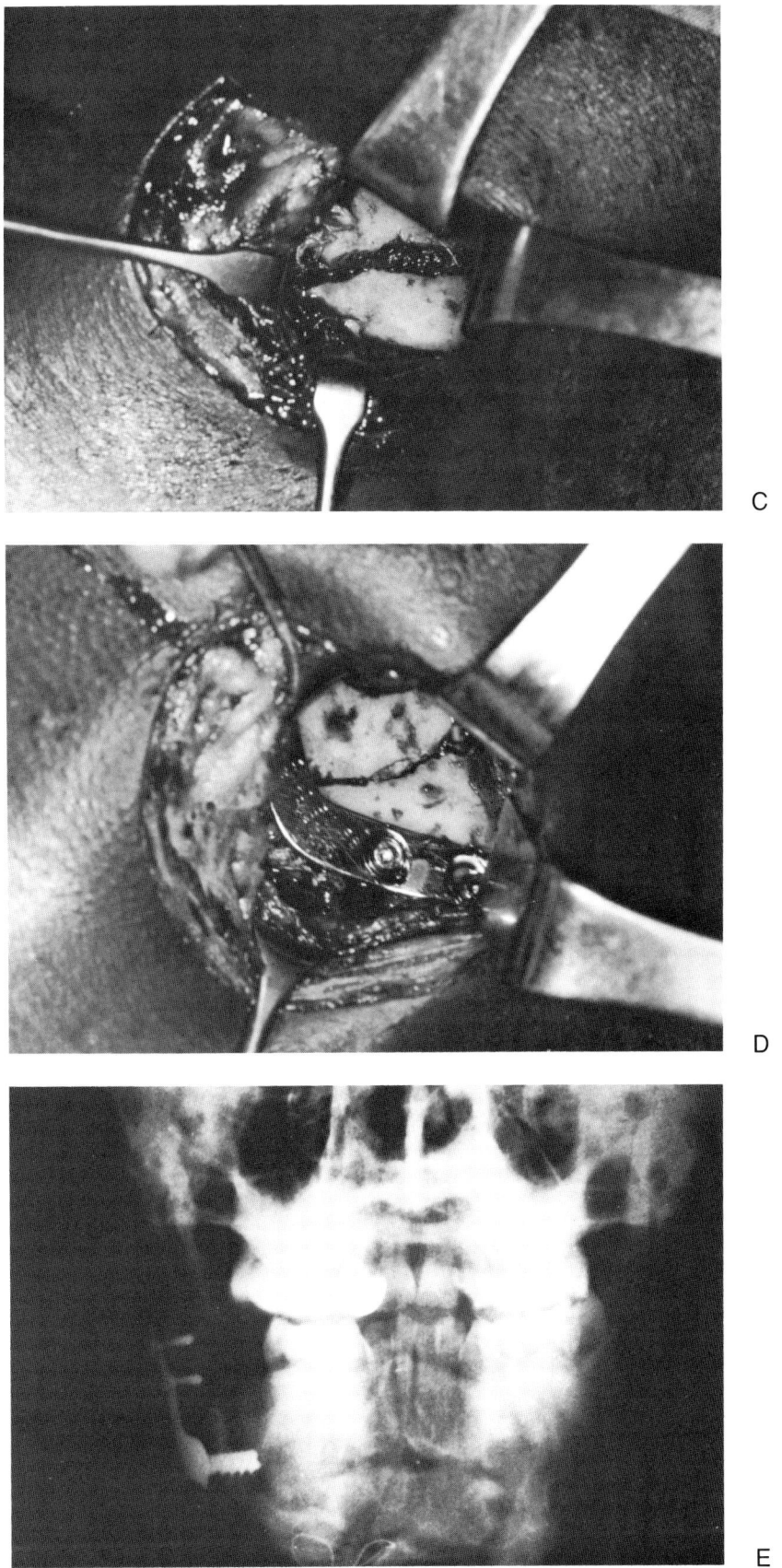

Figure 138. (C) Right-angle fracture segments approached through submandibular incision. (D) Right large-size angled DC plate applied without the need for intermaxillary fixation or arch bars. (E) Postoperative radiograph showing angle plate internally stabilizing accurately reduced mandible fragments.

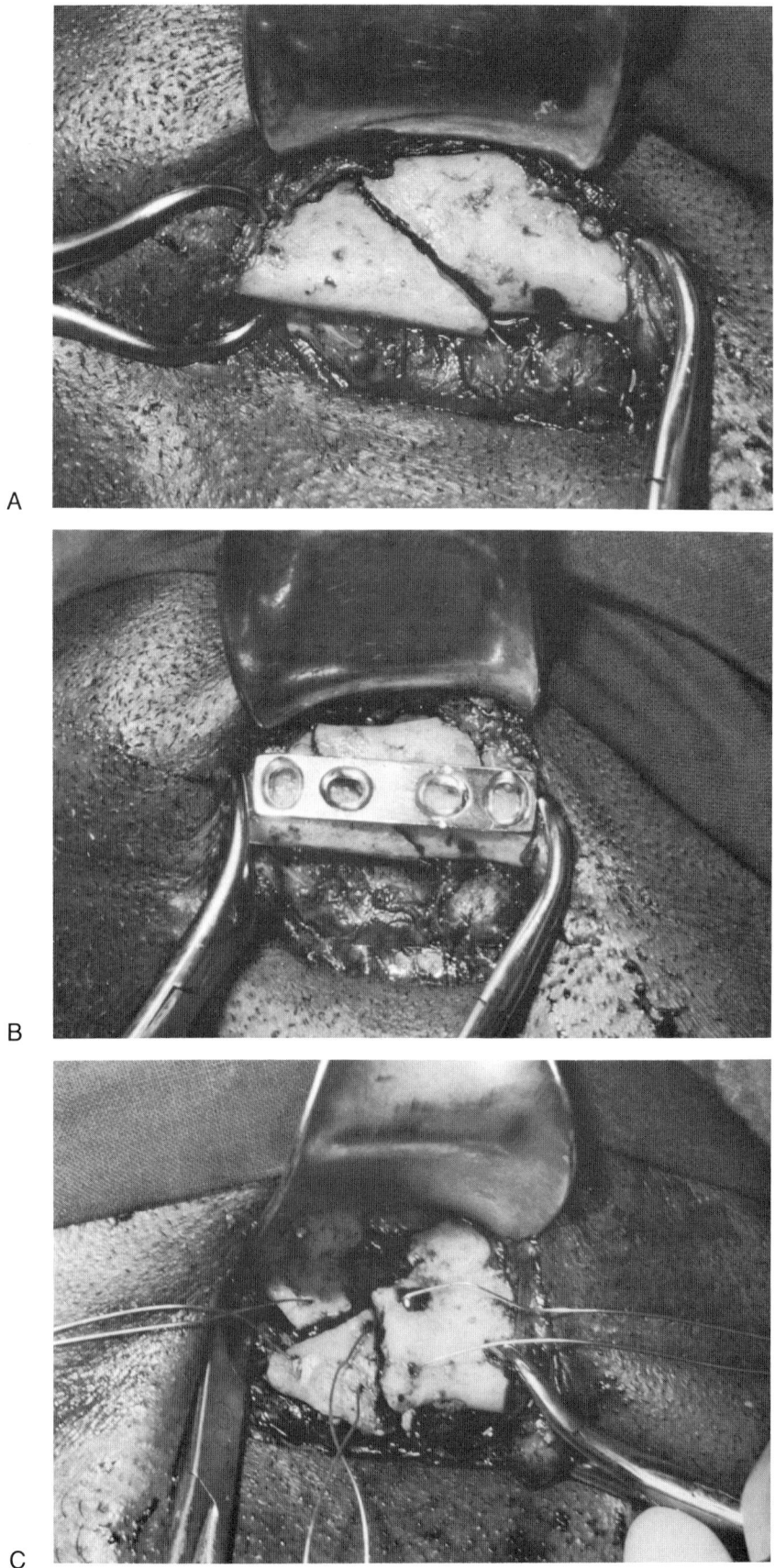

Figure 139. Middle-aged edentulous male with an acute left body and comminuted right angle fractures. (A) Exposure and reduction of left body fracture through submandibular approach. (B) The chosen 90 degree four-hole EDC plate being applied. (C) Wiring-in of triangular bone segment along lower margin of right angle of mandible.

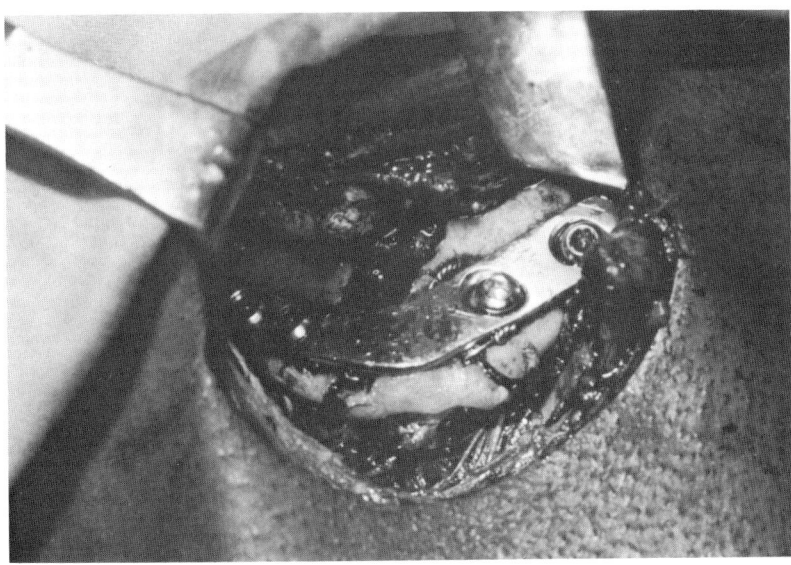

Figure 139. (D) Large, right-angled DC plate bridging wired bone fragment and providing stable internal fixation.

greater potential that patients may sue for medical/legal reasons. Teeth that exhibit crown damage, are devitalized, or have root fractures or overt exposure into the fracture line should be identified and appropriately treated. If dental extraction is relegated to the time of surgery, it should be done with the appropriate instruments and knowledge of extraction technique that will result in a saliva-tight closure, usually utilizing advancement mucosal flaps. The risk of osseous infection increases when excessive periosteal stripping, carried out for operative exposure, leads to devitalized bone fragments. Eburnation leading to bone sequestra and a decrease in the bone purchasing effectiveness by the screws, results if inadequate irrigation is used during bone drilling. Fragment instability tends to prevent the revascularization phase of bone healing and exposes the fracture interfaces to contamination and thereby infection.

The symptoms and signs of bone infection begin similarly to those seen in soft tissue wound infections, accompanied by the gradual development of deep-seated jaw pain on chewing or bimanual manipulation. This may occur before any tell-tale fracture callus signifying fragment instability is seen radiologically. Treatment consists of broad-spectrum, high-dose intravenous antibiotics; of any complicating soft tissue problems by conservative debridement, drainage, and irrigation; and a thorough radiologic search for any teeth or bone fragments involved in the fracture line. If the plate application is still solid, intraoral extraction of the offending tooth, being careful to remove all root tips, or of the devitalized bone fragment, may be all that is required. However, if the internal fixation is no longer stable, it should be removed with curettage and debridement of the fracture segments at the same time and the selection of an external system of fixation to encourage continued fragment healing.

Exposure of the plate is a serious complication because of the potential loss of internal fixation. This uncommon occurrence is usually associated with compound, comminuted fractures where extensive soft tissue damage is a prominent feature. Although at the time of debridement and plastic closure, soft tissue coverage of the plate site may be considered adequate, over the ensuing post-operative days there is a gradual breakdown of the skin or more frequently the thinner mucosal wound. Avoidance of this complication is hampered by the fact that in many patients the prognostic vascular damage is not obvious at the time of the initial trauma. To avoid this problem, early closure of the soft tissue components of compound, comminuted mandible trauma may be performed, even if the definitive bone work needs to be delayed. Soft tissue debridement should not be aggressive unless adequate tissue remains available for plate coverage or its viability is obviously compromised. Copious irrigation with an antibiotic-containing solution as well as systemic antibiotic coverage may minimize the potential for infection at many questionably healthy tissue margins. Adherence to atraumatic soft tissue technique cannot be overstressed, including the use of atraumatic forceps, delicate skin hooks, sharp scapel debridement, multiple fascial, muscle, and subdermal layer closures followed by a noncompromising skin approximation. When an intraoral approach is chosen, the incision should not be too high up on the alveolar ridge in the edentulous patient because of interference with den-

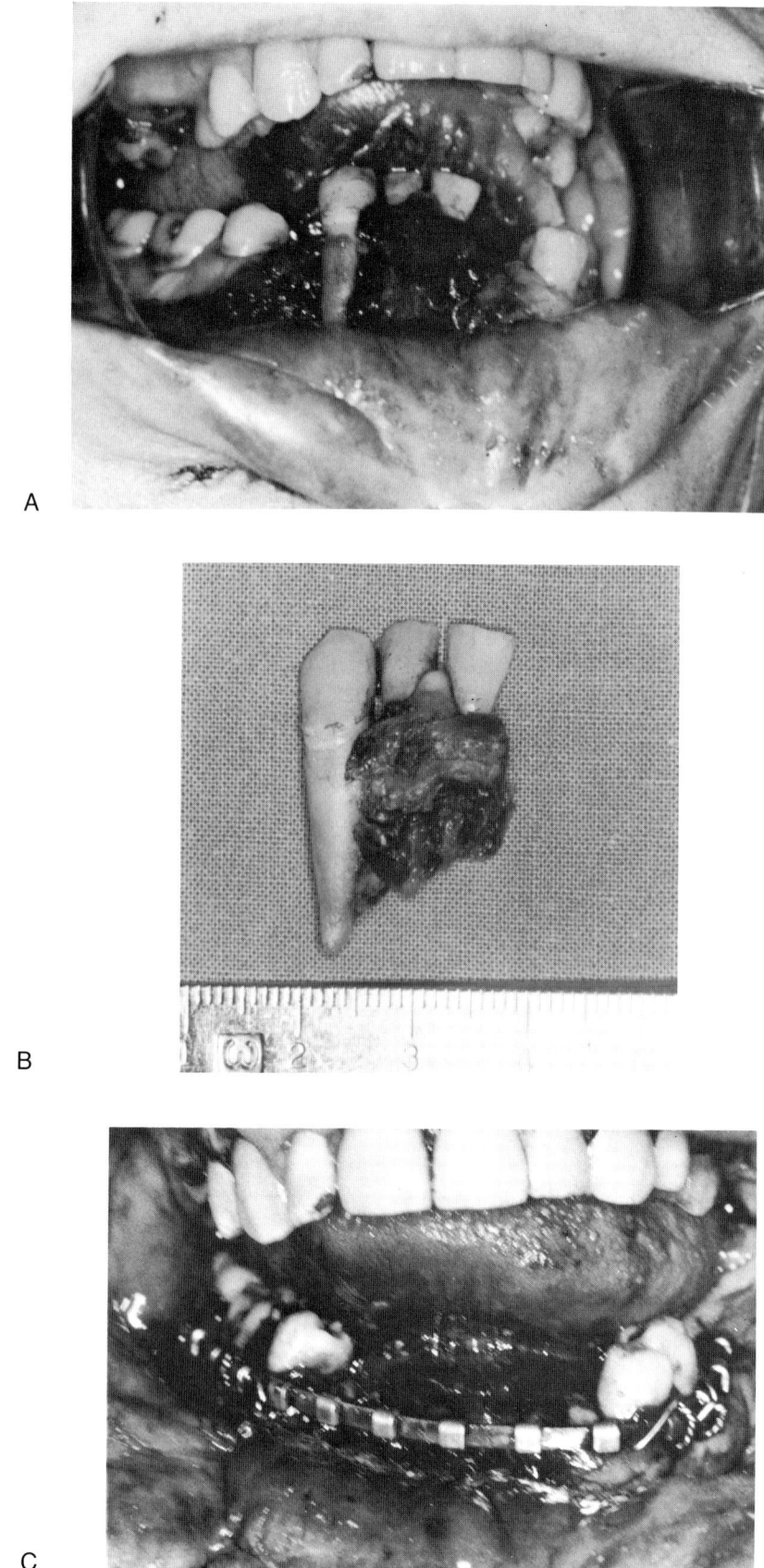

Figure 140. Middle-aged male who sustained a fracture evulsion in the anterior jaw region. (A) Intraoral view showing displaced right canine, lateral, and medial incisors. (B) Teeth within alveolar fragment after removal. (C) Arch bar shown spanning the discontinuity in the dental arch.

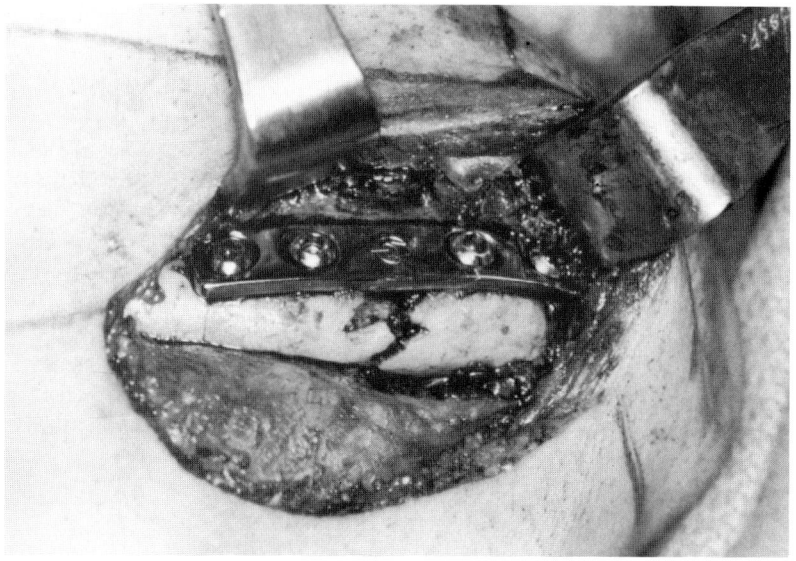

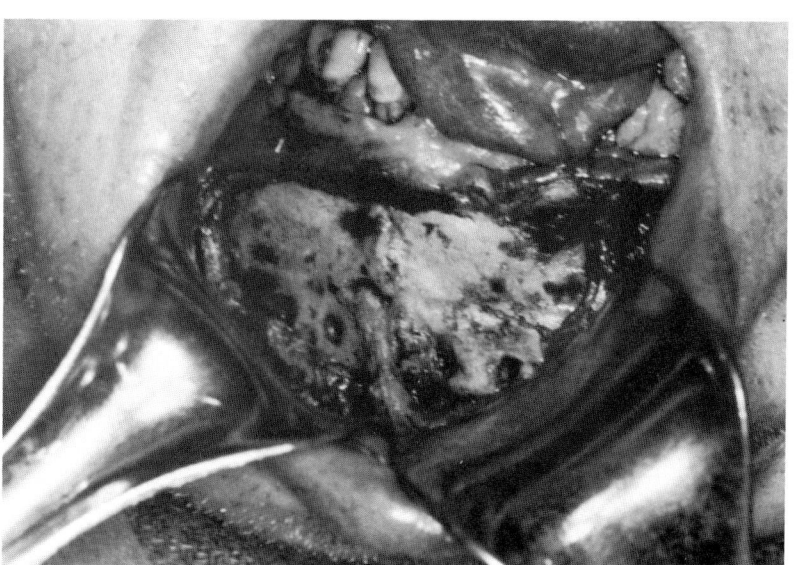

Figure 140. (D) Four-hole EDC plate spans the fracture line beneath the alveolar dehiscence. (E) Intraoral view during patient-elected plate removal shows good bone healing has occurred beneath the evulsion site above. The mandible was clinically stable.

ture wearing, or too low into the buccogingival groove where saliva pooling and subsequent infection due to retained food particles may lead to disruption of the wound.

The approach to treatment of the exposed plate depends on the degree of bone healing and the stability of the osteosynthesis. If it has been adequate to result in sufficient clinical bone healing, the plate can then be easily removed through the soft tissue wound. If bone healing is considered insufficient but the bone fixation is stable enough to avoid crepitus and pain on chewing and there is no radiologic evidence of nonunion, simple soft tissue debridement and removal of any loose screws followed by frequent irrigations and wound care may be tried. These temporizing efforts can often maintain fragment stability long enough to produce adequate clinical healing. With the obvious loss of effective fragment stability, however, both the plate and screws should be removed, the granulation tissue debrided, and the fracture surfaces freshened and an external fixation device applied.

Nonunion is infrequent unless there are associated problems such as wound infection, loss of adequate soft tissue coverage, inadequate plating technique, or poor vascularity of the bone fragments due to traumatic or preexisting local or systematic factors. Patients who have sustained significant multisystem injuries frequently have, due to clinical inexperience of the trauma staff, an unnecessarily and potentially dangerous low priority assigned to their mandibular trauma. Compound wounds can often be relatively easily turned into lesser long-term management problems by temporarily immobilizing several of the stable teeth with circumdental wires and carrying out early soft tissue wound debridement and closure under local anesthesia, or during general anesthesia given the patient for other procedures.

Early wound closure followed by broad-spectrum antibiotic coverage and good oral hygiene decreases the potential for infection at the time of the definitive bone surgery. Attention to the details of the technique of osteosynthesis should prevent inadequate internal fixation and further soft tissue compromise. Postoperative roentgenographic evidence of callus formation should alert the surgeon to the possibility of a delayed union because of a loss of interfragmentary stability. Depending on the degree of apparent clinical bone healing, the fragments may need to be replated or externally stabilized. When delayed union, however, has progressed to clinical or radiologic nonunion, removal of the plate and debridgement of the fibrous scar is necessary. Where there has been loss of sufficient bone such that direct coaptation will result in occlusal imbalance, bone grafting is required. In the absence of infection and with the assurance of good tissue coverage, cores of iliac crest bone marrow can be obtained through a 2-cm stab incision, placed into this gap, and the bone fragments immobilized by an internal SF plate. If this is contraindicated, a traditional iliac crest bone graft and intermaxillary or external pin fixation should be considered.

Malocculusion is usually not a problem of ineffective internal fixation by the plate but rather due to an inaccurate reduction of the bone fragments in relation to the preexisting occlusal planes. Without fixing the alveolar arches into the desired relationship at the start of the plating procedure, it is easy because of the deliberately limited surgical exposure to misjudge the three-dimensional reduction of the fracture fragments. A prerequisite knowledge of dental occlusion and the correct appreciation of the patient's own bite must precede the application of temporary intermaxillary fixation, which is further stabilized by the use of acrylic around the wires and the traction bar. Improved accuracy of reduction is helped by the use of reduction-compression pliers, which make manipulation of the bone fragments easier and help to secure them in the desired position during the critical stages of plate bending and drilling of the screw holes. The two-dimensional bending of the plate must be accurate but with a slight overbend to compensate for the anticipated lingual splaying effect. An inaccurately bent four-hole plate can result in sufficient compressive or torsional forces during application to detract all but the most solidly fixated bone fragments. Difficulties may arise when multiple fragments containing teeth are encountered; however, this is not a contraindication for osteosynthesis, but rather an indication for correctly carrying out this procedure. If malocclusion develops postoperatively, the stability of the osteosynthesis must be checked clinically and radiologically while bony union is not yet complete. Rubber-band-secured intermaxillary fixation may result in successful restoration of the occlusion if the plate is removed at this time. With bone healing completed, however, treatment of the fixed malocclusion involves dental consultation with some modification, if possible, carried out to the involved occlusal planes. Greater bite discrepancies may necessitate functional appliance orthodontics and/or selective osteotomies followed by plating or external fixation.

Nerve injury usually involves the mental and dental nerves or the mandibular branch of the facial nerve. The mental nerve exits from the mandible in an area frequently involved in blunt, penetrating, or osseous trauma. Careful preoperative evaluation and documentation are medical-legal prerequisites. During intraoral approaches, the gingival incision must avoid the region from the canine to the second molar unless the radiologic evidence suggests otherwise, to prevent cutting the nerve as it exits from the mental foramen. Incisions should straddle this area and the approach to the mental foramen should be made in the subperiosteal plane. This bridge of undisturbed mucosa containing the intact nerve branches also serves to protect the nerve branches from inadvertent injury by the assistant's retractors. Usually only the lower 2 cm of the mandible are deliberately chosen for plate application in order to help prevent direct injury to the inferior alveolar nerve as it courses through the bone. In edentulous mandibles, these precautions are especially critical because the absorption that occurs with time usually lowers the alveolar ridge, resulting in a relatively superficial exposure of the mental nerves and dental nerves that are surrounded by less protective bone. The branches of the facial nerve have been thoroughly studied and this information must be respected in the preoperative planning and carrying out of any submandibular incisions. One or more of the many operative techniques, including directly isolating the facial nerve branch exiting from the parotid gland, isolating such a branch distally on its course in the submandibular fascia, or retracting it out of the operative field by branches of the facial vein, should be considered. Rarely, if ever, does reexploration with attempts at microanastomosis of severed smaller branches prove therapeutically successful.

Objectionable scarring, either intraoral or at the skin incision site, is avoidable except in rare circumstances. Intraorally keeping the incisions out of the apex of the buccogingival gutter prevents soft tissue webbing and later prevents entrapped food particles from creating problems in oral hygiene. External incisions can be optimized by adhering to the well-established principles of soft tissue surgery whose tenets include beginning with good hemostasis, reapproximation of the masticatory and platysmal muscle layers and fascial planes, and atraumatic closure of the dermis followed by loose approximation of the epidermis.

Patients complain of being able to palpate the plate, depending on its size, placement, and the amount of overlying soft tissue. When the initial plates were developed they were only scaled-down versions of large long bone plates and consequently were still quite massive in their dimensions. Clinical experience has led to product refinement and the present plates are not as thick or wide; in addition, because of the more anatomically appropriate spacing of the screw holes, plates of shorter lengths can be utilized. These newer, smaller plates are more difficult to palpate and patients state that there is less hot/cold temperature sensitivity associated with them. Because of the amount of overlying soft tissue, palpation of the plate is most frequently observed in the symphyseal and parasymphyseal area; palpation of the plate is more common when the intraoral route is chosen, probably because of the subsequent connective tissue contraction surrounding it. Because of improvements, however, in technique and plate sizing, it is rare for patients to be sufficiently bothered to request removal of the screws and plate.

SUMMARY

The dynamics of bone plate osteosynthesis are based on well-described principles that have been successfully clinically tested on thousands of patients worldwide over the last decade. Further developments in response to evolving clinical needs have resulted in modification of the DC plate, the development of the EDC plate, and the creation of the newer mandibular reconstruction plates. It has been determined through investigation of its effects on bone healing that dynamic compression plating results in an advanced form of healing termed "primary bone healing." This is due to the mechanical advantages of fragment coaptation and compression which result in a histologic acceleration of the earlier phases of bone healing as traditionally reported. At the same time, despite initial concern, the potentially detrimental effects of stress shielding leading to bone resorption and pathologic fractures, have not proven to be significant problems in the mandible region.

With the appropriate instrumentation and adherence to established technique, a minimum of operative time and a low potential risk of untoward results should accompany this therapeutic modality. Each step of the application technique has been well worked out and it is essential for the avoidance of complications that these steps be carried out in the prescribed manner. Very few clinical situations arise now in which the choice of internal plating is not possible, due to the increased number of different-sized and -shaped plates available.

The indications for dynamic or passive bone plate osteosynthesis depend on the complexity of the fractures and the variety of patients in whom they occur. In the case of dynamic bone plate osteosynthesis, the choice revolves about the added advantages for the surgeon that plating can bring to improve the technical aspects of reduction and fixation. In the case of passive bone plate osteosynthesis, the decision to use a plate is predicated on the desire to minimize the patient's discomfort and morbidity. In either case, the rate of infection, nonunion or malunion, nerve damage, or untoward healing sequelae is rare with appropriate attention to indications and use of accepted surgical technique. Bone plate osteosynthesis should not be considered superior to or meant to replace traditional, time-proven maxillofacial techniques; rather bone plate osteosynthesis should be employed, in selected technical and patient-related situations, to provide an additional therapeutic dimension to the treatment of mandibular fractures.[13]

REFERENCES

1. Bagby GE, James JH: The effect of compression on the rate of fracture healing using a special plate. Am J Surg 95:761, 1958
2. Perren SM, Russenberger M, Steinemann LS, et al.: A dynamic compression plate. Acta Orthop Scand (suppl)125:29–41, 1969
3. Müller ME, Allogower MA, Schneider R, et al.: Manual of Internal Fixation. New York: Springer, 1979
4. Spiëssl B: New Concepts in Maxillofacial Bone Surgery. New York: Springer-Verlag, 1976
5. Schenk R: Morphological findings in primary bone healing. Symp Biol Hung 7:75, 1967
6. Heppenstall R: Fracture healing. In Heppenstall R (ed): Fracture Treatment and Healing. Philadelphia: WB Saunders, 1980
7. Levine PA, Goode RL: Mandibular fractures reduction with dynamic compression plates: A new treatment for an old problem. Otolaryngol Head Neck Surg 89:569–574, 1981
8. Strelzow VV, Friedman WJ: Dynamic compression plating in

the treatment of mandibular fractures—early experience. Arch Otolaryngol 108:583–586, 1982
9. Levine PA, Goode RL: Treatment of fractures in the edentulous mandible. Arch Otolaryngol 8:167–173, 1982
10. Schmoker R: Rigid internal fixation of compound fractures of the mandible using a specially designed reconstruction plate. In Jacobs JR (ed): Maxillofacial Trauma: An International Perspective. New York: Praeger, 1983
11. Strelzow VV: Mandibular reconstruction using implantable stabilization plates. Arch Otolaryngol 109:333–337, 1983
12. Strelzow VV: Bone plate osteosynthesis in the treatment of mandibular fractures. In Ward P (ed): Plastic and Reconstructive Surgery of the Head and Neck, Proceedings of the Fourth International Symposium. St. Louis: CV Mosby, 1984
13. Spiëssl B: Rigid internal fixation of fractures of the lower jaw. Reconstr Surg 7:124–127, 1972
14. Michelet FX, Deymes J, Dessus B: Osteosynthesis with miniaturized screwed plates maxillofacial surgery. J Maxillofac Surg 1:79–83, 1973
15. Rudiger B: Stable compression plate fixation of mandibular fractures. Br J Oral Surg 12:13–23, 1974
16. Strelzow VV, Strelzow AG: Osteosynthesis of mandibular fractures in the angle region. Arch Otolaryngol 109:403–406, 1983
17. Strelzow VV: An internal compression plating approach to the management of maxillofacial fractures. In Jacobs JR (ed): Maxillofacial Trauma: An International Perspective. New York: Praeger, 1983

ACKNOWLEDGMENTS

The author gratefully acknowledges Laura Henson and Ellen Takahashi for their editorial assistance and Dr. Robert H.I. Blanks for his helpful review of the chapter.

9 The Mandible: Its Role in Facial Balance

Joseph E. Van Sickels, D.D.S.
Curtis Chilcoat, D.D.S.

The mandible can not be viewed in isolation. Its relationship with the rest of the face must be considered. While there is a certain amount of interpretation as to how one should treat a particular individual, certain guidelines are followed. In general, bony relationships are corrected before purely cosmetic consideration. Establishing a functional occlusion is paramount. The idea of moving the jaws to where they are aesthetically pleasing and having an orthodontist or dentist fix the teeth is not only ludicrous but is also bad practice. The orthodontist and surgeon should be introduced in a coordinated treatment plan. To this end the surgeon must not only understand the intricacies of good occlusion, the tenets of which are beyond the scope of this chapter, but also the orthodontic principles must be understood.

Moving the mandible can have profound effects on the rest of the face. A relatively large nose may look normal or small when the mandible or chin is advanced. Maxillary osteotomies will directly effect the size and shape of the nose. Hence, purely cosmetic rhinoplasties are delayed until after changes in the bony bases are completed. Determining the best procedure for a patient involves the evaluation and integration of patient desires, and aesthetic and cephalometric norms.

AESTHETICS

Pleasing facial aesthetics are the result of a relative harmony between facial structure as opposed to an absolute measurement of size. One cannot treat to a single norm least we make everyone look the same. Racial and family characteristics must be considered. If there is a family characteristic to have a strong chin, then it is best to leave the patient with a slightly strong chin. However, personality traits, rightfully or not, are subconsciously associated with the structural characteristics of one's face. A protruding chin and prominent cheek bones are associated with masculinity and boldness of character. In contrast, the receding or weak chin is most often associated with weakness of character or intellect. Orthognathic surgical procedures are thus aimed at achieving a "balanced" facial form in addition to improving the functional integrity of the masticatory system. When evaluating the face both the frontal and profile views are appraised. Of the two, the frontal should have equal if not greater importance as this is how the patient sees himself.

FRONTAL EVALUATION

Aesthetically the face has been divided into thirds in the horizontal plane. These are: from the forehead to the eyebrows, from the eyebrows to the base of the nose, and from the base of the nose to the chin. In a well-balanced face these should be equal.[1] Patients with small lower jaws will tend to be vertically deficient as well as horizontally deficient. Those with horizontal mandibular excess will tend to look vertically long.

Vertically the face has also been divided. The distance between the medial canthi of the eyes should equal the intercanthal distance of one eye (approximately 3.5 cm)[1] (Fig. 141).

The alar width of the nose will fall within or slightly lateral to vertical lines drawn through the intercanthal areas. In patients with horizontal mandibular excess, the alar width is often normal. In contrast, if a patient has horizontal maxillary deficiency the alar width is frequently constricted.

PROFILE

When one vertically evaluates lower facial height, the face is again divided into thirds. In a balanced profile, the distance from the base of the nose (subnasale) to the junction of upper and lower lips (stomion) is one-third and from the stomion to soft tissue chin (menton) is two-thirds[1] (Fig. 142).

To evaluate a patient from the horizontal aspect

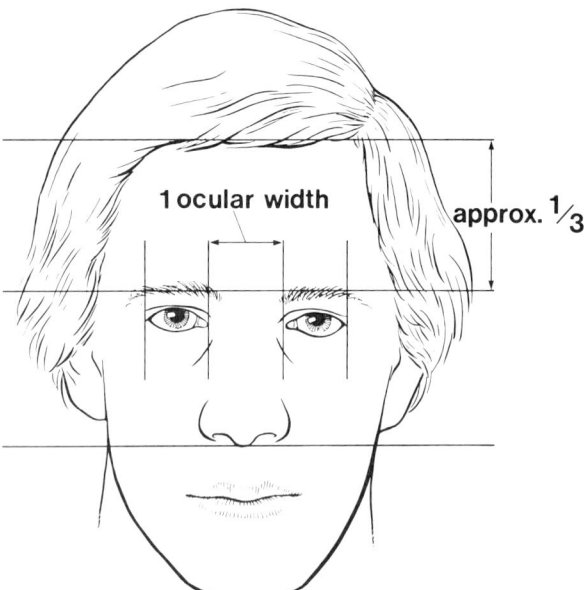

Figure 141. Ideal face, facial thirds and vertical measurements.

the patient is placed so he assumes a natural head position.[2] *Natural head position* is that position assumed while looking directly into one's eyes in the mirror. With the head in this position a vertical line is dropped through subnasale. In the balanced, relatively straight face this line passes near or through soft tissue nasion (junction of forehead and nose) and soft tissue chin (pogonion). The upper and lower lips are slightly anterior to this line. In more protrusive profiles the natural vertical through subnasale is tangent to soft tissue pogonion but anterior to soft tissue nasion.[3]

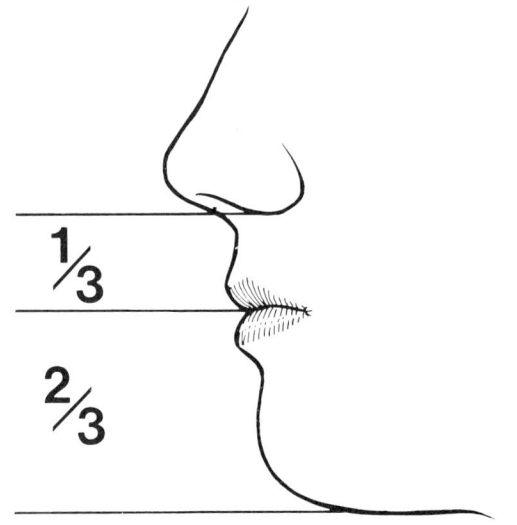

Figure 142. Profile view of facial thirds.

CEPHALOMETRIC ANALYSIS

Standardization of the lateral cephalometric film is performed by utilizing a cephalostat which holds the head in a fixed and reproducible position. The analysis can be divided into four parts: (1) vertical facial measurements, (2) horizontal midface measurements, (3) horizontal lower face measurements, and (4) dental measurements. Most orthodontic texts cover specifically designated anatomic landmarks commonly used.

Cephalometry is a very valuable tool in the evaluation of the relative relationships of the facial skeleton and dentition to the cranium. A series of analysis systems are utilized in presurgical orthognathic evaluation.[1, 4-8] Serial examinations have established accurate values for different age, sex, and racial groups. In most cephalometric analyses, the cranial base (line from sella turcica to nasion) is used to evaluate relative anteroposterior (AP) positions of the maxilla and mandible (the angles SNA and SNB, respectively). Lawrence and coworkers[9] noted that only 7% of Class 2 patients had horizontal maxillary excess. The other 93% had horizontal mandibular deficiency or a combination of maxillary and mandibular deficiency. Recently Ellis and colleagues[10] examined the Class 3 patient. Their study noted that the combination of maxillary skeletal retrusion associated with mandibular skeletal protrusion was the most common combination of skeletal anomalies (30.1%).

SURGICAL CORRECTION OF MANDIBULAR DEFORMITIES

In the last 25 years, many surgical procedures have evolved for the correction of dentofacial deformities. Initially the majority addressed the mandible, frequently with less than optimum results.

Today there are several surgical procedures now available. The subsequent discussion will be limited to the most commonly utilized techniques.

Segmental Surgery

With the close working relationship of orthodontics and oral surgery, segmental surgery is not used as frequently. It may be used in isolation when the maxillomandibular relations are satisfactory, or in combination with other procedures. The anterior subapical osteotomy is frequently used to level a severe Spee's[11] curve. As with all subapical procedures bony cuts should be a minimum of 4 to 5 mm below the apicies of the teeth.[4,11-14]

The posterior subapical osteotomy may be used to upright teeth, close spaces, or correct crossbites. The blood supply with this procedure is very tenuous, and extreme care should be made to detach a minimum of tissue.[11,13,14] Once the dentoalveolar segment is freed from the basal bone, it can be further subdivided to correct segmental deformities. The inferior alveolar neurovascular bundle may be easily injured with this procedure. Frequently it is necessary to unroof the nerve first and then complete the osteotomy. The entire mandibular alveolar bone may be moved *in toto* or in segments. The total mandibular subapical osteotomy was originally described to correct the Class 2 deep bite patient who has a prominent chin.[11,15,16] While the total mandibular subapical osteotomy has its advocates, most surgeons prefer to advance the mandible coupled with a genial setback (Figs. 143A, B, Fig. 144A; Fig. 145).

Ramus Surgery

Subcondylar ramus surgery can be performed either extraorally or intraorally. In general, the extraoral approach allows greater visibility and access to the mandibular ramus. The major advantage of the intraoral approach is obvious—it leaves no facial scar.

An extraoral approach is used when the mandible is repositioned greater than 10 mm, the mandible is asymmetrically shaped, there is vertical shortening of the ramus, or when the patient has had a previous operation.[11]

In contrast, the intraoral approach is used when repositioning the mandible 10 mm or less.[11] Preoperatively it has been suggested to obtain a submental vertex film to determine the posterior angulation of the mandible.[17]

Surgical access with the intraoral approach was generally accepted as being more difficult. In addition, proper positioning of the proximal segment was often a problem. This enhanced the chances for postsurgical movement.[1,11] The term "condylar sag," as coined by Hall and colleagues,[18] specifically relates to the problem of condylar placement and subsequent occlusal stability following the intraoral vertical subcondylar osteotomy.

A recent national survey by Niebergall and associates[19] revealed that because of improved instrumentation and surgical techniques, the intraoral vertical subcondylar osteotomy is now the preferred approach for the correction of mandibular prognathism (when compared specifically to the extraoral approach)[18–20] (Fig. 146).

The sagittal split ramus osteotomy, as first described by Obwegeser[21] in 1952, was complicated by aseptic necrosis and sequestration of the mandibular ramus. Animal studies revealed that complete stripping of the pterygomasseteric sling, performed in order to minimize relapse and facilitate the bony incisions, led to a reduction in blood supply sufficient enough to cause a vascular ischemia of the proximal segment.[22] These findings led to the development of modifications in the sagittal split technique.[23–25] By minimizing the detachment of the pterygomasseteric sling and mucoperiosteum from the proximal segment, bone healing could occur uneventfully.[22]

The sagittal split ramus osteotomy has become a popular technique for both advancement and setbacks, and when performed correctly, the procedure retains the proper position of the ramus and its normal anatomic relationship to the glenoid fossa. In addition, virtually all of the muscular and ligamentous attachments are maintained on the proximal segment allowing for enhanced anterior, posterior, and vertical repositioning of the distal segment (Figure 147).

An analysis of 256 sagittal osteotomies by Turvey[26] revealed the most common intraoperative complications to be: inferior alveolar nerve trauma, proximal segment fractures, and hemorrhage. All of the complications appeared to be related to osteotomy design, and attention to detail. In addition, many authors have reported a significant incidence of postoperative relapse.[27–33] This will be discussed in Postoperative stability, below.

Mandibular Body Surgery

This procedure is performed on the body of the mandible in either a bilateral or unilateral fashion. Sectioning of the mandible anterior to the mental foramen circumvents having to identify and isolate the inferior alveolar neurovascular bundle. Division of the mandibular body posterior to the mental nerve mandates surgically isolating the neurovascular bundle and is therefore a technically more difficult procedure. Both procedures are customarily performed intraorally[11] (Fig. 148A, B).

When mandibular prognathism associated with an anterior open bite is severe, additional surgery in the maxilla or mandibular ramus may be necessary to achieve the desired result.[11]

Because the ostectomized portions of the mandible are anterior to muscles of mastication (i.e., masseter, medial and lateral pterygoids, and temporalis) the effects of these muscles are negligible

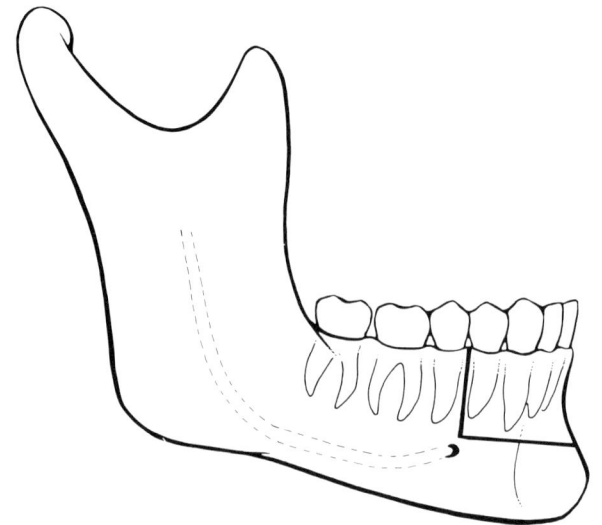
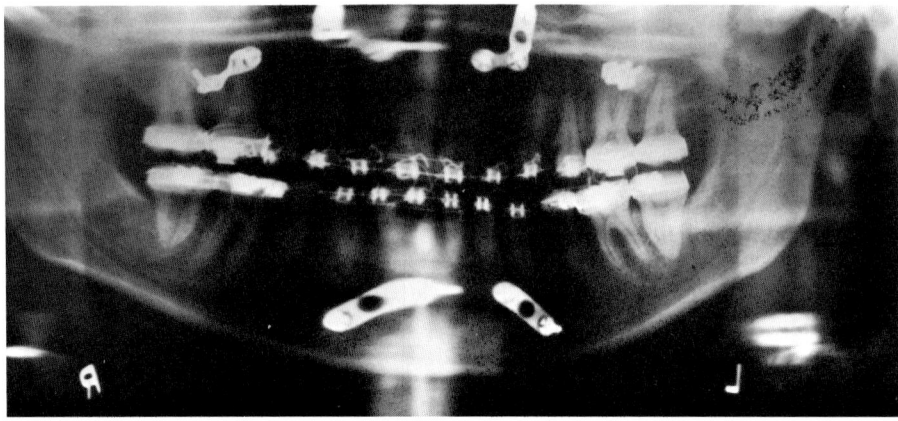

Figure 143. (A) Diagram of anterior subapical osteotomy. (B) Preoperative radiograph. (C) Postoperative radiograph of patient who underwent anterior subapical osteotomy and concomitant maxillary osteotomy.

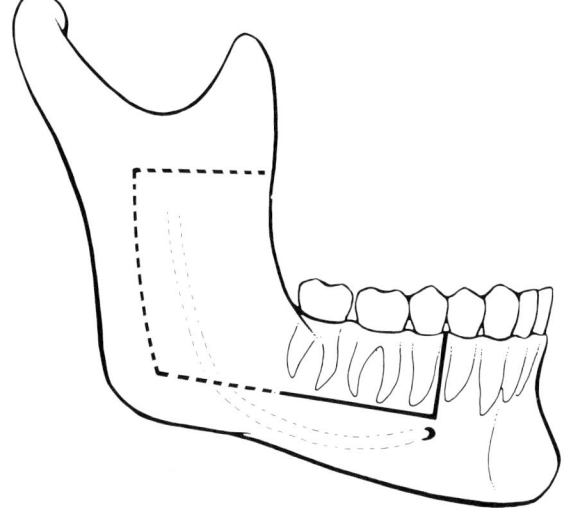

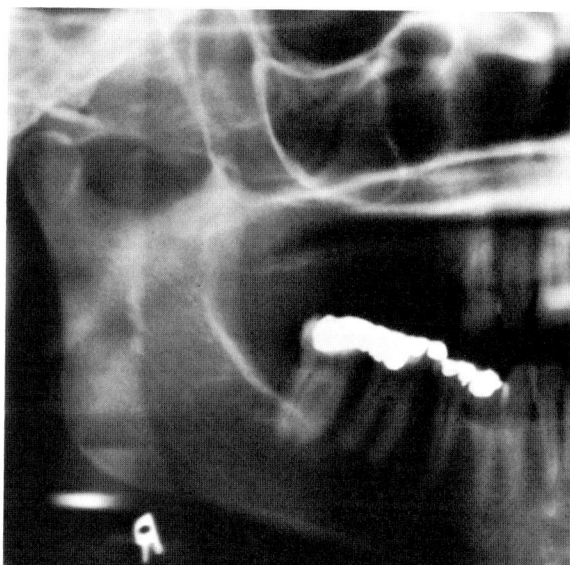

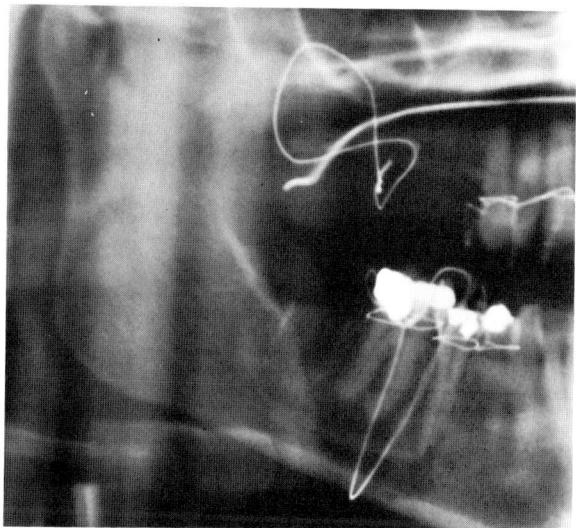

Figure 144. (A) Diagram of posterior subapical osteotomy. (B) Preoperative radiograph, supererupted teeth. (C) Postoperative radiograph, posterior subapical osteotomy.

with resultant enhancement of postoperative stability.[11]

Genioplasty

In order to achieve optimal aesthetic results when performing orthognathic surgery, the chin must often be an independent consideration. Surgical repositioning of the chin can be performed as a single procedure, or as is most often the case, in combination with other procedures. Genioplasties are performed to lengthen, reduce, straighten, or augment the appearance of the soft tissue chin. The chin may be changed by an osteotomy or by alloplastic augmentation. The sliding horizontal osteotomy may increase, decrease, shorten, or, in combination with an autogenous graft, lengthen the lower face. It is much more predictable than an alloplastic graft, and resorption of the bone under alloplastic grafts is not a problem.[3] An alloplastic augmentation is easier to perform than a horizontal osteotomy, however, it has several disadvantages. Resorption of bone and roots of teeth has been a problem.[3,34,35] They are subject to migration, and trauma may dislodge a previously stable implant.[3] Furthermore, especially with large augmentations, the contour is not natural unless they are custom fabricated. Surgically, when performing a horizontal osteotomy, a minimum of soft tissue is uncovered.[3,36,37] Excessive stripping or degloving of the chin results in a hematoma that will give unpredictable results[3,37] (Fig. 149A, B). In addition, excessive stripping has resulted in necrosis of the osteotomized segment.[3,37]

Asymmetry

Factors such as trauma and developmentally aberrant growth pattern often manifest as frontal facial asymmetry. In cases of lateral gnathia a straightening genioplasty provides an excellent result. However, one must assess whether there is a simple lateral gnathia or if a transverse plane problem exists involving the maxilla, mandible, and the bony chin. A correction genioplasty in a patient like this must be considered a masking procedure. It involves careful planning removing a wedge on the long side and often adding bone to the short side[11] (Fig. 150A, B).

Combined Procedures

As discussed in the introductory section of this chapter, dentofacial disharmonies are frequently

112 Surgery of the Mandible

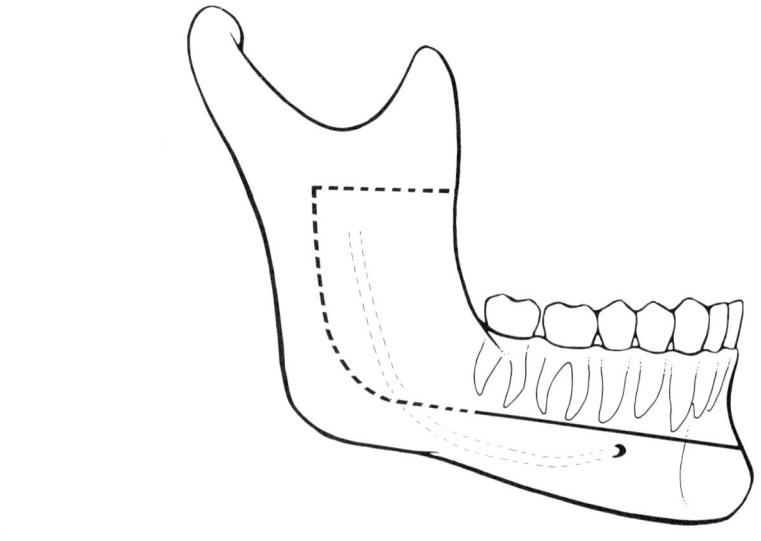

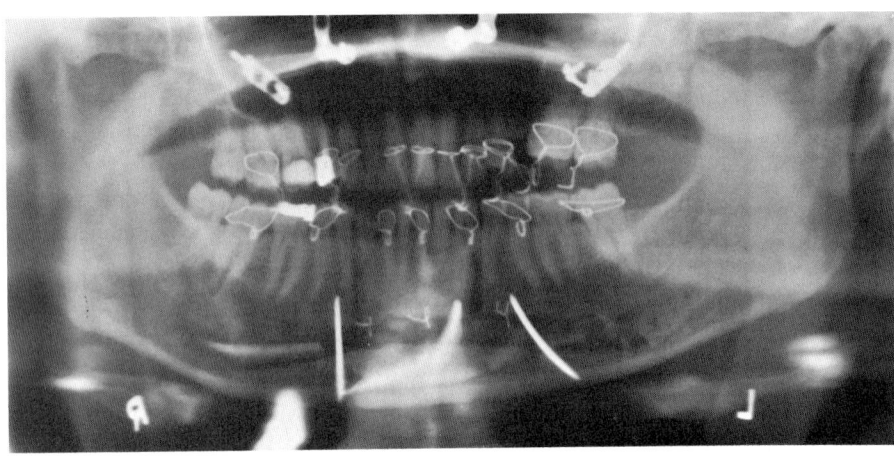

Figure 145. (A) Diagram of total mandibular subapical osteotomy (TMSO). (B) Postoperative radiograph three-piece TMSO, combined with multiple segmental maxillary osteotomy.

not just a single-jaw problem. The extent of a two-jaw deformity will determine whether one or both jaws are moved.

Figure 151 depicts a 28-year-old female with vertical maxillary excess, horizontal mandibular deficiency, and microgenia. Her surgery involved a maxillary impaction with autorotation of the mandible, a further mandibular advancement, and genial augmentation. Total advancement of her chin was 14 mm. A simple procedure involving either one jaw or the other would have been inadequate.

Postoperative Stability

Surgically repositioning the mandible disrupts the natural equilibrium between bone and soft tissue. The natural tendency for this imbalanced system is to return toward its original relationship. Postoperative relapse after mandibular advancement remains one of the most frustrating problems encountered in mandibular surgical procedures and is well documented in the literature.[17,27,30,38] Early and late postoperative relapse should be defined. Early postoperative relapse occurs during intermaxillary fixation, while late postoperative relapse occurs after the release of fixation.

A high mandibular plane angle, tension from stretching of the suprahyoid musculature, anterior-superior rotational advancement of the distal segment, and improper positioning of the condyle are all believed to contribute to relapse.[28–31,33,39,40]

Maxillomandibular fixation alone has proven inadequate in preventing early skeletal relapse after mandibular advancement. Dental compensation; that is, tooth movement within the alveolus, allows for

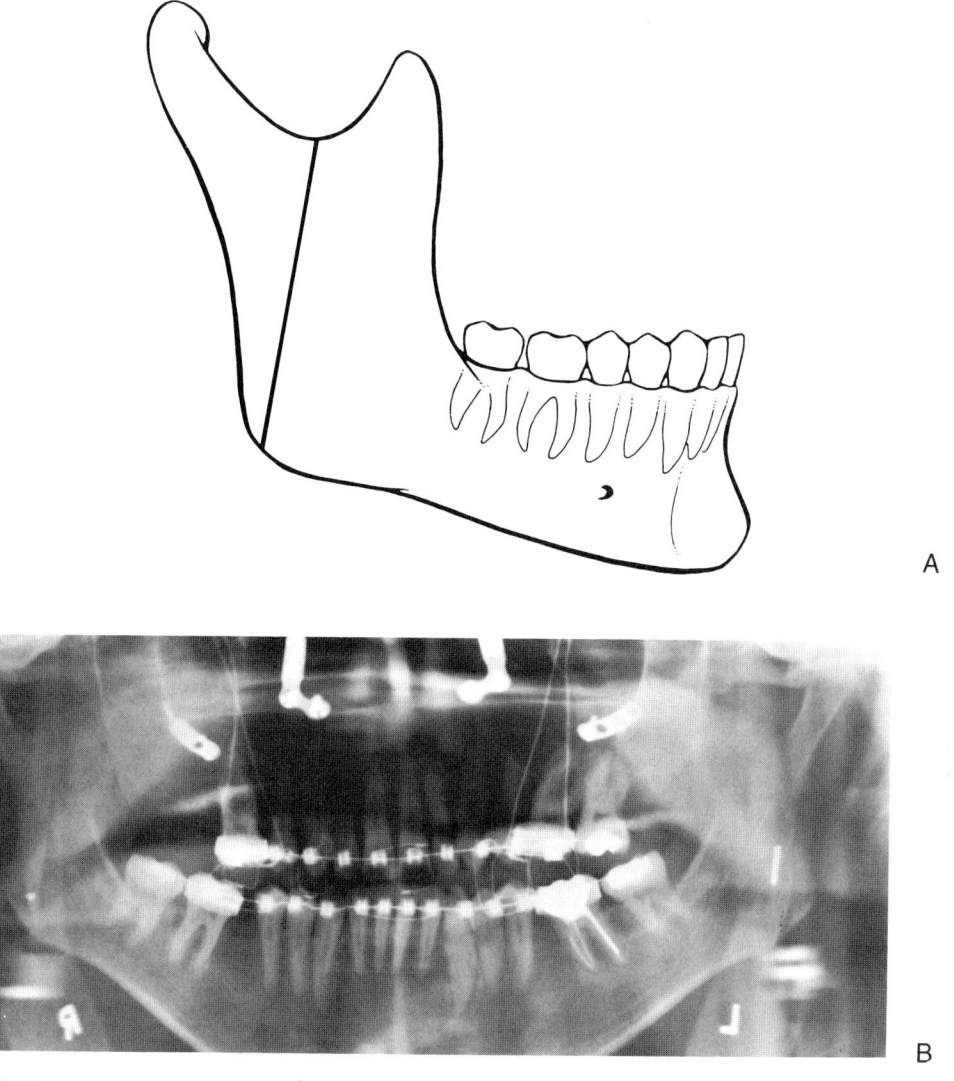

Figure 146. (A) Diagram of subcondylar osteotomy. (B) Postoperative radiograph, bilateral intraoral subcondylar osteotomy combined with maxillary osteotomy.

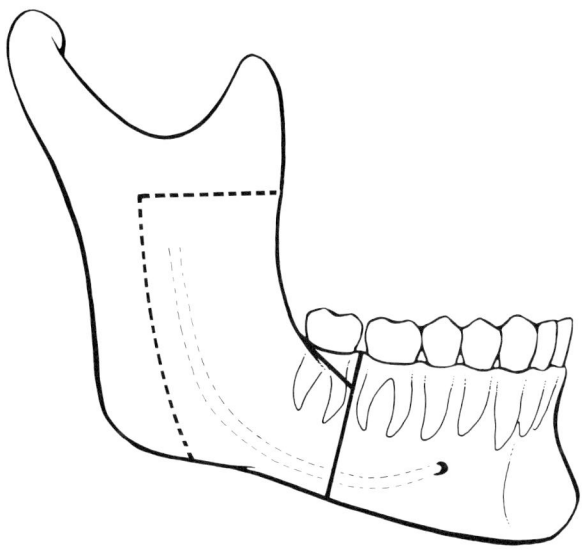

Figure 147. Outline of sagittal split osteotomy.

significant skeletal relapse in spite of the maintenance of stable occlusal relationships.[27,30,31,38]

Attempts to control postoperative relapse include: suprahyoid myotomies, cervicle collars, overcorrection, posterior bite opening splints, and interosseous wiring.[31,33,38–41] However, these techniques have proven less than optimal in significantly reducing the incidence of postsurgical relapse.

Recent studies evaluating rigid transosseous fixation techniques reveal promising preliminary results.[32,42–44] Biocortical screws are utilized to rigidly fixate the proximal and distal segments, eliminating interfragmentary movement.[32,42–45] Advocates of this technique site a more rapid and stronger bony union, early restoration of function, and a significant reduction of skeletal relapse.[42–44] Animal studies lend support, revealing that fracture

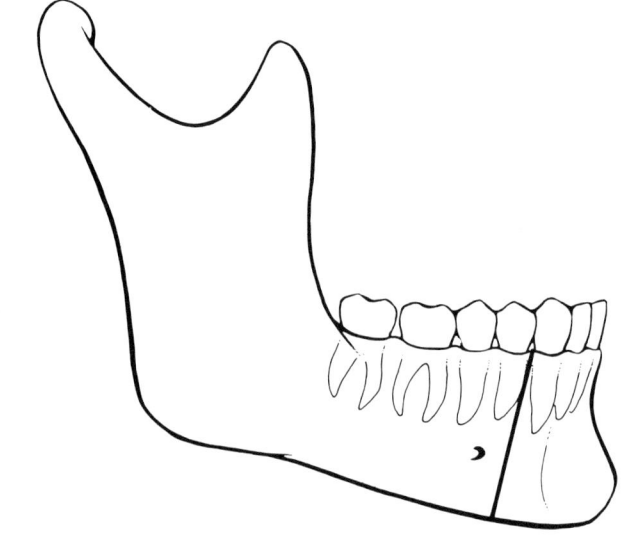

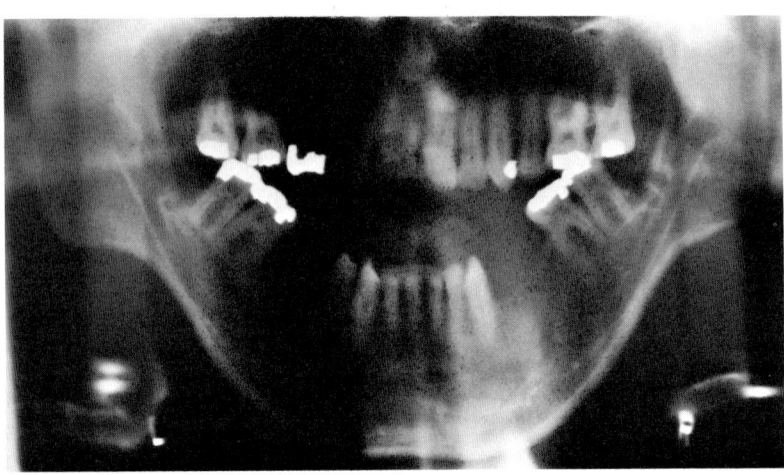

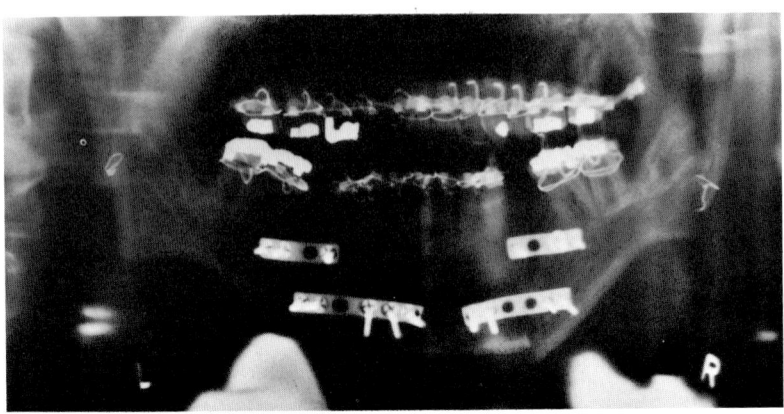

Figure 148. (A) Diagram of body osteotomy. (B) Preoperative radiograph. (C) Postoperative radiograph, bilateral body osteotomies, bilateral extraoral subcondylar osteotomies.

The Mandible: Its Role in Facial Balance 115

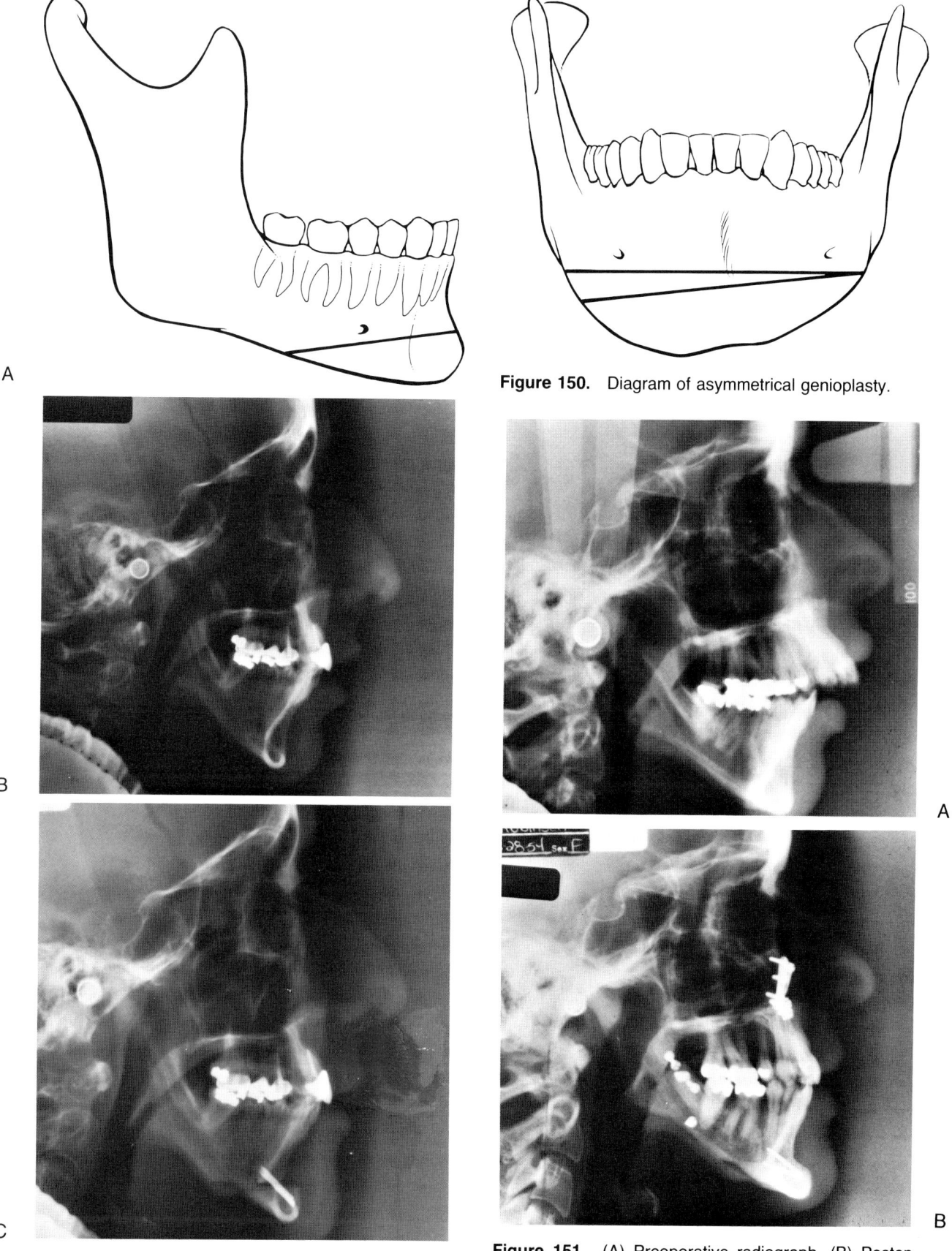

Figure 150. Diagram of asymmetrical genioplasty.

Figure 149. (A) Diagram of genioplasty. (B) Preoperative radiograph. (C) Postoperative radiograph, advanced 6 mm.

Figure 151. (A) Preoperative radiograph. (B) Postoperative radiograph, maxilla moved up, bilateral sagittal split osteotomy advancing the mandible and an advancement genioplasty.

segments in tight contact (0.8 mm gap) heal by primary intention, without the formation of fibrocartilage or callous formation.[46] This also allows for earlier function thus promoting faster healing.[46]

REFERENCES

1. Hinds EC, Kent JN: Surgical Treatment of Developmental Jaw Deformities. St. Louis: Mosby, 1972
2. Moores CF, Kean MR: Natural head position. A basic consideration for the analysis of cephalometric radiographs. Am J Phys Anthropol 16:213, 1958
3. McBride KL, Bell WH: Chin surgery. In Bell WH, Profitt WR, White RP (eds): Surgical Correction of Dentofacial Deformities, Vol. 3. Philadelphia: Saunders, 1980
4. Bell WH, Dann JJ: Correction of dentofacial deformities by surgery in the anterior jaws. Am J Orthod 64:162, 1973
5. Burstone CJ, et al.: Cephalometrics for orthognathic surgery. J Oral Surg 36:269, 1978
6. Khouw FE, Profitt WR, White RP: Cephalometric evaluation of patients with dentofacial disharmonies requiring surgical correction. Oral Surg 29:789, 1970
7. McNamara JA Jr: A method of cephalometric analysis. In McNamara JA Jr, Ribbens KA, Howe RP (eds): Clinical alterations of the growing face. Monograph No. 14, Craniofacial Development, Ann Arbor: University of Michigan, 1983
8. Worms FW, Issacson RJ, Speidel TM: Surgical orthodontic treatment planning: Profile analysis and mandibular surgery. Angle Orthod 46:1, 1976
9. Lawrence LN, Ellis E, McNamara JA Jr: The frequency and distribution of skeletal and dental components in Class II orthognathic surgery patients. J Oral Maxillofac Surg 43:24 1985
10. Ellis E, McNamara JA: Components of adult Class III malocclusion. J Oral Surg 42:295, 1984
11. Epker BN, Wolford LM: Dentofacial Deformities; surgical Orthodontic Correction. St. Louis: Mosby, 1980
12. Bell WH: Revascularization and bone healing after anterior mandibular osteotomy. J Oral Surg 28:196, 1970
13. Bell WH, Gallagher DM: The versatility of genioplasty using a broad pedicle. J Oral Maxillofac Surg 41:763, 1983
14. Scheideman GB, Kawamura J, Finn RA, et al.: Wound healing after anterior and posterior subapical osteotomy. J Oral Maxillofac Surg 43:408, 1985
15. Booth DF, Deitz V, Geanelly AA: Correction of Class II malocclusion of combined sagittal ramus and subapical body osteotomy. J Oral Surg 34:630, 1976
16. Fitzpatrick B: Total osteotomy of the mandibular alveolus in reconstruction of the occlusion. Oral Surg 44:336, 1977
17. Mossey GB: Intraoral oblique osteotomy of the mandibular ramus. J Oral Surg 32:755, 1974
18. Hall JD, Chase CC, Payor LG: Evaluation and refinement of the intraoral vertical subcondylar osteotomy. J Oral Surg 33:33, 1975
19. Niebergall CF, Mercuri LG: Intraoral vertical subcondylar osteotomy, a national survey. J Oral Maxillofac Surg 43:450, 1985
20. Herbert JM, Kent JN, Hinds EC: Correction of prognathism by an intraoral vertical subcondylar osteotomy. J Oral Surg 33:384, 1970
21. Obwegeser H: The surgical correction of mandibular prognathism and retrognathia with consideration of genioplasty. Part I. Surgical procedures to correct mandibular prognathism and reshaping of the chin. Oral Surg 10:677, 1959
22. Bell WH, Schendel SA: Biologic basis for modification of the sagittal split ramus osteotomy. J Oral Surg 35:362, 1977
23. Booth DF: Simplified approach to the sagittal osteotomy. J Oral Surg 34:745, 1976
24. Dal Pont G: Retromolar osteotomy for the correction of prognathism. J Oral Surg 19:42, 1961
25. Epker BN: Modifications in the sagittal osteotomy of the mandible. J Oral Surg 35:157, 1977
26. Turvey TA: Interoperative complications of sagittal osteotomy of the mandibular ramus, incidence and management. J Oral Maxillofac Surg 43:504, 1985
27. Ive J, McNeil RW, West RA: Mandibular advancement: Skeletal and dental changes during fixation. J Oral Surg 35:881, 1977
28. Leonard M: Preventing rotation of the proximal fragment in the sagittal ramus split operation. J Oral Surg 34:942, 1976
29. MacIntosh, RB: Experience with the sagittal osteotomy of the mandibular ramus: A 13 year review. J Maxillofac Surg 8:151, 1981
30. McNeill WR, Hooley JR, Sundberg JR: Skeletal relapse during intermaxillary fixation. J Oral Surg 31:212, 1973
31. Schendel SA, Epker BN: Results after mandibular advancement surgery: An analysis of 87 cases. J Oral Surg 38:265, 1980
32. Souryris F: Sagittal splitting and biocortical screw fixation of the ascending ramus. J Maxillofac Surg 6:198, 1978
33. Wessberg GA, Schendel SA, Epker BN: The role of the suprahyoid myotomy in surgical advancement of the mandible via sagittal split osteotomies. J Oral Maxillofac Surg 40:273, 1982
34. Dann JJ, Epker BN: Proplast genioplasty. A retrospective study with treatment recommendations. Angle Orthodont 47:173, 1977
35. Robinson M, Shuken R: Bone resorption under plastic chin implants. J Oral Surg 27:116, 1969
36. Bell WH, Schendel SA, Finn RA: Revascularization after surgical repositioning of tooth dento-osseous segments. J Oral Surg 36:757, 1978
37. Dechow PC, McNamara JA Jr, Carlson DS, et al.: Advancement genioplasty with and without soft tissue pedicle: An experimental investigation. J Oral Maxillofac Surg 42:637, 1984
38. Epker, BN, Wessberg GA: Mechanisms of early skeletal relapse following surgical advancements of the mandible. Br J Oral Surg 20:175, 1982
39. Epker BN, Wolford LM, Fish LC: Mandibular deficiency syndrome: Surgical consideration for mandibular advancement. Oral Surg 45:349, 1978
40. Steinhauser EW: Advancement of the mandible by sagittal ramus split and suprahyoid myotomy. J Oral Surg 31:516, 1973
41. Singer RS, Bays RA: A comparison between superior and inferior border wiring techniques in sagittal split ramus osteotomy. J Oral Maxillofac Surg 43:444, 1985
42. Paulus GW, Steinhauser EW: A comparative study of wire osteosynthesis versus bone screws in the treatment of mandibular prognathism. Oral Surg 54:2, 1982
43. Spiessel B: The sagittal splitting osteotomy for correction of mandibular prognathism. Clin Plast Surg 9:4, 1982
44. Van Sickels JE, Flanary CM: Relapse associated with mandibular advancement treated by rigid osseous fixation. J Oral Maxillofac Surg 43:338, 1985
45. Jeter TS, Van Sickels JE, Dolwick MF: Rigid internal fixation of ramus osteotomies; A technique article. J Oral Maxillofac Surg 42:220, 1984
46. Reitzik M, Schoorl W: Bone repair in the mandible. A histologic and biometric comparison between rigid and semirigid fixation. J Oral Maxillofac Surg 41:215, 1983
47. Kundert M, Kadjianghelen O: Condylar displacement after sagittal splitting of the mandibular ramus. J Maxillofac Surg 8:278, 1980

10 Surgery of the Chin

Donald L. Steed, D.D.S., M.S.

The chin serves as the foundation for facial harmony and is one of the determinants of the cosmetic appearance of the face. Occupying one-third to one-half of the lower face (Fig. 152), the chin is one of the most obvious facial structures.[1]

In western society a prominent chin (macrogenia) is thought to be "manly" or "athletic," whereas a man with a recessive chin (microgenia) is described as having a "weak chin" which is considered undesirable. In women slight microgenia is thought to be more desirable than is a prominent or pointed "witch's chin."

The position of the chin in relation to the face, its anatomical form, the location of the major nerves to the area, and its excellent blood supply all enhance the versatility of surgical repositioning procedures. These procedures can be performed to modify chin form, thus altering the countours of the overlying and surrounding soft tissues. Dimensional alterations can be made in all three planes, that is, transverse, vertical, and anteroposterior (AP), or any combination of the three, thus allowing correction in the chin area of virtually any deformity. In Figure 153 are depicted alterations that are possible in the vertical and AP planes by performing various osteotomies, ostectomies, and grafts.[2] Possible alterations that can be made in the transverse plane with osteotomy, ostectomy, or an combination of both are shown in Figure 154.[1,3]

GENERAL CONSIDERATIONS

Although a variety of contour and dimensional alterations to the chin area are surgically possible, genioplasties (menoplasties or profileplasties) are not the panacea for all lower facial deformities (see Fig. 153).[1-8] Less than 15% of lower face disharmonies are isolated chin problems; the other 85% relate to the jaws, teeth, and midface. When formulating a surgical course of treatment, function as well as form must be considered. Operations to be avoided are those designed to achieve enhanced physical appearance while masking a correctable functional problem. Before a logical treatment plan is formulated, careful analysis of the entire face, which includes the skeletal, soft tissue, and dental relationship and the upper to lower facial height ratios, must be completed.

The following cases demonstrate that by establishing proper functional occlusion and correcting discrepancies in the size and position of the jaws, chin surgery may be minimized or eliminated.

Case 1–1 (Fig. 155) is a 28-year-old woman who was evaluated for treatment of a deviated chin. Clinically there was a transverse discrepancy in the chin area with the chin-point deviated to the right (Fig. 155A). Skeletal and soft tissue analyses showed slight elongation of the left condylar neck but no AP component. Dental occlusal examination showed a crossbite on the right with the dental midline deviated to the right in the mandible (Fig. 155C). Correction included orthodontic therapy and a subcondylar osteotomy. Surgery was not indicated in the chin. Figures 155B and D are the posttreatment photographs.

Case 1–2 (Fig. 156) is a 23-year-old man who was unhappy with his prominent chin (Fig. 156A). The facial height ratio (vertical component) was within the limits of normal. The skeletal analysis indicated a large mandible (macrognathic rather than macrogenic). The dental/occlusal analysis demonstrated a Class 3 malocclusion (Fig. 156C). Correction for the mandibular AP discrepancy was accomplished by a bilateral ramus osteotomy and by repositioning the mandibular body posteriorly 6 mm. Figures 165B and D are posttreatment facial and occlusal appearances.

Case 1–3 (Fig. 157) is a 24-year-old man who complained of a prominent chin (Fig. 157A). Skeletal analysis (cephalometric) indicated an AP deficiency of the maxilla rather than an AP excess of the mandible/chin. The facial height ratio showed a slightly short lower face. Soft tissue evaluation showed a retrusive upper lip, a prominent nose, and mid-face sallowness. There was a Class 3 dental relationship. To correct the AP and vertical discrepancies, surgery included a Le Fort 1 advancement osteotomy and a rhinoplasty as a second procedure. Figure 157B shows the postoperative facial harmony achieved without surgery of the chin or mandible.

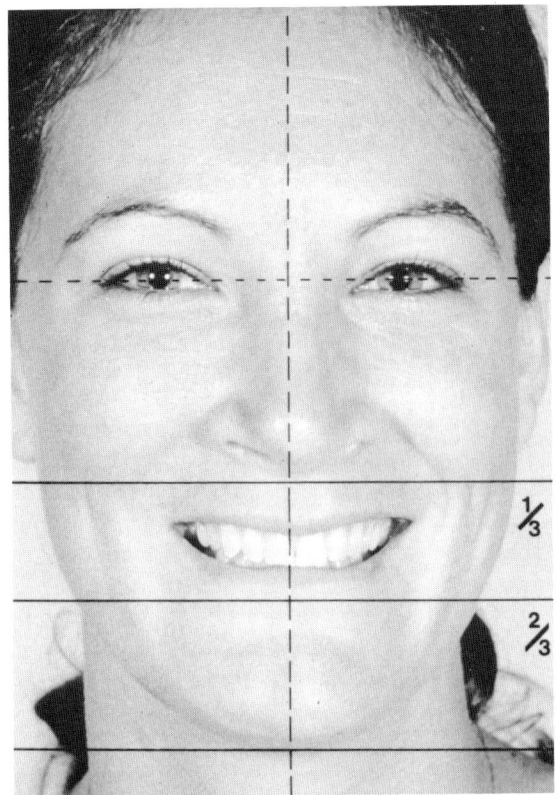

Figure 152. Occupying one-third to one-half of the lower face, the chin is one of the most obvious facial features.

Case 1–4 (Fig. 158) is a 25-year-old man who wanted a chin augmentation to correct a "weak chin." He had an obvious receding chin and a deep mentolabial groove suggestive of microgenia (Fig. 158A). The skeletal analysis showed an AP deficient mandible *(retrognathia)* and the dental workup showed an accompanying Class 2 malocclusion. Treatment indicated was orthodontics to level and aligh the teeth and surgical advance of the mandible to correct the micrognathia/microgenia and the Class 2 malocclusion (Fig. 158B).

ANATOMIC CONSIDERATIONS

A brief survey of anterior mandible and osteology is appropriate. Normally the mental protuberance lies in the midline with two mental tubercles on each side. From each tubercle there is a ridge of bone that extends posteriorly to blend into the prominent external oblique ridge of the ramus.[9] The thickness of the bone below this ridge is approximately 10 to 15 mm with thick lateral and medical cortical plates. The mental foramina are located on or just above this line and below the root apexes of the first or second premolar teeth.

The mandibular canal just proximal to the mental foramen curves inferiorly. Therefore, to preserve the integrity of the inferior alveolar neurovascular bundle, osteotomy incisions in this area should be located at least 3 mm below the foramen. Above the mental protuberance are located two shallow depressions called the *incisive fossae*.[9] The roots of the four incisor teeth are superior to the incisor fossae and the mentalis muscles originate from the fossa and insert into the skin of the chin. When an intraoral approach is planned for surgical procedures on the chin, the mentalis muscle should be transected rather than stripped from the bone to facilitate muscle layer proximation when closing the surgical site. The cuspid or canine teeth roots form the lateral border of the incisor fossae. It is expeditious to measure and record the length of the cuspid teeth from the panographic radiographs. To avoid devitalizing the teeth, osteotomy incisions should be made at least 3 mm below the apex of the teeth. The most notable structure on the medial surface of the anterior body of the mandible are the genial tubercles which serve as attachments for the genial muscles.[9] Since the major blood supply to the pedicled osteotomized segment will necessarily come from this area, the surgeon should attempt to preserve the muscle attachments on the medial side. The soft tissue thickness overlaying the chin at the midline mental protuberance should measure 12 ∓ 2 mm in whites and 14 ∓ 2 mm in blacks.[2]

IMPLANT MATERIALS FOR AUGMENTATION

Prior to World War II, homogenous and heterogenous bone, ivory, and various metals were the only materials available for grafting countour defects. After World War II and through the 1960s, acrylics and silicone rubber became the alloplastic materials of choice.[3]

Sialastic

Because Sialastic chin implants may be placed with relative ease from either an intraoral or extraoral route, they were probably the most popular alloplastic augmentation material of the 1960s and into the early 1970s.[10–13] The two main disadvantages encountered with the use of Sialastic chin implants are (1) the tendency for slippage or migration if they are not secured to the bone, and (2) severe erosion into the underlying bone.[1,3,14,15] Fig-

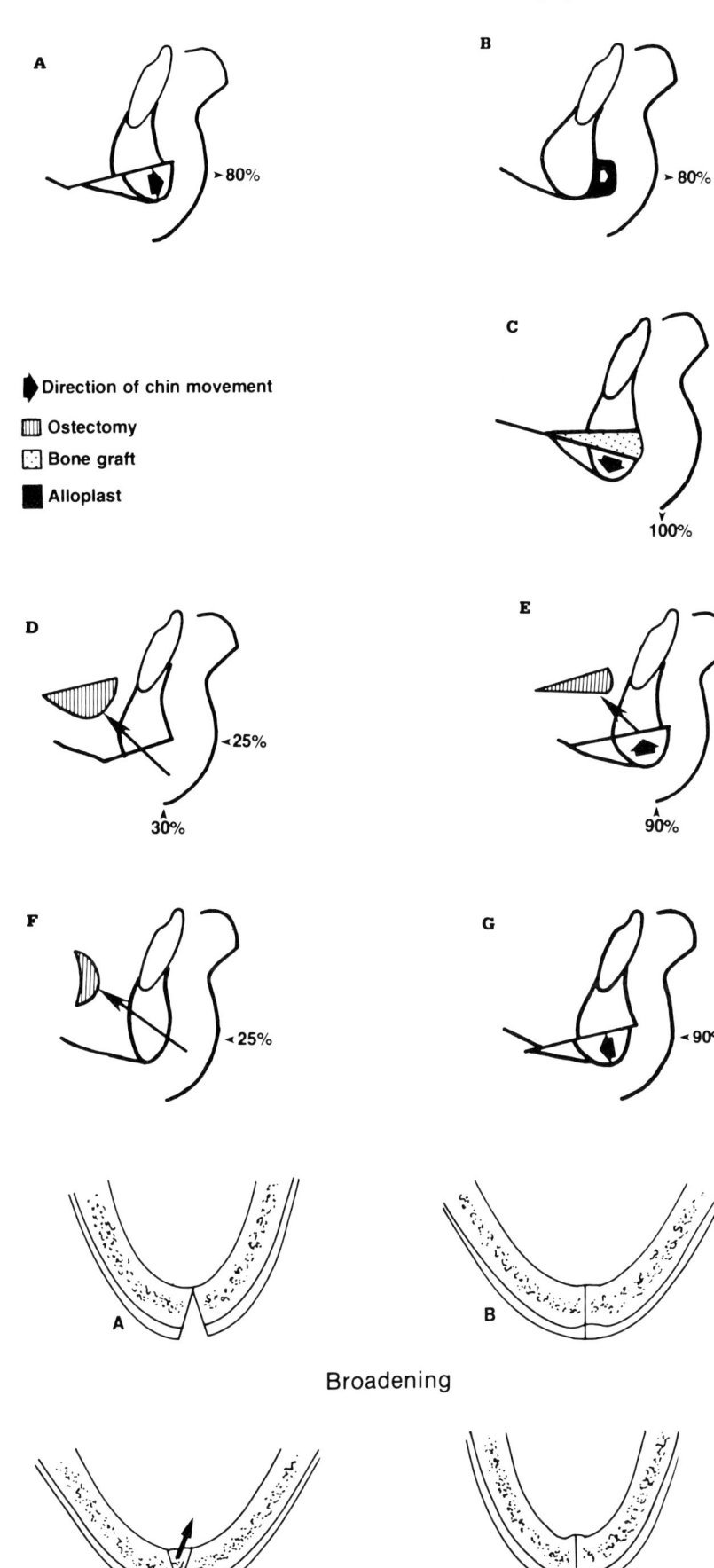

Figure 153. Average soft tissue change expressed as percentage of hard tissue movement. (A) Osseous sliding advancement osteotomy. (B) Alloplastic augmentation. (C) Osseous vertical augmentation (downgraft). (D) Vertical reduction osteotomy. (E) Vertical wedge reduction osteotomy. (F) Anterior reduction osteotomy. (G) Osseous sliding AF reduction osteotomy. (From Wolford LM, Hilliard FW, Dugan DJ: Surgical Treatment Objectives: A systemtic Approach to the Prediction Trac. St. Louis: Mosby, 1985. With permission.)

Figure 154. Methods of broadening and narrowing the bony chin by wedge excision.

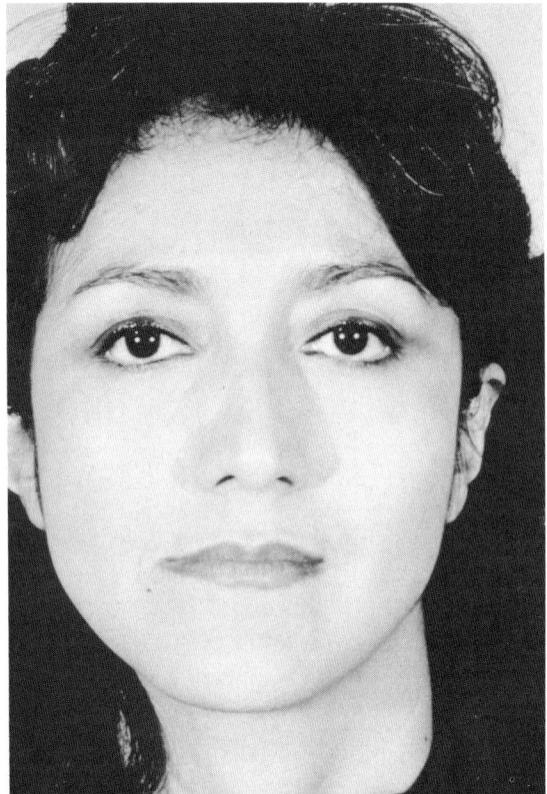
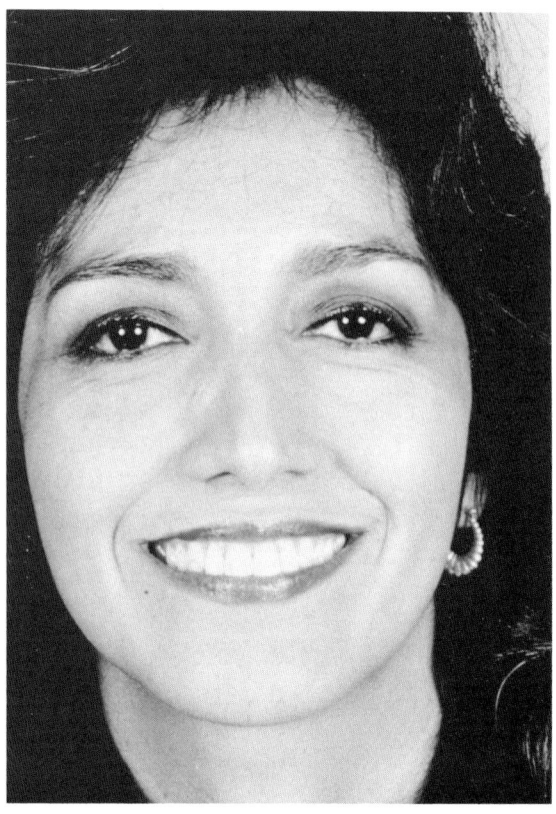
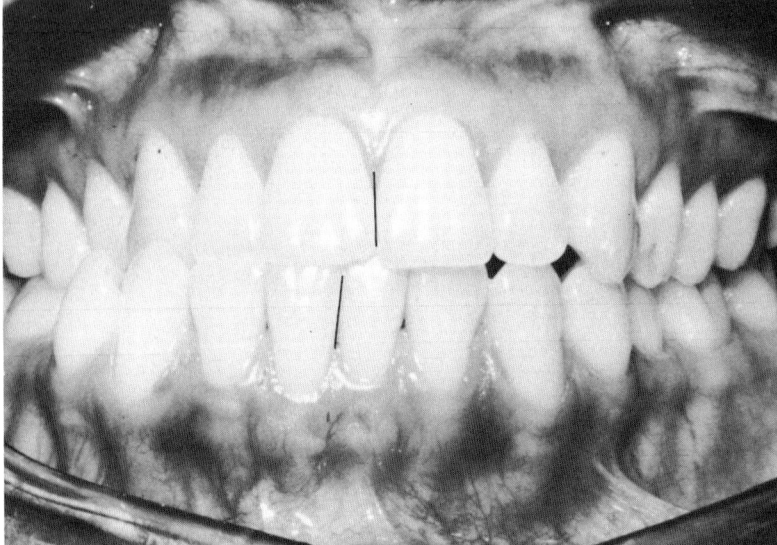

Figure 155. (A) Twenty-eight-year-old woman with the chin deviated to the right. (B) Postoperative orthodontic therapy and subcondylar osteotomy. (C) Abnormal dental occlusion with deviation of mandible to right.

ure 159 is a lateral skull radiograph showing marked erosion extending through cortical bone 6 months after placement of a medium-sized Sialastic chin implant. To prevent further erosion into the roots of the teeth, the implant was removed.

Proplast

Proplast is a porous alloplastic material prepared from Teflon, fluorocarbon polymer, and vitreous carbon fibers with characteristics that permit in-

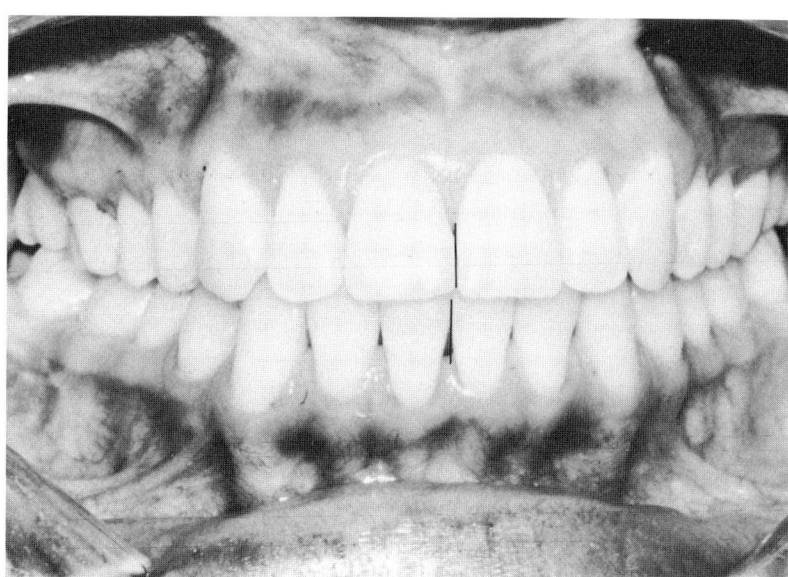

Figure 155. (D) Reestablishment of normal dental occlusion following surgical orthodontic and surgical therapy.

growth of the host tissues, thus stabilizing the implant and minimizing erosion into the underlying bone.[1,16–19] Proplast can be carved to any form or contour at time of surgery and has been used as bone and soft tissue onlay augmentation grafts, and in conjunction with sliding osteotomies to eliminate notching at osteotomy sites.

Hydroxylapatite

Hydroxylapatite is an alloplastic material with chemical composition similar to bone which has recently received attention as a bone substitute in granular form.[20–23] A personal conversation in January 1985 with Dr. D.R. Melisch confirmed that while currently being used to fill in bone defects, hydroxylapatite is presently under clinical investigation in a porous block form for both augmentation and graft material for discontinuity procedures.

Autogenous Bone and Cartilage

Autogenous bone is most useful in vertical augmentation as an interpositional graft. Autogenous bone and cartilage grafts used in augmentation as onlay grafts have two disadvantages: (1) they vary unpredictably in the amount of resorption that occurs, and (2) a second surgical site is required to harvest the graft.[1,3]

PLANNING THE NEW POSITION OF THE CHIN

The cliche "well-planned surgery goes well" is especially true in surgical movements of the chin and jaws. Accurate prediction of the end result are possible when cephalometric tracings of the existing structure are made and when cutouts or patterns are moved to represent known dimensional changes that occur with movement of hard tissue.[2,24–31] When one or more facial components is to be moved surgically, a working knowledge of cephalometric points, planes, angles, and distances is needed to plan the most aesthetic position of the components (Fig. 160; Table 10–1). The literature is not replete in number of analyses suggested to assess facial balance and harmony,[2,32–46] but if all other facial structures and the occlusion are acceptable and only the chin contour is to be surgically modified, analysis is simplified.

Cephalometric prediction planning for chin surgery described below is indentical to that described by Wolford and co-workers.[2] The chin position must be evaluated in both the AP and vertical planes, and if a transverse problem is apparent, an additional posteroanterior (PA) skull film analysis is indicated. The analysis is started by positioning acetate tracing paper over a true lateral skull radiograph with modification for viewing soft tissue outlines.[3,47] The soft tissue outline is traced first (the normal range of soft tissue thickness of the lips and chin measuring 11 to 14 mm). Desirable soft tissue thickness of the upper lip, lower lip,

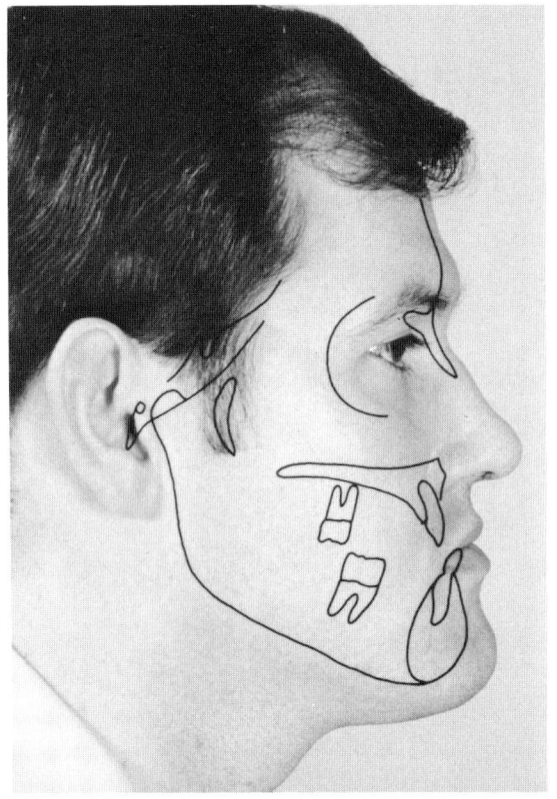
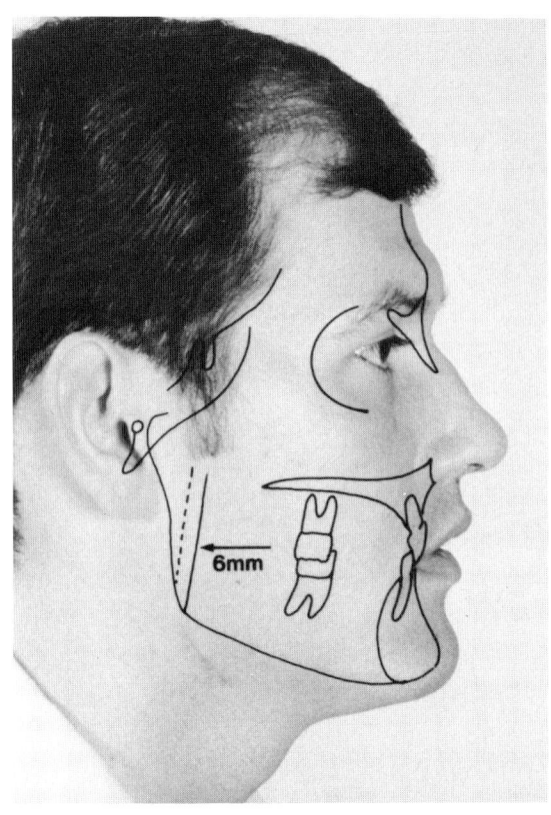

Figure 156. (A) Twenty-three-year-old man with prominent chin and malocclusion. (B) Lateral facial appearance following bilateral ramus osteotomy and repositioning of the mandibular body posteriorly approximately 6 mm. (C) Abnormal dental occlusion.

and chin is a 1:1:1 ratio. Bony anterior craniodentofacial structures are traced next, that is, the anterior nasal spine, anterior maxilla, maxillary central incisor, anterior mandible, and mandibular central incisor. Next, the soft tissue glabella, subnasale, and pogonion are located and marked. A line is then drawn from the glabella to subnasale and extended downward to below the chin area. A second line is drawn from subnasale to the soft tissue pogonion (Fig. 161A). For normal chin projection, the angle thus formed by the intersection of these two lines should measure 11 ∓ 4 degrees.

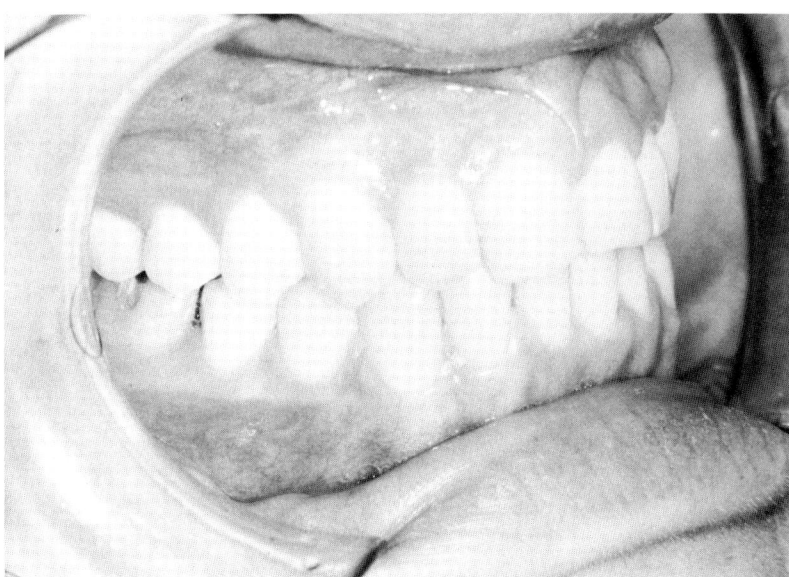

Figure 156. (D) Normal dental occlusion achieved after surgical therapy.

Figure 161B shows a marked decrease in angle which would indicate the need for a reduction genioplasty in the AP plane, whereas in Figure 161C there is a much larger angle which would indicate retrogenia. Correction could be accomplished with an advancement or augmentation genioplasty in the AP plane.

If the diagnosis of AP chin deficiency is made as in Figure 161C and if surgical correction is planned for an advancement genioplasty, the diagnostic cephalometric tracing can be used to accurately determine the new chin position for the optimum aesthetically balanced result. For example, if the glabella-subnasale-pogonion angle is 21 degrees, then a second line can be scribed to intersect the glabella-subnasale line at subnasale to create an ideal 11 degree angle. This, then, is the location of the new soft tissue pogonion. If the distance from the original soft tissue pogonion to the new soft tissue pogonion is 5 mm, and the soft tissue moves 80% of the distance the graft moves (see Fig. 153), then the graft must be moved 6.25 mm in order to accomplish a 5-mm change of the soft tissue (Fig. 161D). If the chin is too large in the AP plane and is to be corrected by a posterior sliding osteotomy, similar calculations can be used, allowing for the soft tissue to move 90% of the total move of the bone. In the case of an ostectomy, the soft tissue moves only 25% of the total distance of the bone movement (see Fig. 153).

The vertical position of the chin is related to the anterior dental height of the mandible. The lower anterior dental height is a measurement from the incisal edge of the central incisor to the menton. The average height is 40 ∓ 2 mm in women and 44 ∓ 2 mm in men.[2] Another useful vertical measurement is the lower anterior soft tissue height. This is a measurement of a line from soft tissue menton to stomion (the point where the lips meet). The average length is 51 ∓ 3 mm for men and 48 ∓ 3 mm for women (Fig. 162).[2] When the analysis indicates a vertical excessive chin and when a measured amount of bone is removed by wedge ostectomy, ostectomy, or recontour shave ostectomy (see Fig. 153), a prediction tracing can be made to reconstruct the hard and soft tissue.[2]

SURGERY

Surgery on the chin usually requires a general anesthetic. Alloplastic implants for augmentation

Table 10–1. Cephalometric Landmarks

A (subspinale): The point of greatest concavity of the maxilla between anterior nasal spine and maxillary dental alveolus
ANS (anterior nasal spine): The most anterior point of the nasal floor
B (supramentale): The point of greatest concavity of the mandible between mandibular dental alveolus and pogonion
FH (Frankfort): Anatomic porion—orbitale plane
Ga (glabella): The most prominent point of the forehead
Go (gonion): The point located by bisecting the angle formed by tangents to the posterior border of the ramus and inferior border of the mandible
Me (menton): The most inferior point on the mandibular symphysis
Me' (soft tissue menton): The most inferior point on the soft tissue of the chin
N (nasion): The point formed by the frontonasal suture
Or (orbitale): The most inferior point of the orbital rim
Po (pogonion): The most anterior point on the mandibular symphysis
Pr (porion): The most superior point on the curvature of the bony ear canal (internal auditory meatus)
S (sella): The midpoint of sella turcica
Sn (subnasale): The most posterior superior point on the nasolabial curvature

124 Surgery of the Mandible

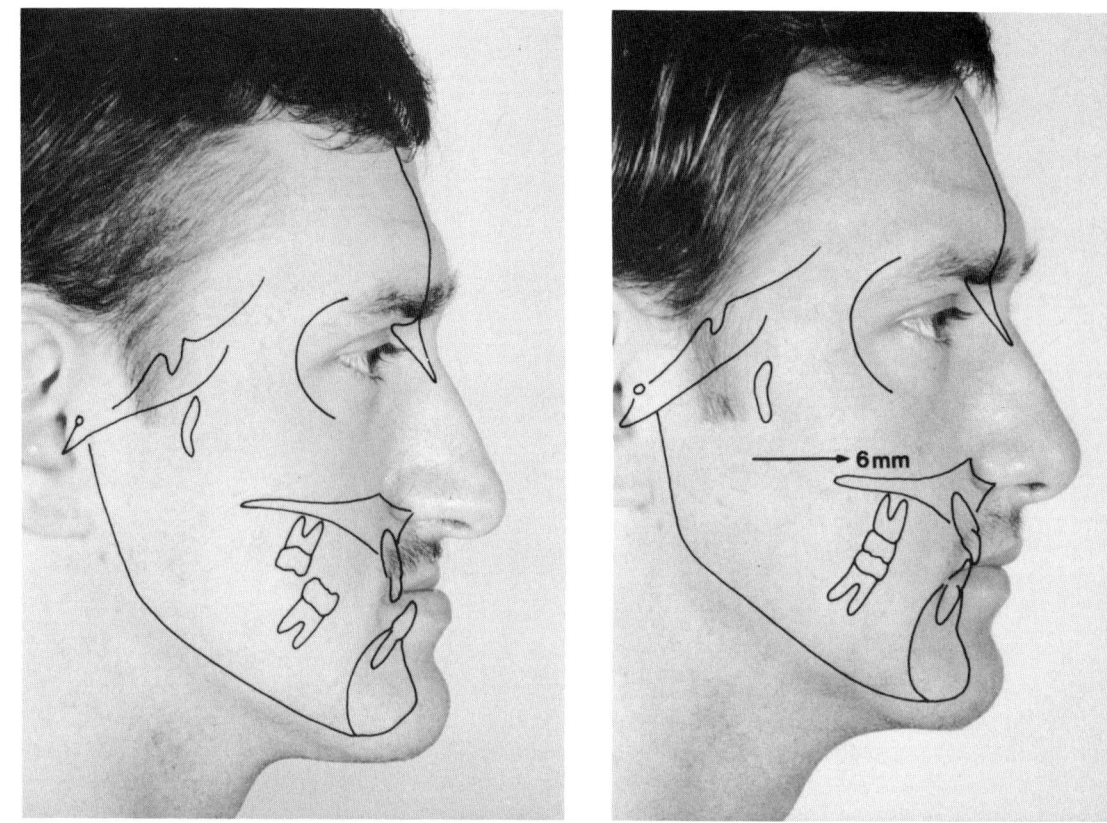

Figure 157. (A) Twenty-four-year-old man with prominent chin due to an anteroposterior deficiency of the maxilla. (B) Postoperative facial harmony achieved without surgery of the chin utilizing LeForte 1 advancement osteotomy and rhinoplasty.

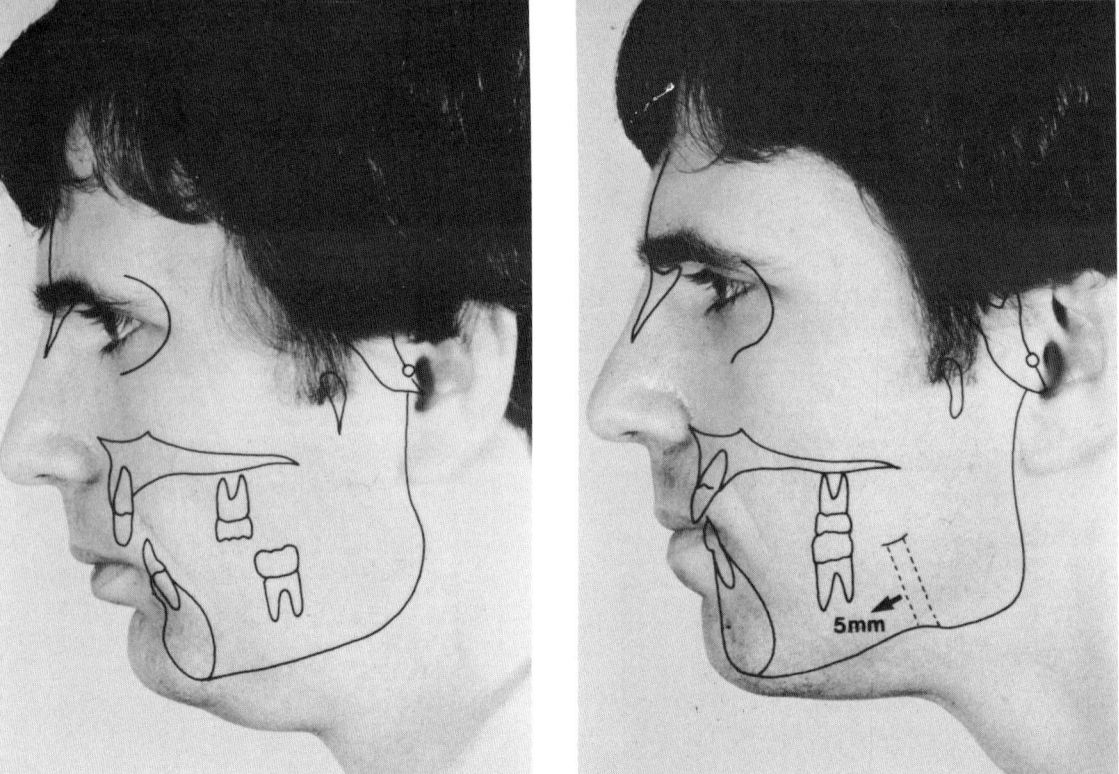

Figure 158. (A) Twenty-five-year-old man with receding chin and deep mentolabial groove. Skeletal analysis showed an anteroposterior deficient mandible and a Class 2 malocclusion. (B) Appearance in occlusion following orthodontic therapy and surgical advancement of the mandible.

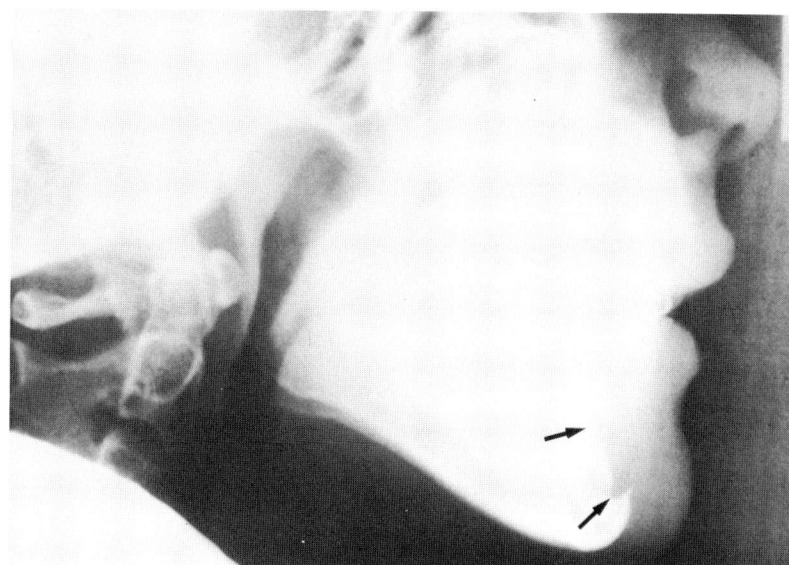

Figure 159. Lateral skull radiographs showing marked erosion extending through cortical bone 6 months after placement of a medium Silastic chin implant (arrows.)

procedures can be accomplished on selected patients under local anesthesia with sedation. The intraoral approach is the most frequently used. The mucosal incision is placed 6 to 10 mm on the lip side of the vestibule. The incision extends from premolar to the premolar on the opposite side (Fig. 163A). The mentalis muscles are transected and the incision is carried through the periosteum to bone. The periosteum is reflected superiorly to visualize the bony prominence over the roots of the teeth. The mental foramina and nerves are located and the mental prominence is degloved of its periosteum and muscle attachments. The planned osteotomy, midline, and two other vertical reference lines are scribed into the cortical surface of bone with a power saw or rotating handpiece (Fig. 163B). The bone cuts are made with a reciprocating saw while retracting the mental nerve and soft-tissue flap. The saw cuts must be 3 to 4 mm below the mental foramen. Once the inferior segment is completely sectioned, it should be mobilized along with its pedicle which will include the geniohyoid and digastric muscles and the enveloping periosteum (Fig. 163C). Holes are drilled at three points in the proximal and distal segments. The pedicled segment is moved to its measured position and fixed into the position with 24 or 26-gauge stainless steel wire (Fig. 163D). Lag screws, pins, or plates can also be used to stabilize the inferior segment. A mimimum of a two-layer closure is recommended (Figs. 163E, F) and a pressure bandage is placed (Fig. 163G).

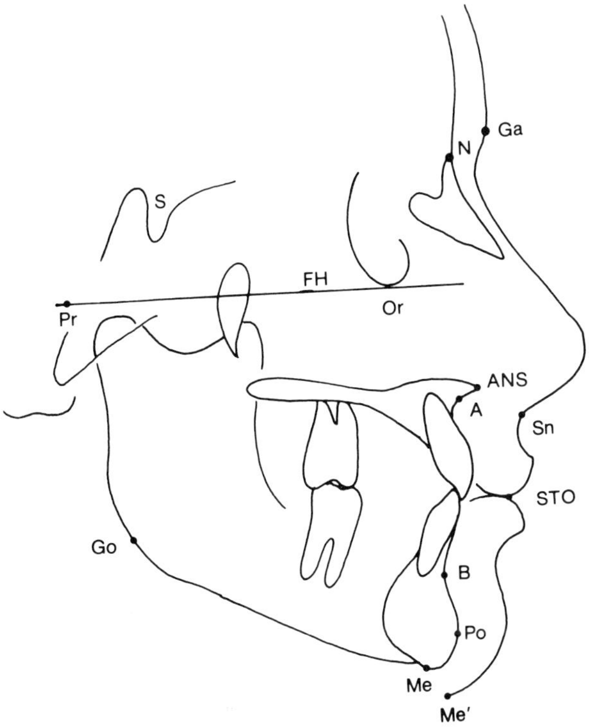

REPORT OF CASES

To illustrate results of various surgical procedures in the chin region, five cases are presented. Case 2–1 is a 27-year-old man with a Class 1 occlusion. Although facial height ratio was good, the patient had AP chin excess or macrogenia (Fig. 164A). Figure 164B shows the result of a reduction genioplasty by an osseous sliding reduction osteotomy. Figure 164C shows the surgical reduction and the contouring of the sharp edges.

Case 2–2 is a patient who had an obvious long lower face in both the vertical and AP plans (Fig.

Figure 160. Cephalometric landmarks (*Abbreviations:* STO= ; other abbreviations as in Table 10–1).

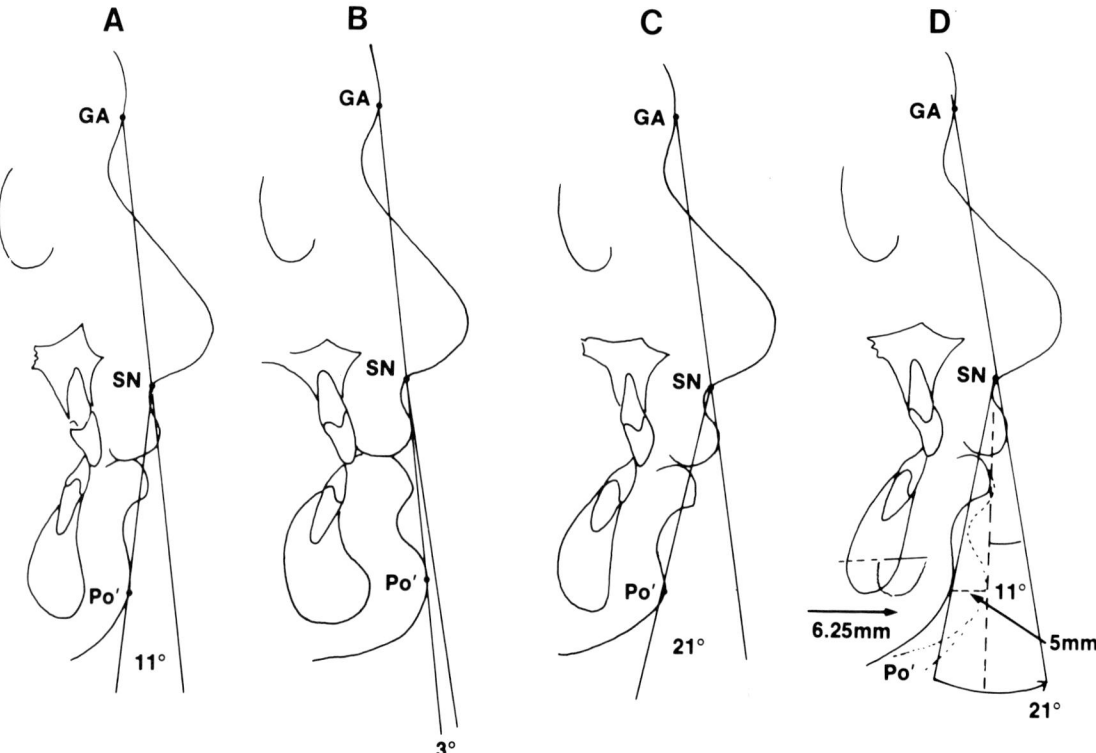

Figure 161. (A) Normal chin projection angle from subnasale to the soft tissue pogonion is approximately 11 degrees. (B) A marked decrease in this angle to 3 degrees would indicate the need for a reduction genioplasty in the anteroposterior plane. (C) A larger angle of 21 degrees indicating a need for an advancement or augmentation genioplasty in the anteroposterior plane. (D) The proposed surgical therapy to correct the abnormality seen in (C) by drawing a line from the abnormal intersection point to a normal 11 degree angle indicating that the mandible should be moved forward 6.25 mm to accomplish a 5-mm change in the soft tissue.

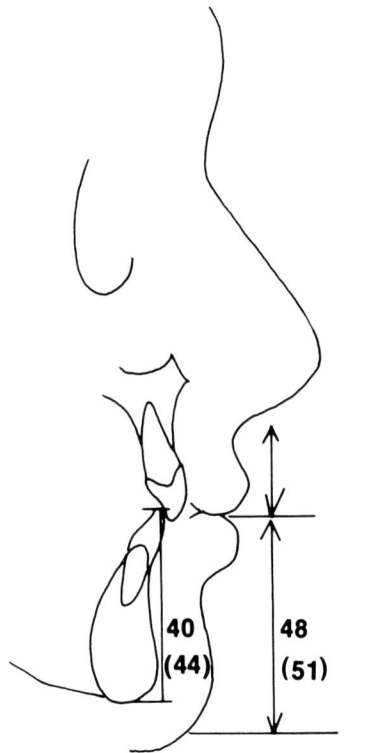

Figure 162. Measurement of a line from soft tissue menton to stomion indicating an average height of 48 mm for women and 51 mm for men. The lower anterior dental height is a measurement from the incisal edge of the central incisor to the menton; and the average height is 44 mm in men and 40 mm in women.

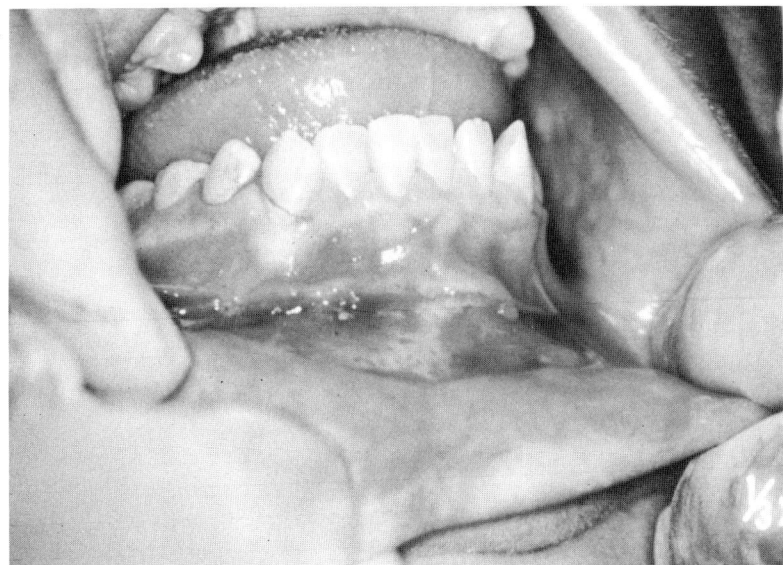

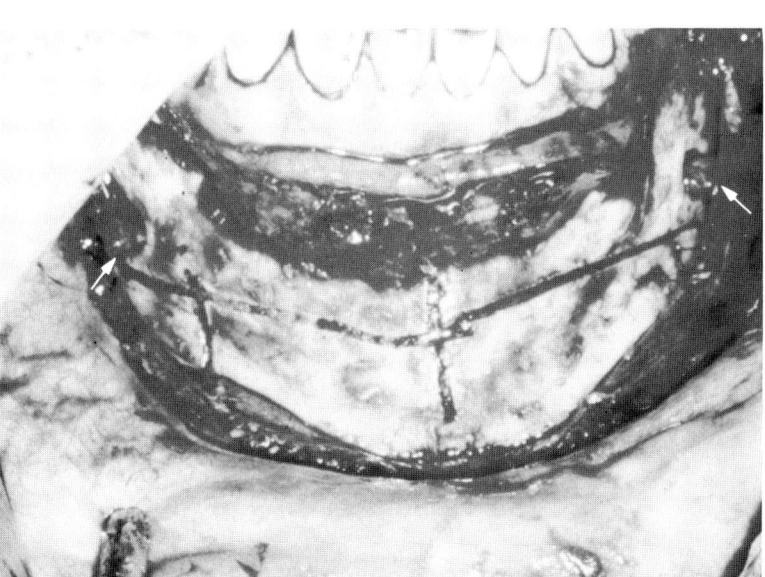

Figure 163. (A) Surgical procedure of mentoplasty. An incision intraorally extending from the premolar to the premolar on the opposite side. (B) The plan osteotomy midline and other vertical lines are scribed onto the cortical surface of bone with a power saw. (C) Once the inferior segment is sectioned it is mobilized along with the pedicle.

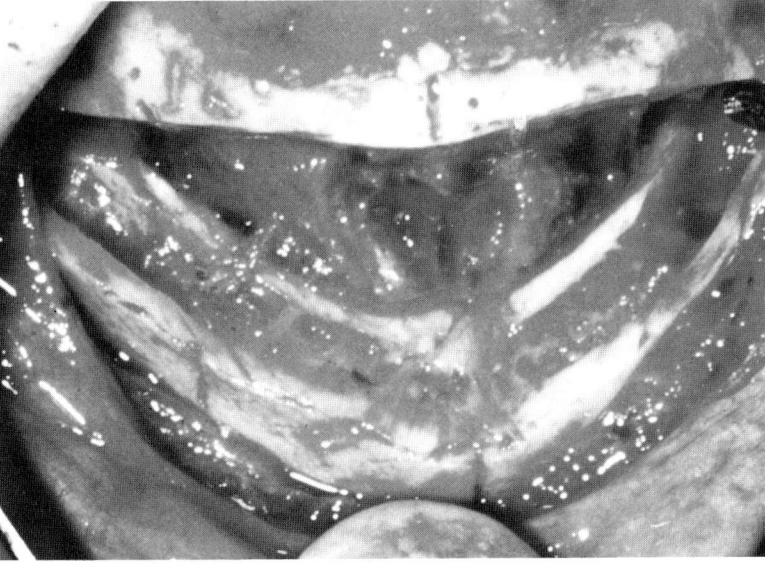

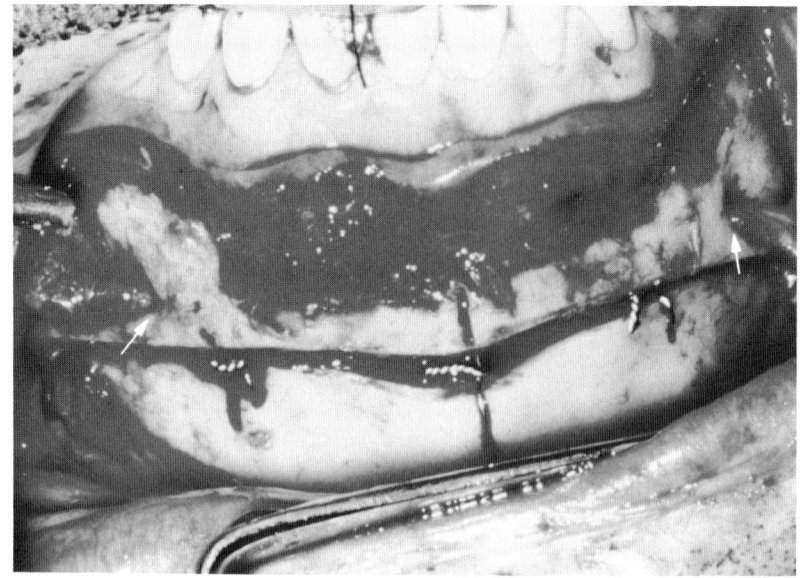

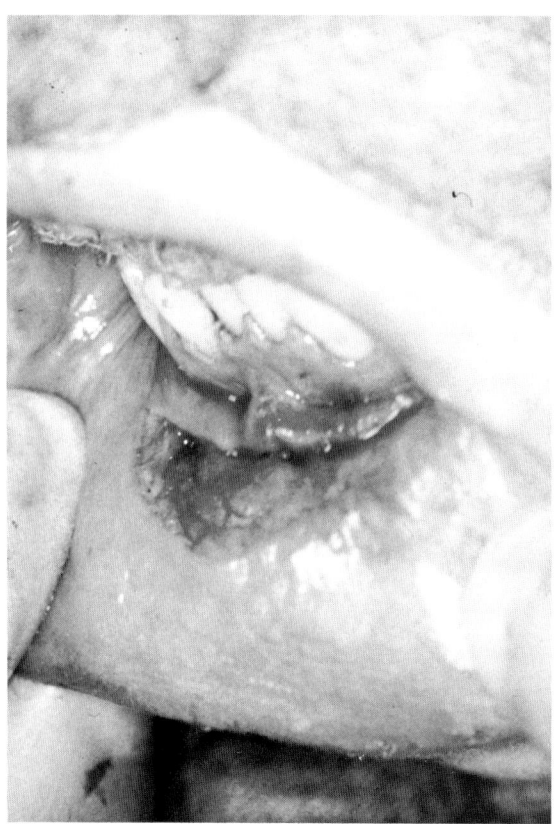

Figure 163. (D) The pedicle segment is moved to its measured position and fixed with stainless steel wire. (E) Two-layer closure.

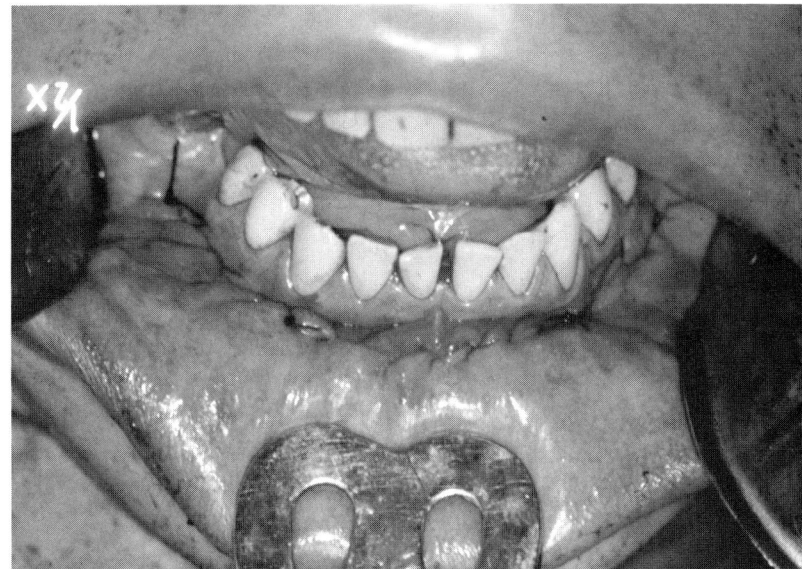

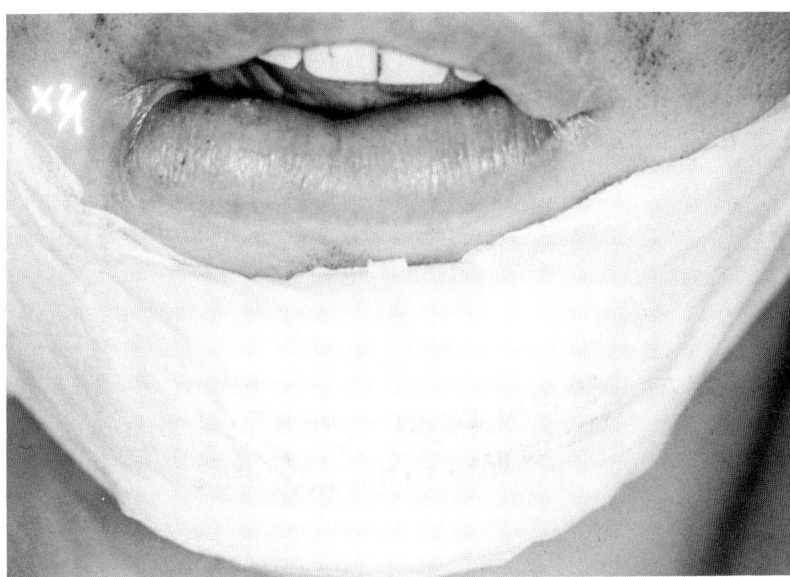

Figure 163. (F) Mucosa closed. (G) Pressure bandages placed on the chin to obliterate the sulcus.

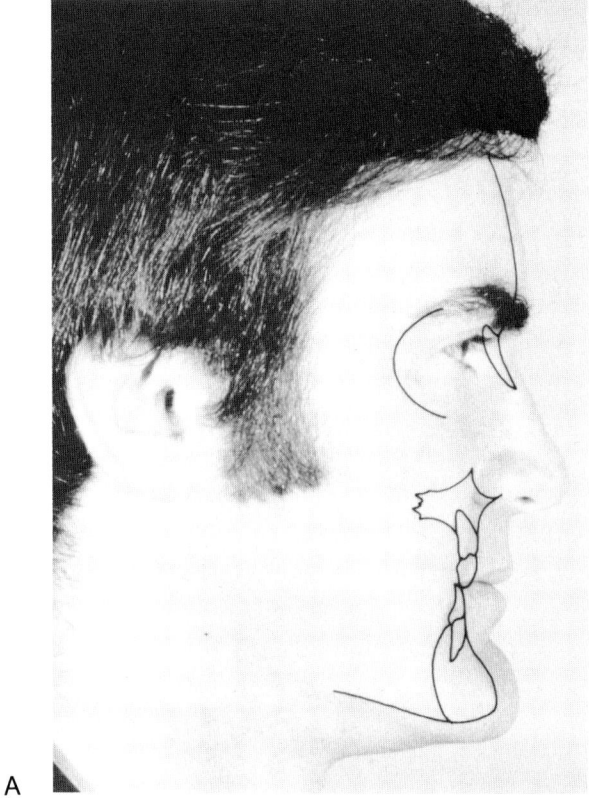
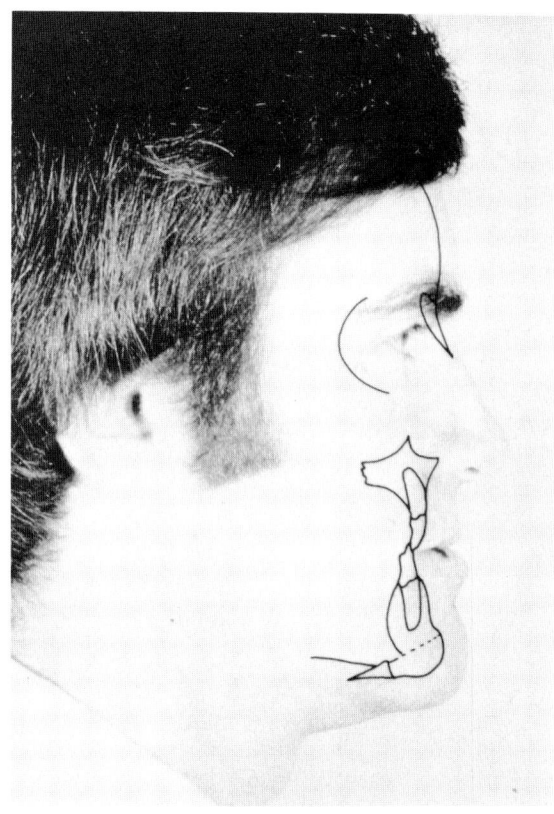
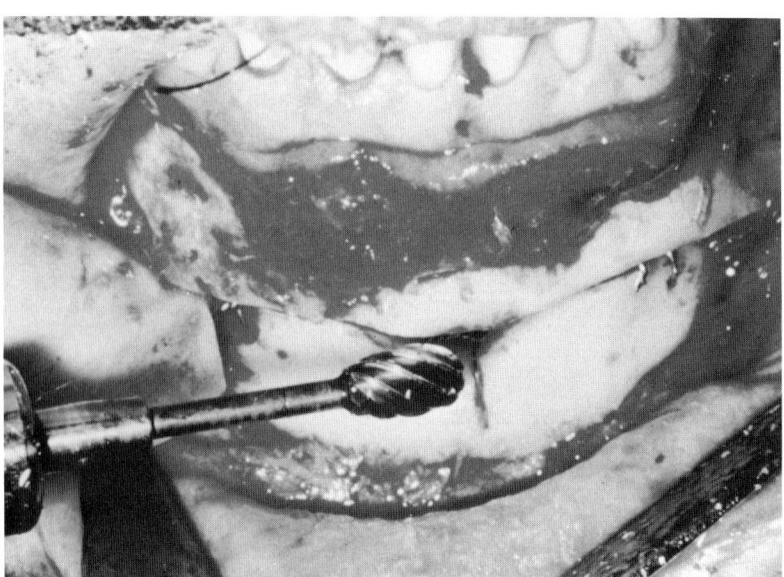

Figure 164. (A) Twenty-seven-year-old man with Class 1 occlusion and good facial height ratio. However, the patient had an anteroposterior chin excess. (B) Results of a reduction genioplasty by sliding osseous reduction osteotomy. (C) Surgical reduction and contouring of sharp edges of the sliding reduction osteotomy.

Surgery of the Chin 131

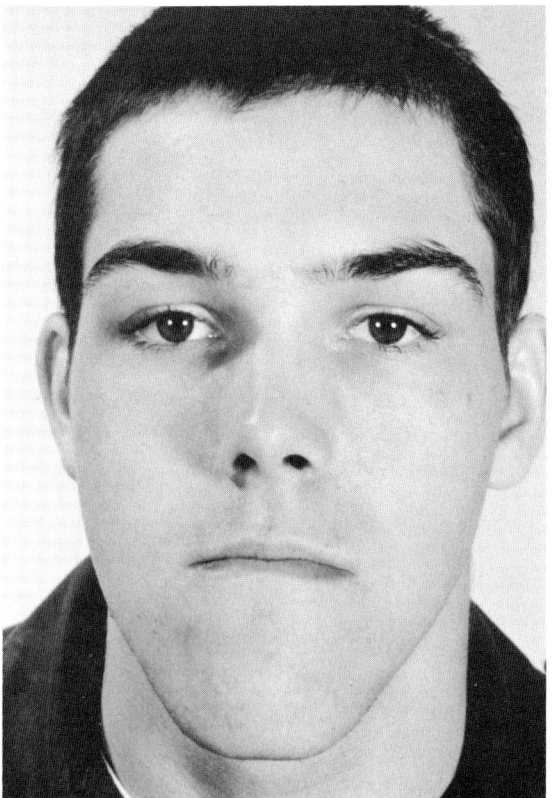
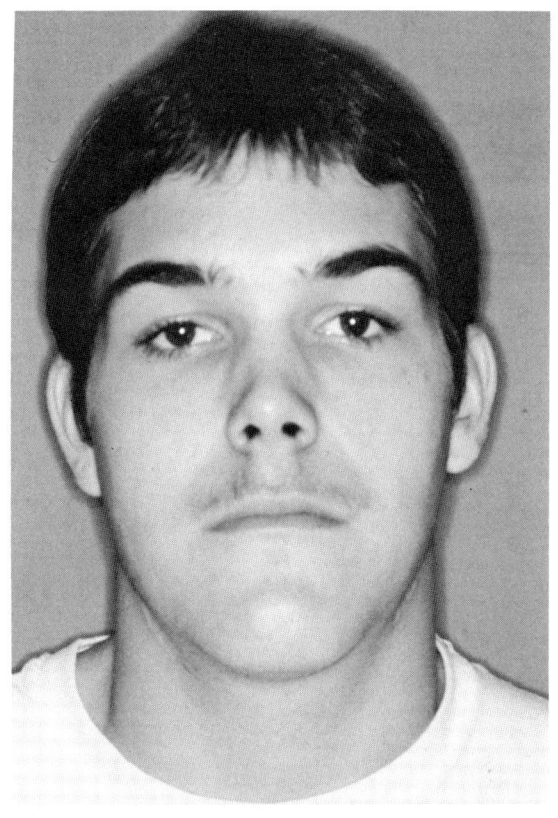
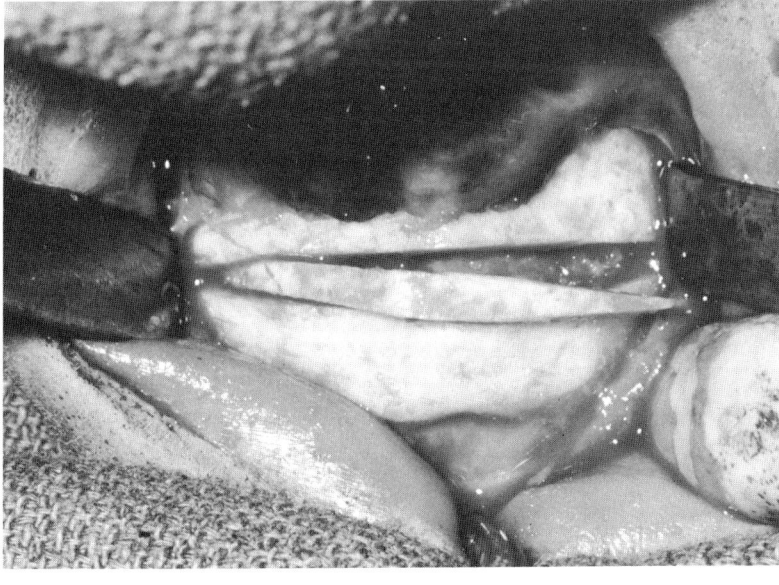

Figure 165. (A) Male teenager with an obvious long lower face in the vertical and anteroposterior planes. (B) Demonstrating results from vertical wedge excision, reducing the facial vertical height. (C) Operative photograph showing vertical wedge prior to its removal.

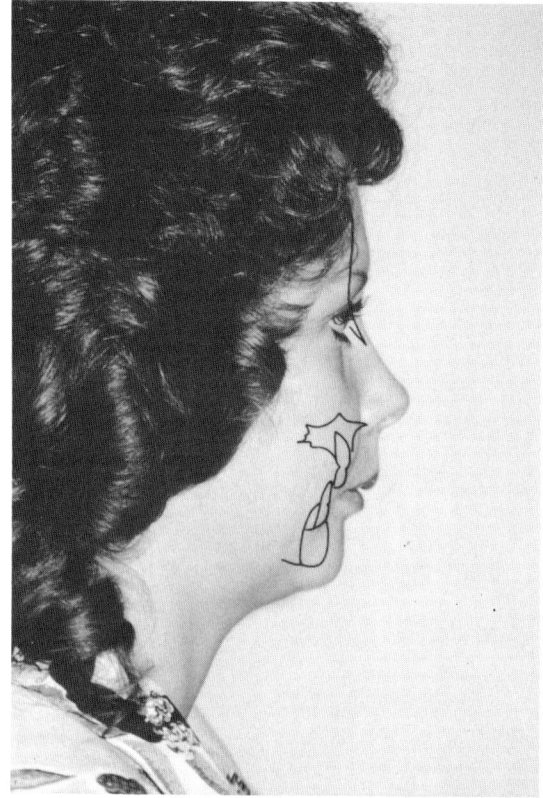
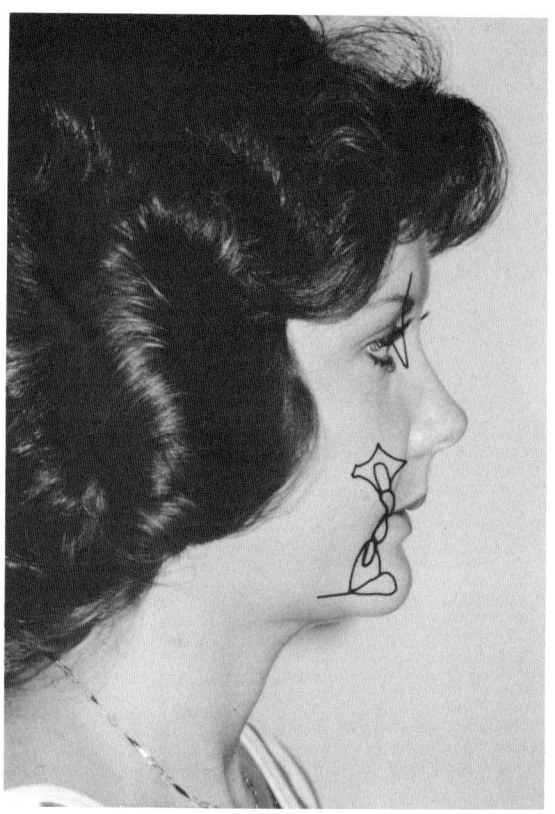
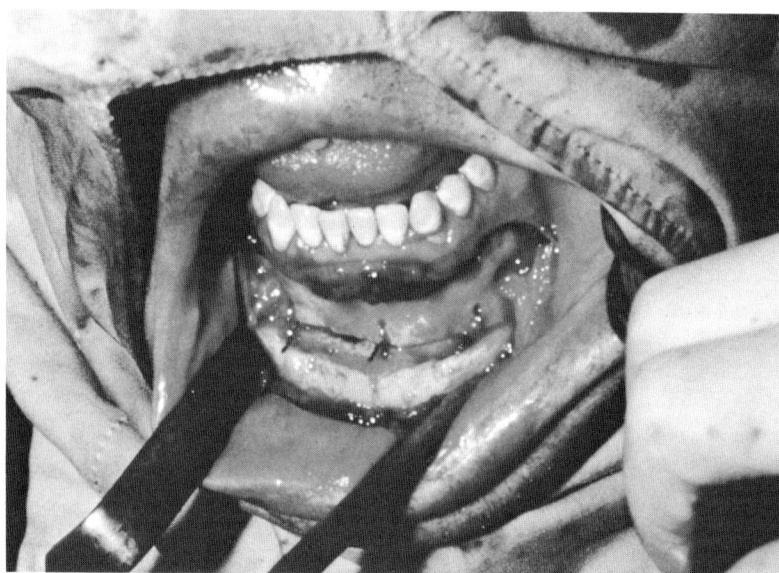

Figure 166. (A) Young woman with Class 2 occlusion but with good function. She has an anteroposterior deficient chin. (B) Long-term follow up of the patient who was treated with an anterior advancement sliding ostectomy. (C) Intraoperative photograph of the secured advanced inferior mandibular segment.

Surgery of the Chin 133

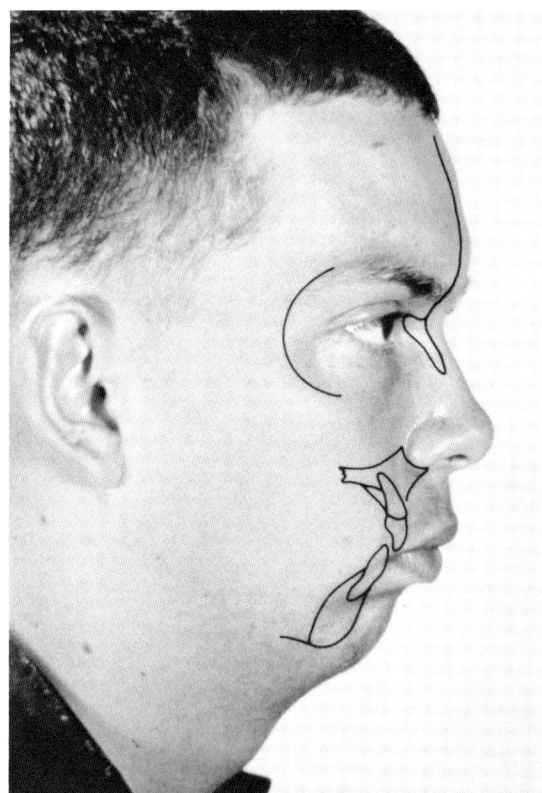
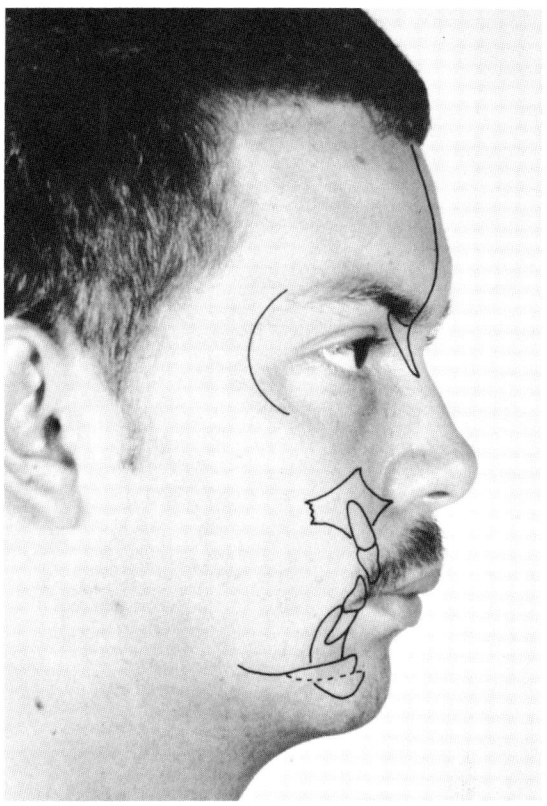

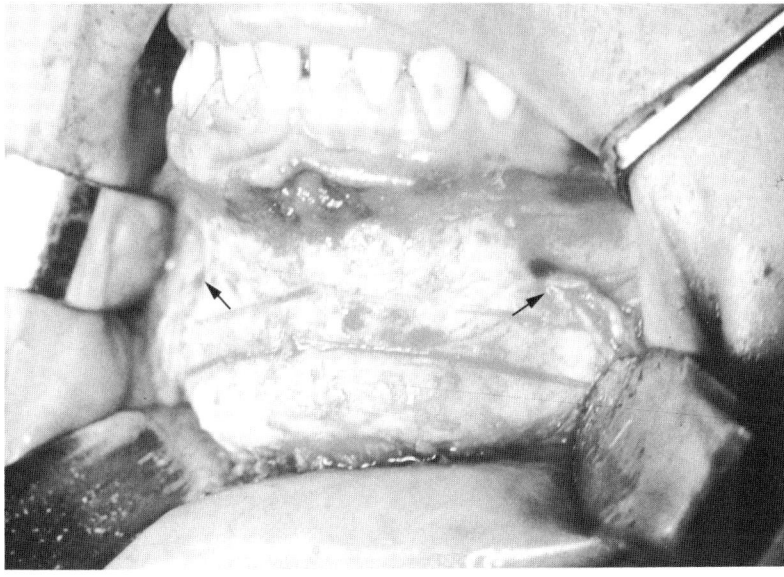

Figure 167. (A) Young male following 4 years of orthodontic therapy. The teeth are now in a Class 1 relationship. There is still an anteroposterior mandibular deficiency. (B) Satisfactory profile change accomplished by a double advancement sliding osteotomy. (C) Proposed osteotomy lines marked on the bone surface.

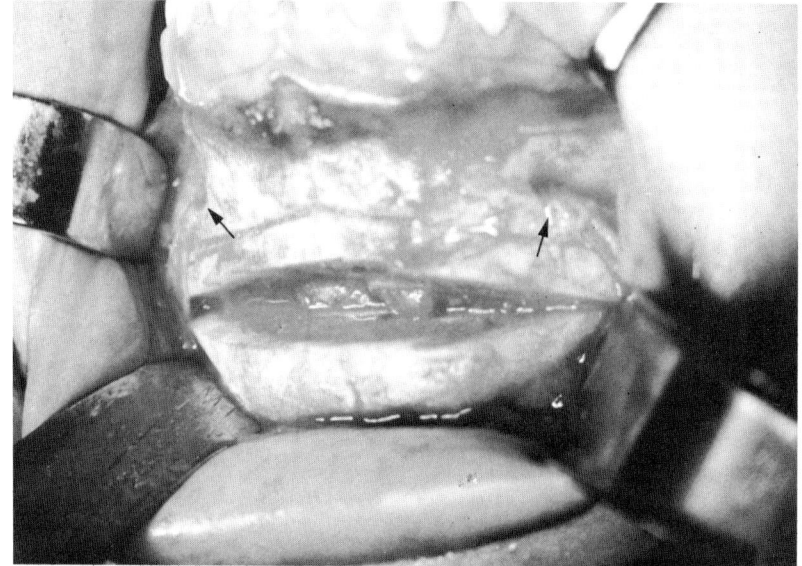

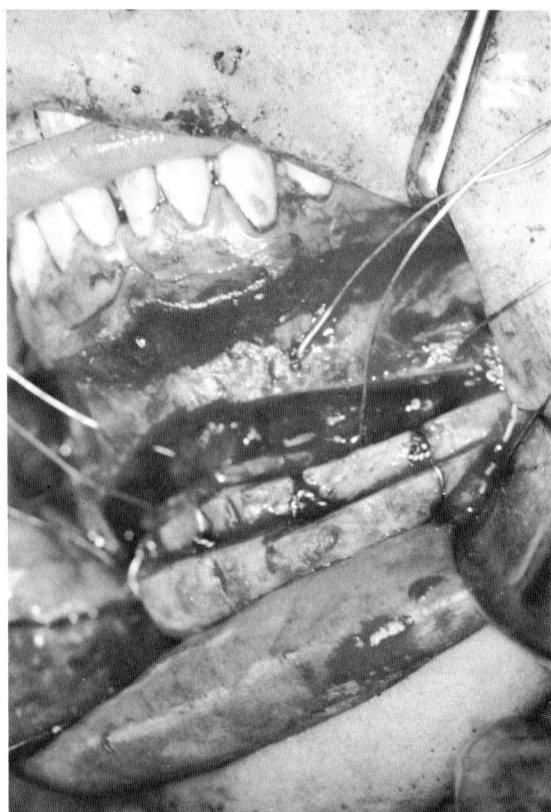

Figure 167. (D) First inferior bone cut. (E) First inferior bone segment advanced and secured with wire and the second bone cut, completed, ready for advanccement and wiring.

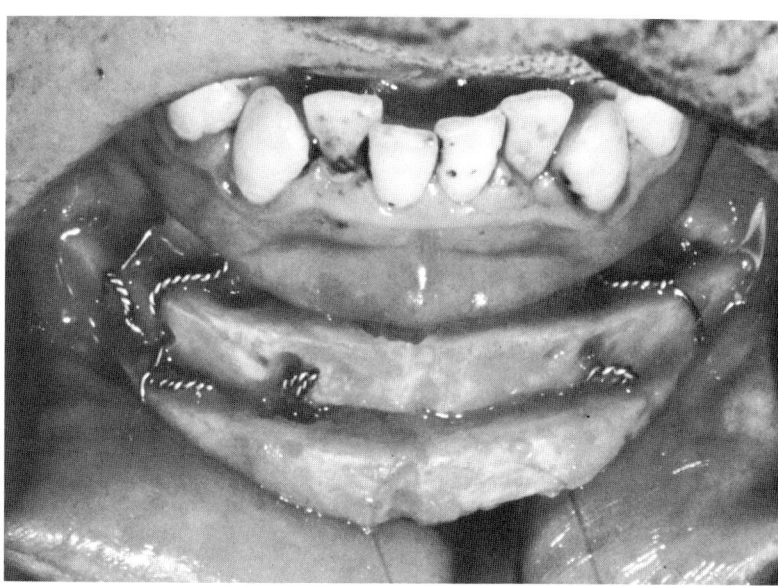

Figure 167. (F) Wired double segments of the final results at the time of surgery.

165A). Figure 165B demonstrates the results obtained by removing a vertical wedge which reduced the facial vertical height yet maintained the good contour of the chin point with its soft tissue attachment. By sliding the inferior segment posteriorly, the chin was reduced in the AP plane also. Figure 165C shows the vertical wedge ready for removal.

Case 2–3 is a young woman who had a Class 2 occlusion but with good function. She had an AP-deficient chin (Fig. 166A). Figure 166B shows the long-term follow-up of this patient who was treated with an anterior advancement sliding ostectomy. Figure 166C is a photograph of the secured advanced inferior segment.

Case 2–4 is a patient who had been treated by an orthodontist for 4 years. The teeth had been brought into a Class 1 relationship without the benefit of a mandibular advancement to correct the AP deficiency (Fig. 167A). Satisfactory profile change was accomplished by a double advancement sliding osteotomy (Fig. 167B). Figure 167C shows the proposed osteotomy lines marked on the bone surface. Figures 167D and E are the first and second bone cuts. Figure 167F shows the wired double segments while Figure 167B is the 6-month follow-up photograph.

Case 2–5 is a young man who had also been treated by orthodontists, although satisfactory occlusion was obtained, there was an AP deficiency in the chin region (Fig. 168A). Figure 168C is a photograph taken at surgery showing the placement of a proplast augmentation graft. Figure 168B depicts profile change that resulted.

CONCLUSION

Facial surgery is a blend of both art and science. Guided by formal scientific training, an artistic eye, and skilled hands, the surgeon can predict the outcome with each patient.

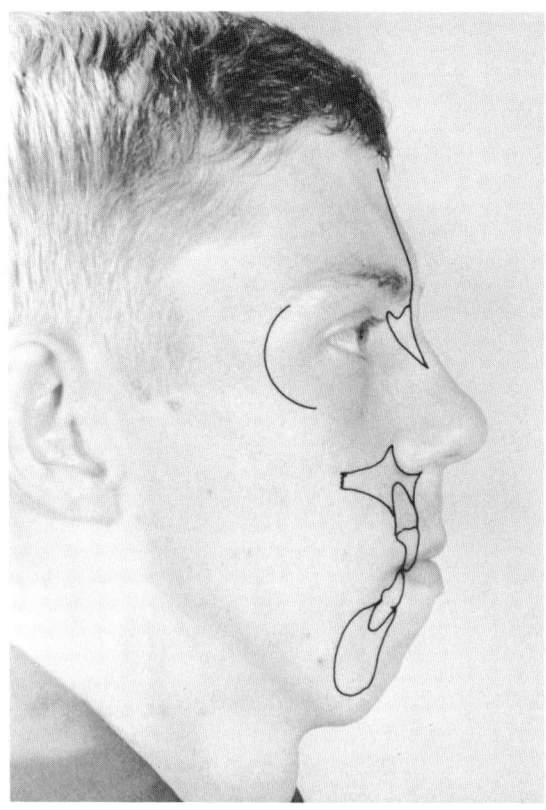
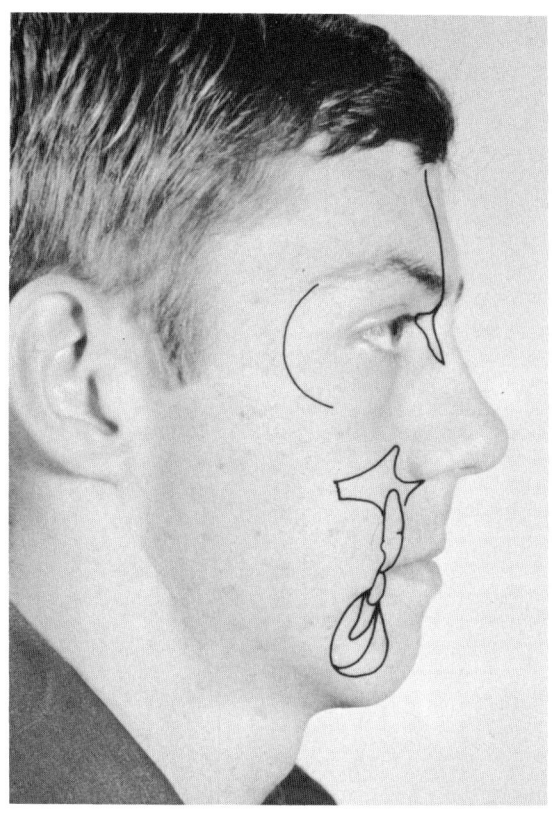
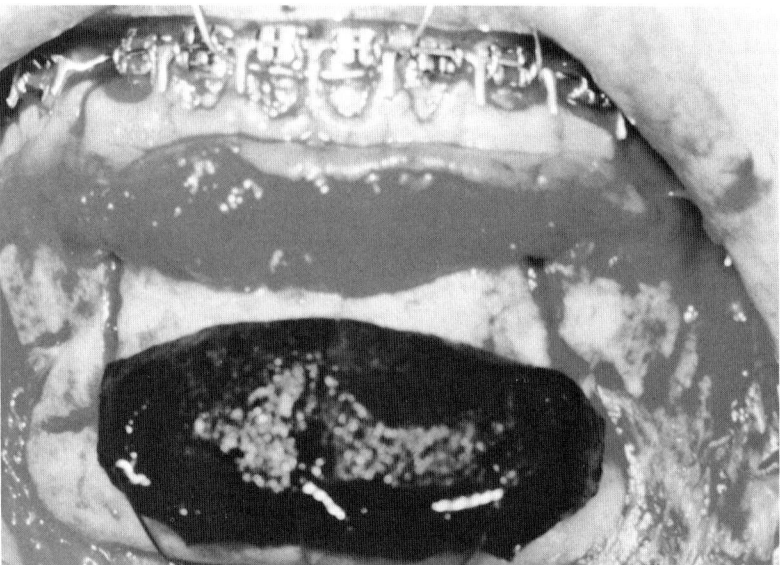

Figure 168. (A) Young male with satisfactory occlusion after orthodontic therapy but with a remaining anteroposterior deficiency in the chin region. (B) Profile change resulting from placement of a Proplast augmentation graft. (C) Intraoperative photograph showing onlay of Proplast graft onto anterior mandible through intraoral incision.

REFERENCES

1. Bell WH, Proffitt WB, White RP: Surgical Correction of Dentofacial Deformities. Philadelphia: Saunders, 1980, pp 1210–1219
2. Wolford LM, Hilliard FW, Dugan DJ: Surgical Treatment Objectives: A Systematic Approach of the Prediction Tracing. St Louis: Mosby, 1985
3. Hinds EC, Kent JN: Surgical Treatment of Developmental Jaw Deformities. St Louis: Mosby, 1972
4. Hinds EC, Kent JN: Genioplasty: The versatility of the horizontal osteotomy. J Oral Surg 27:690–700, 1969
5. Bell WH, Dann JJ III: Correction of dentofacial deformities by surgery in the anterior parts of the jaw. Am J Orthod 64(2):162–187, 1973
6. Gonzales-Ulloa M, Stevens E: Rose of chin correction in profileplasty. Plast Reconstr Surg 41:477–483, 1968

7. Hohl TH, Epker BN: Macrogenia: A study of treatment of results with surgical recommendations. Oral Surg 41:454–467, 1976
8. McDonnell J, McNeill W, West R: Advancement genioplasty, a retrospective cephalometric analysis of osseous and soft tissue changes. J Oral Surg 35:640–647, 1977
9. Crafts RC: A Textbook of Human Anatomy. New York: Ronald Press, 1966
10. Junghans JA: Profile reconstruction with Sialastic chin implants. Am J Orthod 53:217–226, 1967
11. Brown JB, Fryer MP, Ohlwiler DA: Study and use of synthetic materials, such as silicone and Teflon, as subcutaneous prostheses. Plast Reconstr Surg 26:264–279, 1960
12. Meyer RA, Gehrig JP, Funk EC, et al.: Restoring facial contour with implanted silicone rubber. Oral Surg 24:598–603, 1967
13. Parks ML: Chin implants with a newer plastic compound. Arch Otolaryngol 75:429–434, 1962
14. Robinson M, Shuken R: Bone resorption under plastic chin implants. J Oral Surg 27:116–121, 1969
15. Steed DL: Rapid resorption of bone beneath Sialastic chin implant. Read before the Air Force Society of Clinical Surgeons, San Antonio, TX, September 19, 1970
16. Kent JN, Homsy CA, Gross BO, et al.: Pilot studies of porous implant in dentistry and oral surgery. J Oral Surg 30:608–615, 1972
17. Kent JN, Homsy CA, Hinds EC: Proplast in dental facial reconstruction. Oral Surg 39:347–356, 1975
18. Homsy CS, Kent JN, Hinds EC: Materials for oral implants—biological and functional criteria. J Am Dent Assoc 86:817–823, 1973
19. Dann JJ III, Epker BN: Proplast genioplasty: A retrospective study with treatment recommendations. Angle Orthod 47:172–181, 1977
20. Jarcho M, Kay JF, Guman KL, et al.: Tissue, cellular and subcellular events at a bone-ceramic hydroxylapatite interface. J Bioenerg Biomembr 1:79–87, 1976
21. Rejda BV, Peelen JCJ, DeGroot K: Tricalcium phosphate as a bone substitute. J Bioenerg Biomembr 1:93–101, 1977
22. Denissen HW, VanDijk HJA, Gehring AP, et al.: Preparation of densely sintered calcium hydroxylapatite (CHA). New Orleans: International Association for Dental Research Meeting Abstract No. 613, 1979
23. Denissen HW, DeGroot K: Immediate dental root implants from synthetic dense calcium hydroxylapatite. J Prosthet Dent 42:551–556, 1979
24. Gonzales-Ulloa M: Quantitative principles in cosmetic surgery of the face (profileplasty). Plast Reconstr Surg 29:186–198, 1961
25. Khonw FE, Proffitt WR, White RP: Cephalometric evaluation of patients with dentofacial disharmonies requiring surgical correction. Oral Surg 29:789–799, 1970
26. Firmin F, Caccaro P, Converse J: Cephalometric analysis in diagnosis and treatment planning of craniofacial dysostoses. Plast Reconstr Surg 54(3):300–311, 1974
27. Worms FW, Isaacson RT, Speider TM: Surgical orthodontic treatment planning: Profile analysis and mandibular surgery. Angle Orthod 46:1–15, 1976
28. Myer L: A cephalometric guide to the diagnosis of midface hypoplasia at the Le Fort II level. J Oral Surg 35:21–24, 1977
29. Legan HL: Soft tissue cephalometric analysis for orthognathic surgery. J Oral Surg 38:744–751, 1978
30. Burstone CJ, James RB, Legan H, et al.: Cephalometrics for orthognathic surgery. J Oral Surg 36(4):269–277, 1978
31. Scheideman GB, Bell WH, Legan HL, et al.: Cephalometric analysis of dentofacial normals. Am J Orthod 78:404–420, 1980
32. Tweed CH: The Frankfort-mandibular plane angle in orthodontic diagnosis, classification, treatment planning and prognosis. Am J Orthod 175–230, 1946
33. Tweed CH: Frankfort-mandibular incisor angle (FMIA) in orthodontic treatment planning and prognosis. Angle Orthod 24:121–138, 1954
34. Holdaway RA: Changes in relationship of points A and B during orthodontic treatment. Am J Orthod 42:176–187, 1956
35. Downs WB: Analysis of the dentofacial profile. Angle Orthod 22:142–151, 1956
36. Riedel RA: An analysis of dentofacial relationships. Am J Orthod 43:103–119, 1957
37. Moowees CFA, Kean MR: Natural head position: A basic consideration for analysis of cephalometric radiographs. Am J Phys Anthropol 16:213–234, 1958
38. Steiner CC: Cephalometrics in clinical practice. Angle Orthod 29:8–16, 1959
39. Steiner CC: Cephalometrics for you and me. Am J Orthod 39:729–736, 1959
40. Ricketts RM: Cephalometric analysis synthesis. Angle Orthod 31:141–149, 1961
41. Hambleton RS: The soft-tissue covering of the face as related to orthodontic problems. Am J Orthod 50:405–520, 1964
42. Tweed CH: Clinical Orthodontics. St Louis: Mosby 1966
43. Merrifield LL: The profile line as an aid in critically evaluating facial aesthetics. Am J Orthod 52:804–822, 1966
44. Burstone CJ: Lip posture and its significance to treatment planning. Am J Orthod 53:262–284, 1967
45. Holdaway RA: A soft tissue cephalometric analysis and its use in orthodontic treatment planning. Am J Orthod 84(2):1–11, 1983
46. Powell N, Humphreys B: Considerations and components of the aesthetic face. Fac Plast Surg Int Q 1–68, 1984
47. Bean J, Kramer JR, Khouw FE: A simplified method of taking radiographs for cephalometric analysis. J Oral Surg 28:675–678, 1970

11 Augmentation Mentoplasty
G. Richard Holt, M.D.

Augmentation mentoplasty is a cosmetic procedure. It has no real functional aspect and the recommendation to perform this procedure should be presented within this context. This procedure is based on the premise that all alloplastic material with a high degree of biological tolerance can be inserted into the premandibular region to change (and improve) the facial appearance through the achievement of better facial harmony. The evaluation of the patient with mandibular insufficiency via precise cephalometric techniques has been presented in Chapter 9. However, for those surgeons who do not have the training in utilizing these techniques, a simple method of determining the effects of augmentation can be applied utilizing the lateral facial photograph (Fig. 169). Here, a line is formed from the region of the nasion to the vermillion of the lower lip. If the mandible is deficient in its anterior projection, it will not reach to that vertical line. Thus, agumentation may be helpful to improve this relative facial disharmony.

However, if a Class 3 malocclusion exists, then the patient should be evaluated by an oral surgeon for the possibility of orthognathic surgery (mandibular osteotomies) to restore neutrocclusion as well as improving the facial disharmony of the retrognathic mandible. In the case of the patient who does not desire orthognathic surgery, then augmentation mentoplasty is a viable option.

Quite a number of alloplastic materials have been utilized for the augmentation of the chin, but only a few have survived the test of time and long-term acceptance by the tissues. It is important that the surgeon realize that there are at least two aspects of tissue compatibility that allow an implant to remain in place in the region of the chin. First, the implant material must have a low tissue reactivity—it must not be completely bioinert, though, because a foreign body reaction capsule around the implant is desirable and necessary. Second, the implant design has to closely fit the curvature of the anterior mandible so that the forces presented to it through the muscular actions of chewing, talking, and smiling do not distract if from its position on the mandible.

The three most commonly used biomaterials for chin augmentation in the author's experience are Silastic, Proplast, and Supramid. Each of these materials has its own properties and reaction to it by the recipient soft tissues. Silastic implants (medical grade silicone) are usually a solid core of material that have been fabricated to match the usual curvature of the anterior mandible and yet are flexible enough to bend to accommodate individual variations in the mandible's curvature. The implant can be sculpted from a solid block of silastic but is usually utilized in the form of a prefabricated implant in several different sizes. The Proplast implant is fabricated from a block of carbonaceous material which is spongelike (many tiny air pockets) and soft enough to carve with a scalpel blade. If this implant is utilized, it must be impregnated with an antibiotic solution before inserting it into the recipient site. This process involves the filling of the implant's air spaces with an antibiotic solution by applying alternating positive and negative pressures with a large syringe. This process improves the implant's success rate by decreasing the chance for infection originating within the "dead space."

The Supramid implant is created by rolling or folding a length of Supramid sheeting into a cylindrical shape and securing it in this shape with permanent sutures. The implant can then be cut and trimmed with scissors to the desired shape. It may be first inserted into a subcutaneous pocket in the abdomen or supraclavicular fossa to allow it to become impregnated with fibrous tissue before implanting it into the chin, or it can be implanted *de novo*.

These different biomaterials also have somewhat different types of incorporation into the soft tissues of the chin. The silicone implant is incorporated into the soft tissues by the formation of a fibrous capsule around it. On the other hand, Proplast and Supramid are penetrated by strands of scar tissue which invade the dead space network of these nonsolid implants; this tends to fix these implants more rigidly in the tissues than the Silastic. An additional aspect of the Proplast is that the carbonaceous material of which it is composed is to a small degree biodegradable and taken up by tissue

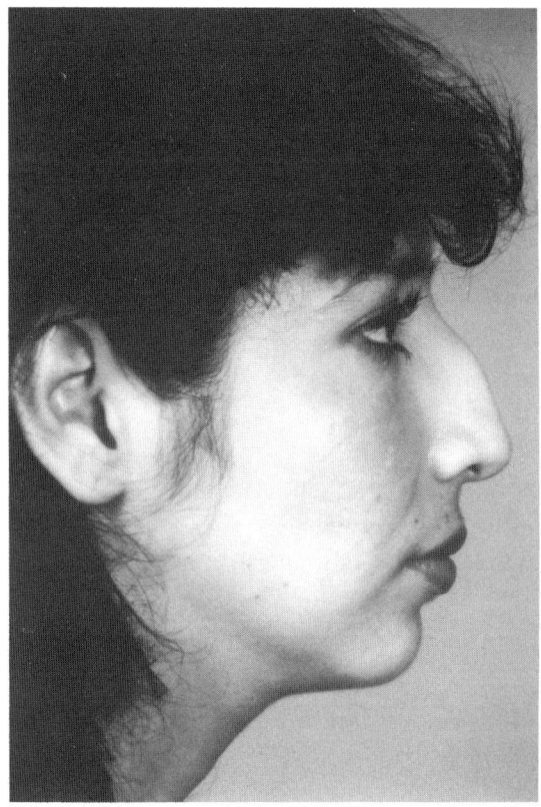

Figure 169. Patient with nasal hump deformity and a concomitant recessed chin. She was in neutrocclusion.

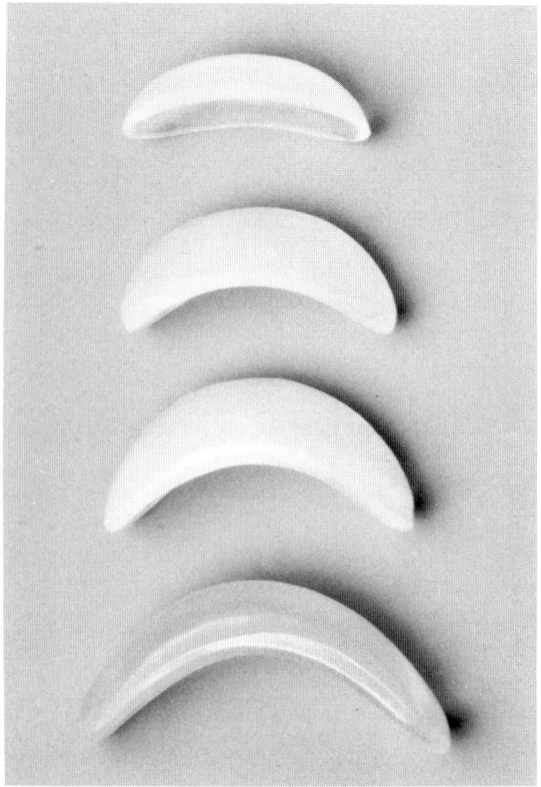

Figure 170. Four sized of Silastic chin implants: small, medium-small, medium, and large.

macrophages. This does not significantly alter its size and shape unless an acute inflammation intervenes which increases the macrophage activity in the wound. If this inflammation is widespread, the tissues might be darkened due to uptake of the carbon compounds.

It is the author's choice to use a preformed Silastic implant, sized to fit the individual patient's needs (Fig. 170). The following description of the augmentation mentoplasty will be given for use of the Silastic implant.

SURGICAL TECHNIQUE

This procedure may be performed in conjunction with a septorhinoplasty or as an isolated procedure. If performed with a reduction septorhinoplasty, it is commonly held that the addition of a chin implant will slightly decrease the amount of reduction of the nasal hump projection than if a chin implant is not used. Using this philosophy, the chin implant should be placed first, and the alterations of the nasal anatomy then performed using the new anterior chin projection as a guide. On the other hand, the experienced rhinoplastic surgeon is able to develop a surgical plan for both the septorhinoplasty and chin implant, integrated the two procedures, and carry out the nasal surgery first. In this case, the intranasal incisions should be completely sutured first and the nose packed before beginning the chin implant procedure. The surgical team should then change gloves and gown and a clean set of instruments should be utilized for the chin surgery.

This procedure is normally carried out under local anesthesia using equal amounts by volume of 1% lidocaine with 1:100,000 epinephrine and 0.75% Marcaine. The addition of Marcaine gives a longer-lasting anesthetic effect, which is particularly important when performed as an outpatient procedure. This local anesthetic is injected into the gingivobuccal sulcus as well as locally into the soft tissues to the chin. The mental nerves can be directly blocked by locating the mental foramina approximately 15 mm below the canine teeth. In the author's practice, a short-acting barbiturate, Brevital, is injected intravenously before the local injections are begun, to achieve a pain-free and amnesic period. During the procedure, any patient discomfort can be alleviated by additional local injections and titrated doses of intravenous analgesics and sedatives.

Elective antibiotic coverage is begun several hours preoperatively by giving the patient 500 mg ampicillin or amoxicillin orally. This is supplemented with parenteral ampicillin, 500 mg given intravenously during the surgical procedure. The ampicillin or amoxicillin is continued postoperatively for 3 days. If the patient is sensitive to penicillin, then erythromycin is utilized; the oral form given is erythromycin ethyl succinate, 400 mg four times a day with meals.

Preparation of the patient's skin and lips involves the use of a noniodine detergent (Phisohex) which is rinsed off the face with normal saline. The patient is placed in a semi-Fowler's position to maximize the patient comfort and to increase visualization of the lower buccal sulcus by the surgeon. This position also is less threatening to the patient as far as saliva and intraoral irrigation fluid control during the procedure is concerned.

If the lip and chin are injected before the prepping and draping of the patient is performed, there is a sufficient time lapse to allow the epinephrine to provide small vessel hemostasis. This will be seen in the blanching of the lip mucosa and skin of the chin. This procedure requires that a surgical assistant perform intraoral suctioning as well as retraction of the lower lip tissues. Finally, the patient's preoperative photographs must be placed in a position convenient to the surgeon for frequent viewing.

The standard incision for the author is an intraoral one, placed slightly up on the lower lip, away from the gingivobuccal sulcus (Fig. 171).

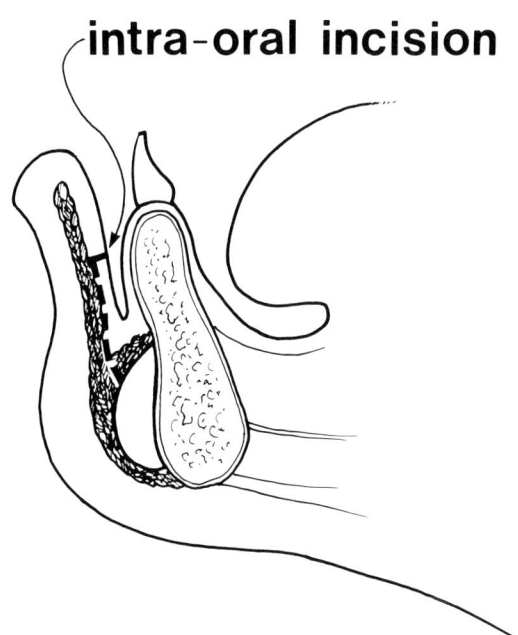

Figure 171. Intraoral incision, placed well up on the lower lip to facilitate three-layer closure of the wound.

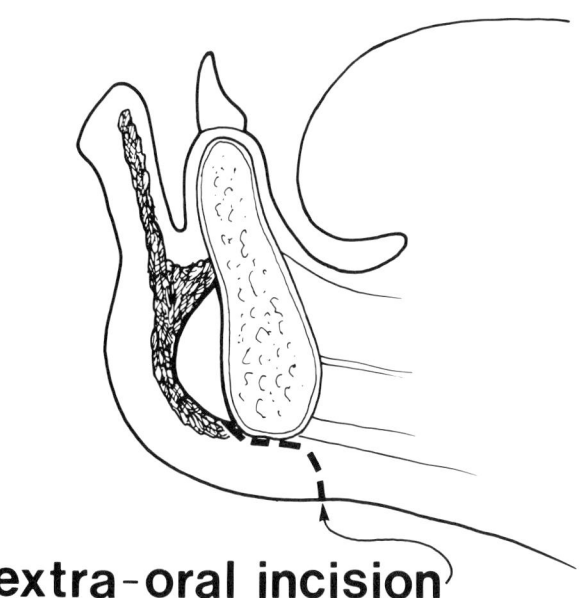

Figure 172. Extraoral or submental incision placed in a curvilinear fashion just behind the inferior bony prominence of the chin.

Placing the incision up on the lip provides sufficient tissue for a multilayered closure as well as preventing the pooling of saliva which could affect the muclsal closure. The mucosal incision is slightly curvilinear and is horizontal in position. This incision is carried down to the level of the chin-labial muscles, which are then separated in an anterior-posterior (vertical) direction within the midline raphe. This technique of two dissections placed at right angles to each other allows for a three-layer closure and makes the implant pocket more secure.

Another alternative approach is to make an external submental incision just beneath the bony prominence of the chin (Fig. 172). While many surgeons prefer this approach, the author utilizes it only when a submental lipectomy is also being performed. However, the slightly curvilinear incision is well camouflaged and is only visualized when the patient's head is tilted backward. Using this approach, the skin and subcutaneous tissues are sharply incised and separated, followed by blunt dissection up over the chin using Metzenbaum scissors and finger dissection to form a pocket anterior to the periosteum. At this stage, the remainder of the pocket preparation for the implant is similar to the intraoral approach (Fig. 173 and 174).

The main objective of the soft tissue pocket preparation is to form a pocket just slightly larger than the size of the intended implant. This pocket is formed superficial to the anterior mandibular periosteum—if placed subperiosteally the implant will erode the cortex and migrate posteriorly. The

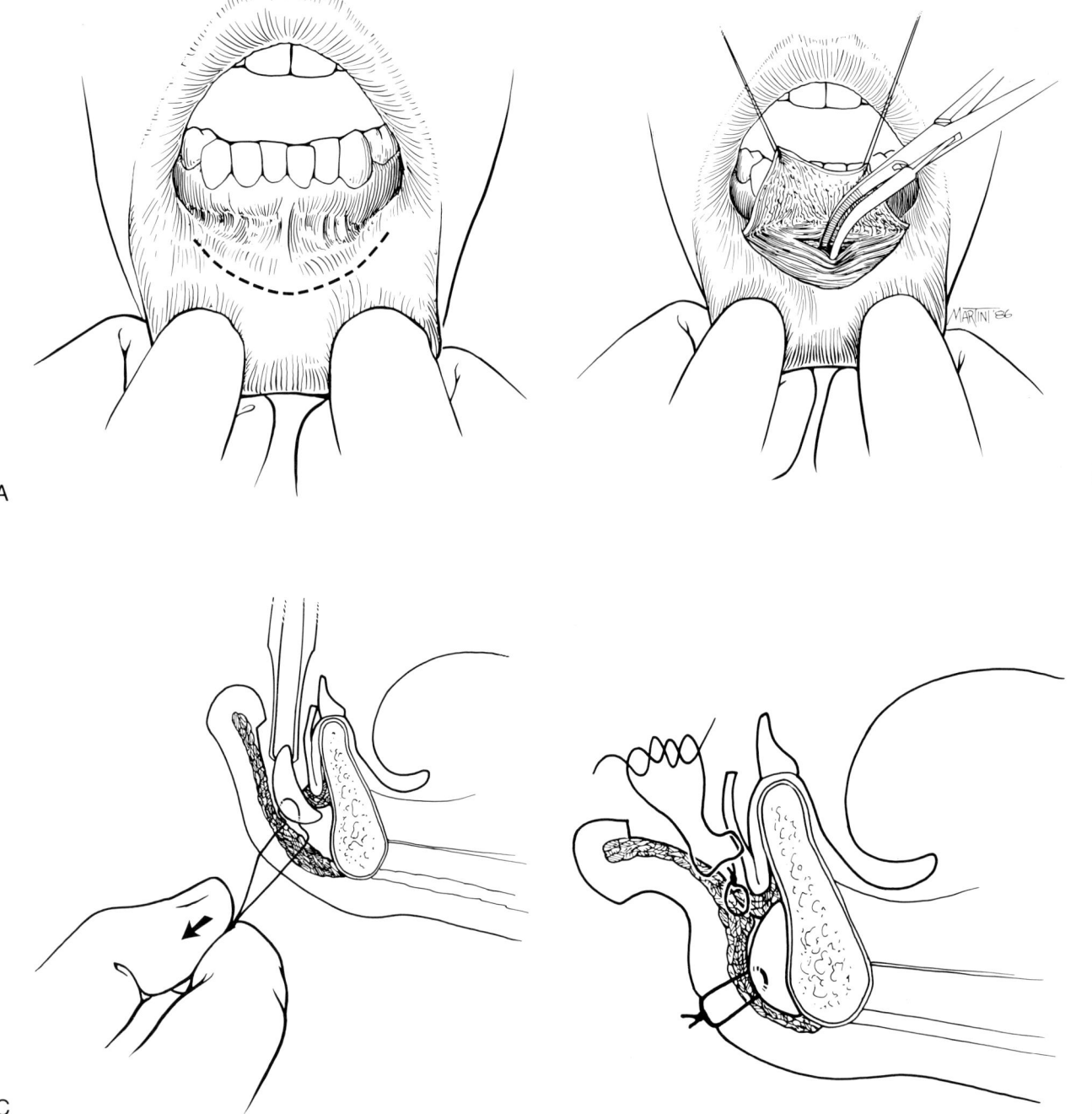

Figure 173. Intraoral chin implant procedure. (A) Incision. (B) Opening mentalis muscles in midline with blunt dissection. (C) Position of implant and guide sutures in lateral view. (D) closure in three layers.

pocket should be formed symmetrically on both sides of the midline so as to prevent a malposition of the implant. It is quite difficult to reposition the implant once scar healing has occurred. Using a combination of blunt finger and scissor dissection, the submuscular pocket is formed. Hemostasis is achieved under direct visualization using point (unipolar) cautery or wet-field (bipolar) cautery. A completely dry field is required since any hematoma formation may jeopardize the implant retention. In this respect it is important to insist that the patient refrain from taking any medication containing aspirin or aspirinlike compounds for 1 week prior and 1 week following surgery.

Once the pocket is formed, the implant can be inserted to test the size and position of the pocket.

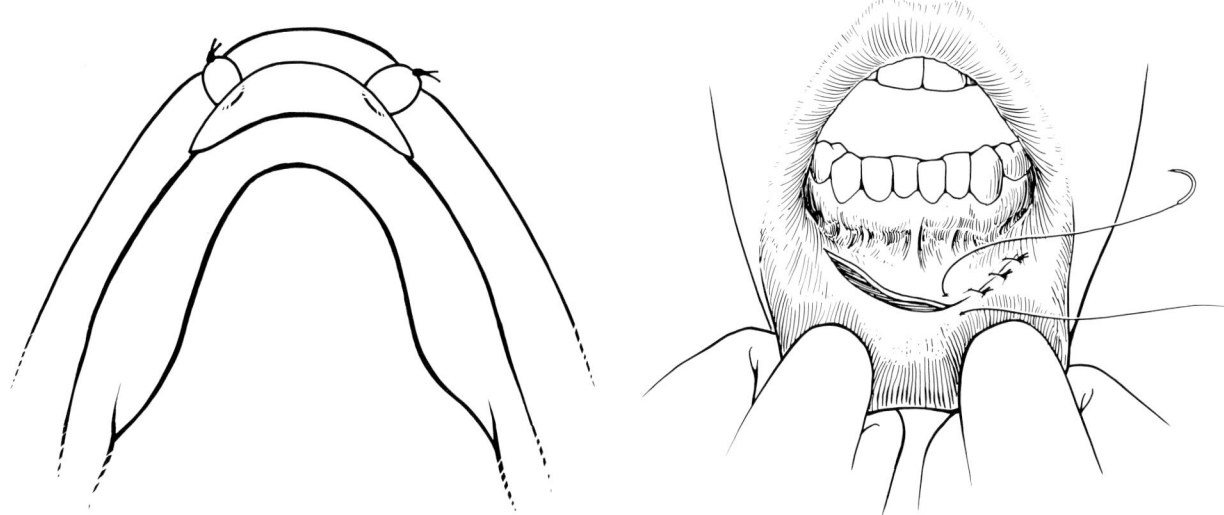

Figure 173. (E) Axial view of stay sutures to secure the implant position. (F) Closure of lip incision with running suture.

All potential contamination such as dust and powder should be washed free from the implant, gloves, and instruments. Each time the implant is handled it should be washed and placed in saline for temporary storage. Finally, once the implant is judged to be in the best location, the pocket should be irrigated copiously.

In testing the pocket by inserting the implant, the borders can be palpated and marked with a surgical pen to determine if the position is correct and symmetrical. In most patients the pocket will be sufficiently close to the size of the implant that the "fit" will be snug. However, if the implant tends to wander or move within the pocket, "stay" sutures can be placed to maintain the implant in its desired position. One, two, or three Prolene sutures can be placed in the midline and lateral chin. The sutures are first placed through the skin and into the pocket; the implant is then "skewered" when it is in the best position. The suture is then brought out through the skin and tied over a soft stent. If placed correctly, the sutures will guide the implant into its proper position and maintain it there. If placed incorrectly these sutures will hold the implant in a malposition. As with most cosmetic and reconstructive facial surgery, considerable spacial awareness is required to visualize and to place both the implant and the stay sutures. However, the approximate position of the implant can be drawn preoperatively onto the black and white photographs to guide the surgeon during the procedure to ensure the correct placement of the implant.

The intraoral incision should be closed in at least three layers; muscular and submucosal layers with Dexon, Vicryl, or PDS; and the mucosa with chromic catgut. This intraoral approach must be closed in a water-tight fashion so that saliva does not contaminate the deep tissues. An extraoral incision can also be closed in the three layers but using Prolene for the skin. The intraoral wound is not drained, but if a concomitant submental lipectomy has been performed, an extraoral incision should be drained for 24 h.

Splinting the chin is a very important aspect for the postoperative procedures. The skin can be cleansed of its natural oils and a firm elastic dressing applied from the mid-cheek to the upper neck in a criss-cross manner to immobilize the chin and lower mandible. The author immobilizes the chin for 72 postoperatively. This allows for early formation of a fibroblastic response around the implant. The immobilizing dressing is removed and the position of the implant checked. If the position of the implant is fine, a light dressing of hypoallergenic tape can be applied for several days to remind the patient that perioral motion should be minimized. An additional aspect of the dressing technique should be emphasized; namely, that the tape should be placed tightly across the lower lip below the vermillion border to compress the labial sulcus and prevent saliva pooling in the region of the incision. As soon as the dressings have been removed, the patient can begin gentle salt water irrigation of the oral cavity.

The main complications of this procedure include implant, infection, malposition, and extrusion. Impending implant extrusion is usually seen as increased tenderness and swelling at the implant site

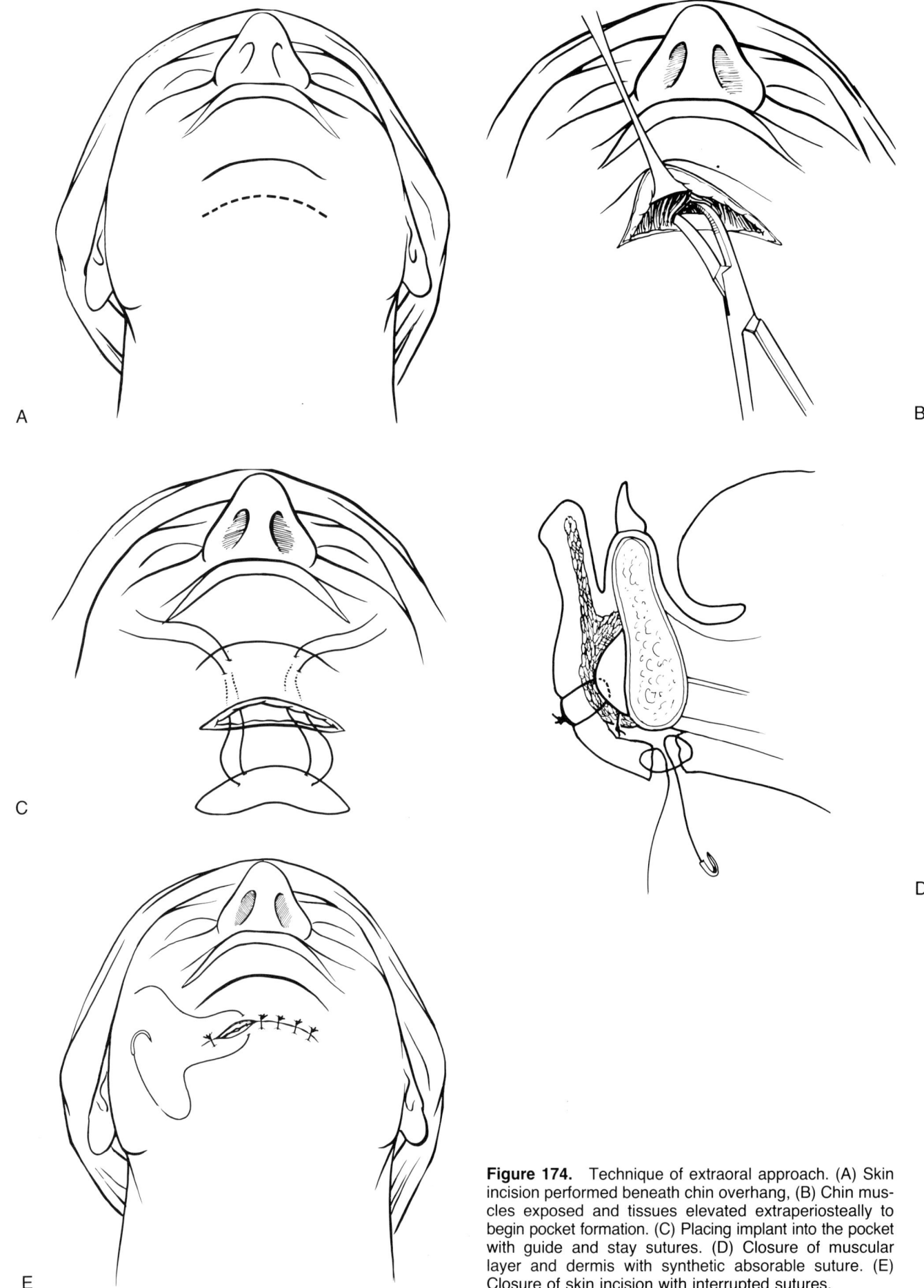

Figure 174. Technique of extraoral approach. (A) Skin incision performed beneath chin overhang, (B) Chin muscles exposed and tissues elevated extraperiosteally to begin pocket formation. (C) Placing implant into the pocket with guide and stay sutures. (D) Closure of muscular layer and dermis with synthetic absorbable suture. (E) Closure of skin incision with interrupted sutures.

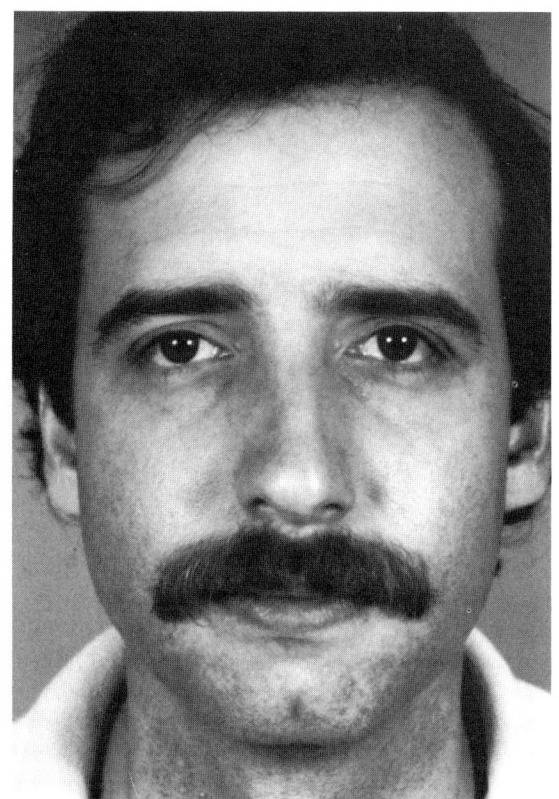

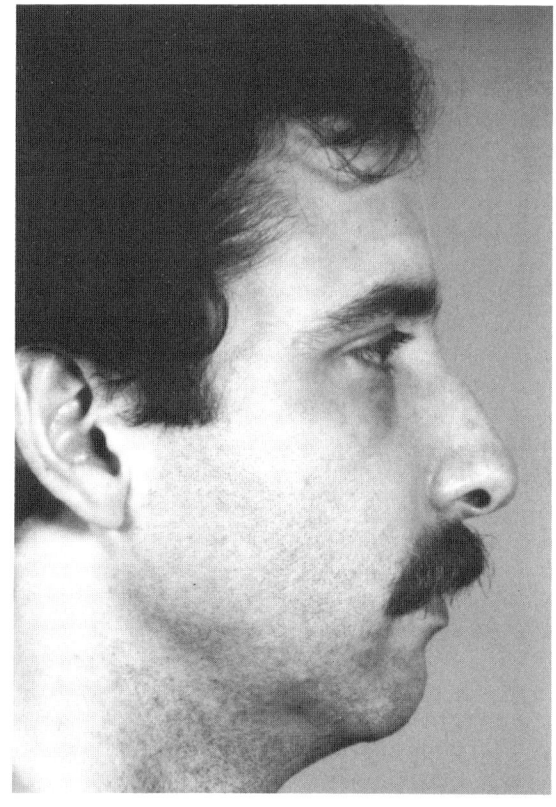

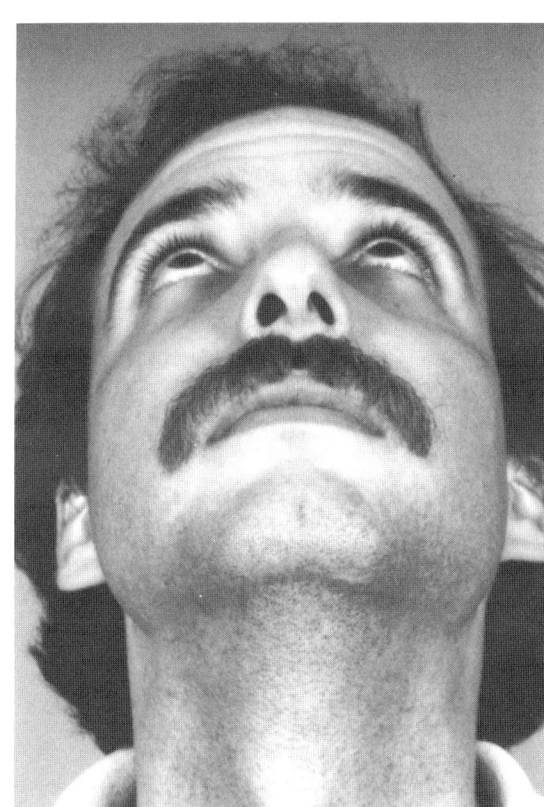

Figure 175. Preoperative views of patient with nasal hump deformity, deficient chin, and Class 1 occlusion.

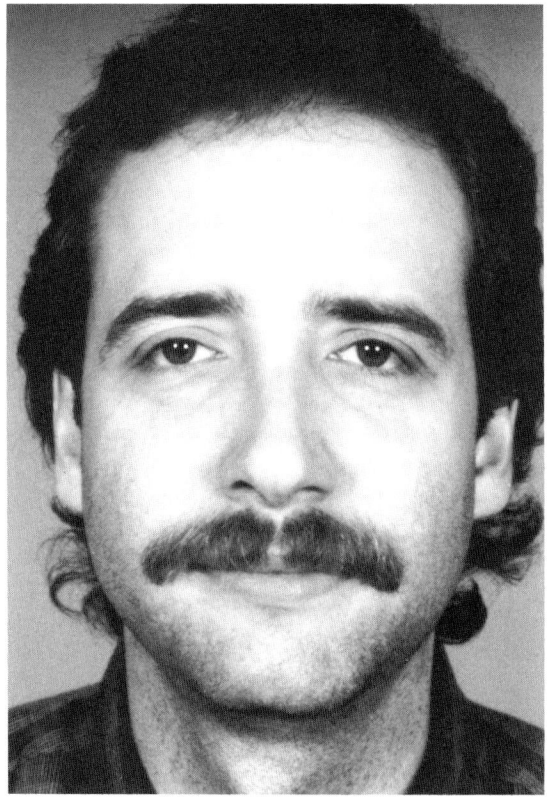

D

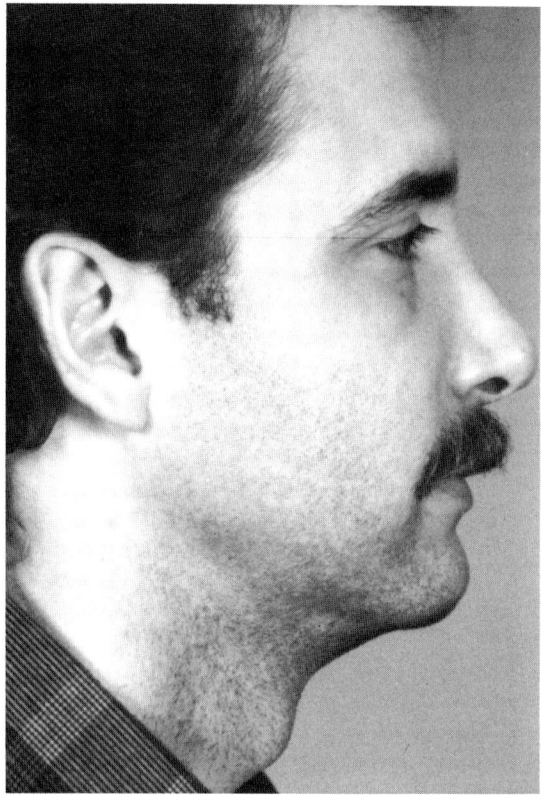

E

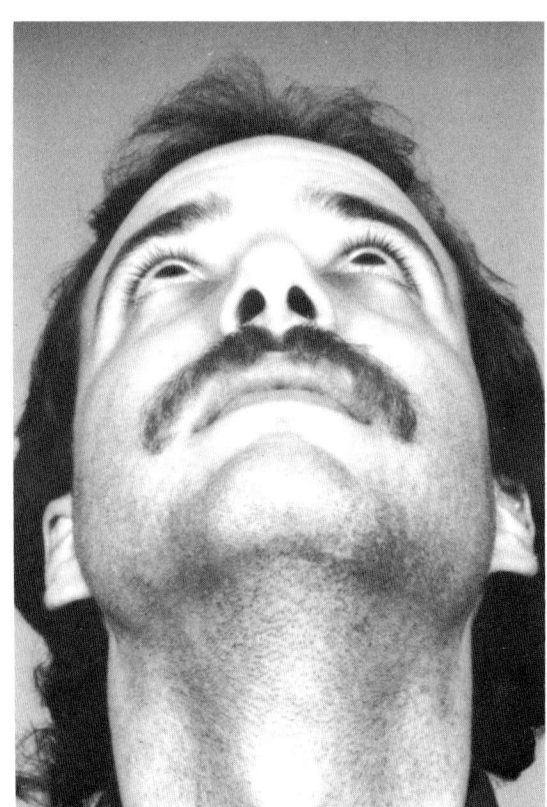

F

Figure 175. 15 months after reduction septorhinoplasty and extraoral insertion of medium-small Silastic chin implant. Note obliteration of chin dimple after insertion of implant.

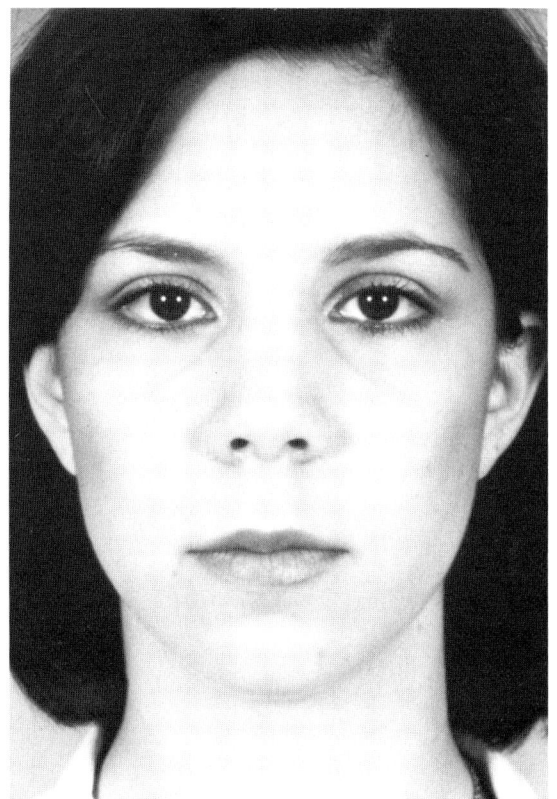
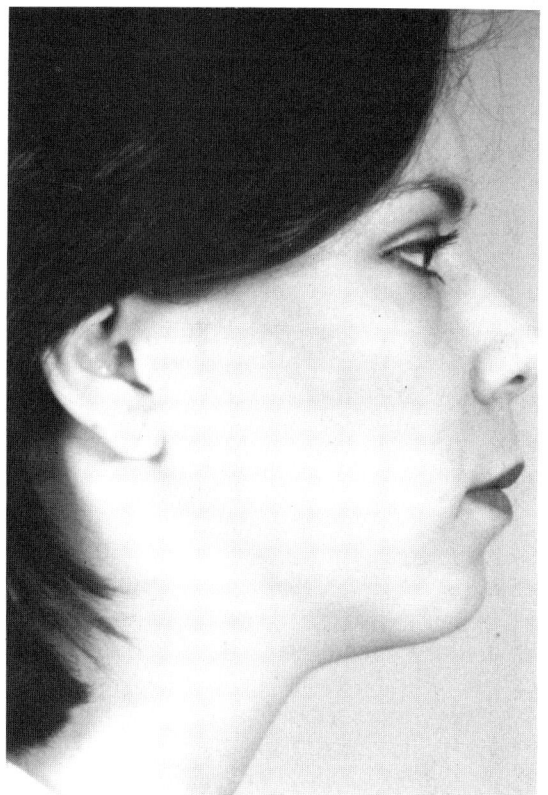
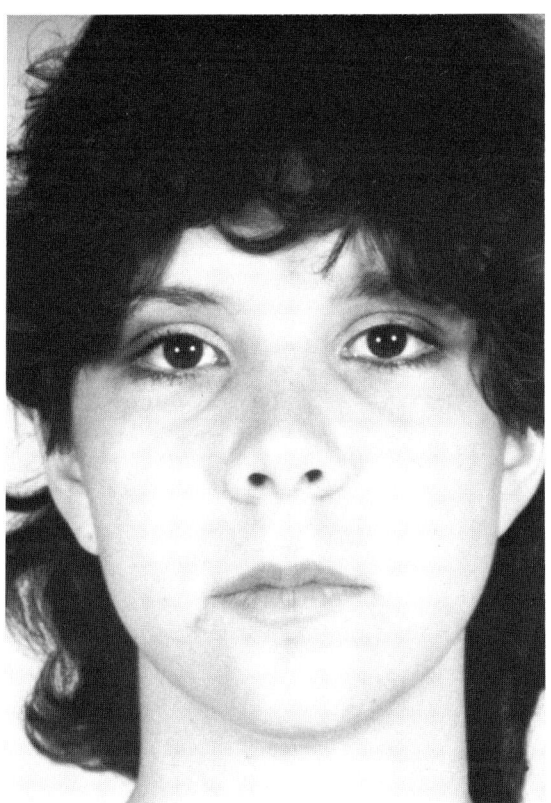
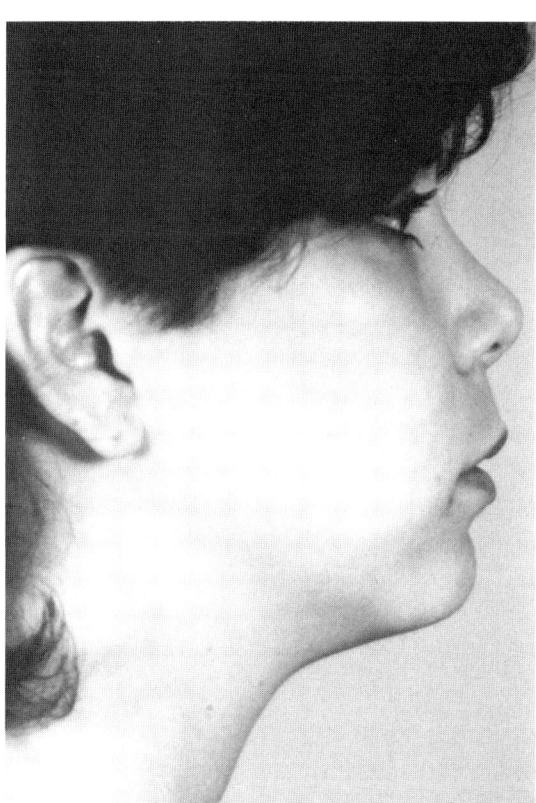

Figure 176. (A, B) Preoperative view of patient with flat, broad nose, mild chin recession, and Class 1 occlusion. (C, D) 12 months after septorhinoplasty and intraoral placement of small Silastic chin implant.

and early dehiscence of the incision. If diagnosed early, broad-spectrum antibiotics can be initiated and the incision resutured under local anesthesia. However, this therapy often is not successful and the implant should be removed under these circumstances. The author does not immediately replace the implant but rather allows the wound to heal and then reevaluates the clinical appearance with the patient before recommending further surgery.

Infection is most commonly seen due to inattention to proper techniques when handling the prosthesis and closing the wound, or when a hematoma has formed. It is very difficult to manage these conditions and the implant usually has to be removed. However, conservative measures should first be tried.

Malposition of the implant may be iatrogenic in etiology or may be due to an inadvertent injury on the patient's part in the postoperative period. The most common reasons for the movement of the implant, in the author's experience, include retching and vomiting by the patient (causing excessive motion of the chin muscles), an external blow or bump to the chin (often administered by the patient's children), and significant talking and chewing too early in the postoperative period. Most of these can be avoided by the preoperative counseling of the patient and explanatory patient educational material. If malposition is present and infection is absent, the author prefers to reoperate under local anesthesia with intravenous sedation, and reposition the implant. This almost always achieves a satisfactory result.

SUMMARY

When performed for the proper indications and using proven surgical techniques, augmentation of the chin with alloplastic material can be a very successful means of improving facial harmony (Figs. 175 and 176). When performed in conjunction with a reduction septorhinoplasty, the total appearance of the face can be improved. However, attention must be paid to the surgical details of the procedure and the appropriate postoperative care must be provided. Complications can often be prevented, but if they do occur, they should be dealt with immediately.

BIBLIOGRAPHY

1. Beekhuis GJ: Augmentation mentoplasty with polyamide mesh: Update. Arch Otolaryngol 110:364–370, 1984
2. McCarthy JG: Microgenia: A logical surgical approach. Clin Plast Surg 8:269–278, 1981
3. Powell N, Humphreys B: The five major aesthetic masses of the face—the chin. In Proportions of the Aesthetic Face. New York: Thieme-Stratton, 1984, pp 35–39
4. Snyder BG, Courtiss EH, Kaye BM, et al.: New chin implant for microgenia. Plast Reconstr Surg 61:854–861, 1978

12 Reconstruction of the Mandible

G. Richard Holt, M.D.

Surgical procedures to remove tumors of the mandible and to repair mandibular fractures have been dealt with in the preceding chapters. This chapter will deal with the various means of reconstructing the mandible following any cause that leads to discontinuity. The major causes of mandibular discontinuity include tumor resection, loss from trauma, unsuccessful healing of a mandibular fracture, osteonecrosis following radiation therapy, and atrophy due to aging and demineralization. A wide variety of forms of mandibular reconstruction will be presented to give the reader a breadth of exposure to the many techniques that are being utilized by head and neck surgeons today. For greater depth in any technique, the reader is referred to the References section at the end of the chapter.

TYPES OF RECONSTRUCTION

An interesting variety of materials has been utilized to provide restoration of continuity to the mandible following loss of substance and space. These materials include the alloplastics, the metallic reconstruction bars, autogenous bone, and free and pedicled composite bone flaps. Each of these will be discussed in detail in this chapter.

Autogenous Bone Grafts

Autogenous bone grafts, used either by themselves or in conjunction with another form of mandibular reconstruction, represent the present mainstay of grafting and reconstructive techniques. Such grafts provide a nonantigenic source of osseous support with the potential for forming new bone by the proliferation of precursor cells to osteoblasts. Cortical bone by itself is not capable of osteoneogenesis but does serve as a good structural support until osteoclastic and enzymatic absorption of its matrix occurs. When cortical bone is resorbed, either new bone or fibrous tissue is formed in its place depending on whether periosteum is present or whether soft tissue is in direct apposition to its surface. Sources of cortical bone for reconstruction in the head and neck include the scapular spine, thoracic rib, and iliac crest. These sources represent the most commonly utilized sites for obtaining strictly cortical bone.

Perhaps a better source of free autogenous bone for the reconstruction of defects of the mandible is the bone-containing marrow or cancellous bone. In most adults there are very few flat bones that still contain marrow, so cancellous bone is usually obtained from the iliac wing between the two parallel cortical surfaces. The technique for obtaining this graft will be discussed in Autogenous Bone Grafts, below. Cancellous bone is so useful in mandibular reconstruction because of its potential to produce osteoblasts that will lay down new bone within the matrix of the graft. It is felt that much of the substance of the cancellous bone graft will remain intact during the first several months after grafting, during which time the old osteocytes will not survive, although their channels will be taken over by the new osteocytes. In addition, a small amount of new bone matrix with new osteocytes will be formed at the periphery of the graft. This process appears to occur in the cancellous bone graft whether periosteum is present on the graft or not.

Cortical bone is useful as a graft when some strength and stability of the graft is required—it can be wired in place or attached to a reconstruction plate and will maintain its stability for months and even years. However, it can be expected to lose up to 60% of its integrity and volume over the first several years it is in its new recipient site. An additional drawback with the cortical graft is that it is fairly brittle at first and can be fractured easily with a direct blow to the region of the graft. For this reason most cortical grafts are not utilized by themselves in mandibular reconstruction but rather serve as a trough or tray to hold cancellous bone in the proper position.

Cancellous bone by itself is a very soft, poorly fixable bone graft and not capable of handling any extent of external force. It is therefore not utilized as a mandibular spacer wired in position without some additional fixation support such as an internal tray, reconstruction plate, or external fixation device. This graft has the ability to achieve osteoneogenesis even in the soft tissues of the mandibular region so long as it is in contact with the ends of the recipient mandibular segment(s), and when fixation of the mandible is achieved by some other means, bony union is likely to occur.

While the iliac crest is the favored place to obtain cortical and cancellous bone grafts, the ribs are also source of material. In adults, the ribs tend to be somewhat brittle and easily fractured, while in younger adults there is a tendency for them to be softer, probably because of larger marrow-containing compartment. While intact ribs have been utilized for mandibular reconstruction, it is more common practice to split the rib or to wedge the inner table to conform to the curvature of the mandible and to insert portions of cancellous bone to conform the the "splint" of the rib. As will be discussed in Autogenous Bone Grafts, below, the obtaining of a rib has a somewhat more morbid potential than does the technique of iliac crest harvesting.

Another technique for utilizing autogenous bone involves the harvesting of the patient's mandible and treating it to rid it of whatever disease process is involved initally. This might involve curetting out the interior of the mandible to form a trough for cancellous bone from the iliac crest or subjecting the mandibular segment to freezing or irradiation. The latter two techniques are usually utilized in those patients in whom a malignancy involving the mandible is resected, and the cell-killing procedure is carried out while the patient is still under anesthesia. The main advantage to this use of the patient's own mandible is that it is nonantigenic and has the exact anatomic conformation. Disadvantages include the fact that the bone is usually nonvital and success depends on the replacement and remodeling of the bone by the cancellous graft.

Formal Appliances and Metallic Reconstruction Bars

As was stated in the preceding section, most cancellous grafts are not utilized alone but are combined with some other form of fixation, stabilization, and space formation. The most common devices for this task include metallic trays and metallic reconstruction bars. The other function that these appliances play in the reconstruction of the mandible is to maintain the proper distance between the proximal and distal fragments of the mandible to be reconstructed. While some surgeons attempt to provide a space maintenance with these devices in preparation for future secondary reconstruction, the truth is that they often cause so much foreign body reaction unless used in conjunction with a bone graft that this procedure is being minimized in clinical practice.

Many types of metallic appliances have been proposed in the past and currently in the literature, including those made of stainless steel, vitallium (chrome-cobalt alloy), titanium, and other precious metals. Most mesh trays are currently being produced from either vitallium or titanium, and serve to bridge the gap between the ends of the mandible and to hold the cancellous bone grafts in the proper shape and position during the bone remodeling process. These trays are usually secured to the mandibular segments with steel wires or lag screws. The trays are meshed in their configuration to allow ingrowth of the budding vascularization from the surrounding soft tissues, which is necessary for the nourishment and support of the process of osteoneogenesis.

The second form of metallic device frequently used in mandibular reconstruction is the *reconstruction bar*. This bar is long and narrow and contains predrilled holes that allow the insertion of wires or screws anywhere along its length to secure the bar to the mandibular segments as well as to the bone graft. These bars are malleable and can be either preformed to fit a certain segmental configuration of the mandible or bent at the time of surgery to conform to the particular need of the surgery at hand. Some bar devices are similar to the compression plates utilized in the repair and stabilization of mandibular fractures. In providing compression, these bars encourage the formation of a bony callous rather than the more fibrous union that often occurs with conventional mandibular reconstruction. As a drawback, however, the bars are bulky and often are removed electively, or frequently when they become syptomatic. Another reason for removing the bar is to allow the remodeling mandibular graft to begin accepting more loading forces and align its healing along the lines of stress and function.

Alloplastic Materials

Most alloplastic materials, with the exception of stainless steel and the rare metals, have been the subject of some negative comments in regard to their utilization in mandibular reconstruction because of their high antigenicity and failure rate. However, some authors have reported rather good results with certain allogenic materials including polyurethane and Dacron mesh, Silastic, and Teflon. Other materials such as plaster of paris and hydroxylapatite have been implicated in a process that encourages new bone formation in the region of placement of these grafts. The success of alloplastic grafts is greatly compromised in the reconstruction of a mandible by previous radiation therapy, and for that reason their greatest application has been in the reconstruction of mandibles injured by trauma or after resection of benign tumors. Another important requirement of the alloplastic graft implant is that abundant, well-vascularized soft tissue overlie the defect as exposure, and extrusion of these implants occurs commonly with inadequate soft tissue coverage.

Occasionally, reconstruction will be done in a patient with the use of an alloplastic implant coupled with an autogenous bone graft to provide new bone as well as functioning as a spacing device. However, the end-result is that the implant usually require removal in order to give the best osseous result.

Free Composite Grafts

Since the development of modern techniques of microvascular surgery, medical ingenuity has focused on the utilization of free tissue flaps that incorporate a bony segment in the reconstruction of defects of the head and neck. One of the first free composite flaps to be used was the dorsalis pedis-metatarsal flap. Since then, the two most commonly used flaps were developed, namely, the latissimus dorsi-rib flap and the deep circumflex iliac-crest flap. Both of these two latter flaps are compound flaps, including the overlying skin, muscle, and bone components, with the vascular pedicle reattached to a convenient large vessel group in the head and neck region. These free flaps are not for the casual head and neck surgeon to use in the reconstruction of mandibular defects; rather, the surgical skills required to successfully perform free flaps operations are learned during a long period of acquisition of laboratory skills, prior to utilizing the technique in a patient care setting.

Pedicled Composite Flaps

In contrast to the free flap procedure outlined above, which requires reanastomosis to artery and vein in the head and neck recipient site, pedicled composite flaps remain attached to their feeding blood supply during the healing phase. The advantage here is that the components of the flap, including the skin, muscle, and attached bone fragments, remain vascularized during the most risky time of transplantion, that is, until the the overlying skin and mucosa heal. Several flaps have become popular with head and neck surgeons for utilization in mandibular reconstruction, including the trapezius, pectoralis major, and latissimus dorsi myoosteocutaneous flaps. These flaps incorporate scapular spine and rib, respectively, for the osseous component. These flaps can be utilized for both immediate and secondary reconstruction, and provide the advantages of reconstructing a soft tissue defect prior to bony reconstruction, and bringing in non-irradiated tissue to improve the chances of bone graft survival.

IMMEDIATE VERSUS DELAYED RECONSTRUCTION

Unfortunately, there are no hard and fast rules that govern the choice of immediate versus delayed reconstruction of the mandible. Because of this uncertainty, most surgeons develop a patient-by-patient decision-making technique that takes into account each patient's individual needs and his particular circumstances. However, certain consistent factors occur frequently enough that some general rules or guidelines may be developed for the head and neck surgeon when making the decision for immediate or delayed reconstruction. In most patients, it is unwise to attempt primary reconstruction in a heavily irradiated area unless a vascularized graft is utilized, either free or pedicled. The nutritional considerations of the patient must also be considered; for example, the situation of the cachectic patient in negative nitrogen balance is not conducive to good healing of the involved area.

Essentially, the patient who has had a resection of the mandible secondary to a benign tumor, such as a cementifying fibroma, is an excellent candidate for immediate reconstruction. Patients with benign lesions are usually younger and therefore in better physical and nutritional condition. A more definite consideration is that the younger patient is likely to be gainfully employed and have a greater requirement for the social and economic ramifications of adequate speech and swallowing. Using the same reasoning, reconstruction of a failed mandibular fracture repair should be performed as soon as feasible if there is no evidence of active infection.

While gunshot wounds usually occur in the younger patient, these constitute a different category for consideration of reconstruction than the younger patient with a benign tumor or fracture. Most low-caliber missiles (i.e., .25 or .32 caliber) are not likely to cause a large loss of mandibular substance, and under most conditions of healing the patient with wounds inflicted by such missiles will not require mandibular reconstruction. Conversely, the mandible that has been severely damaged by high-velocity missiles (i.e., .223 and 30-06 caliber) will also have serious soft tissue damage in the immediate vicinity of the wound that must be dealt with before reconstruction can be attempted. Since the kinetic energy of the missile entering the tissues is directly proportional to the mass of the missile but exponentially proportional (to the factor of 2) to the velocity of the missile, it can be seen that high-velocity missiles can inflict the greatest damage. Significant soft tissue repair and healing must be accomplished prior to reconstructing the mandible in cases of gunshot wounds caused by high-velocity missiles.

In cases of malignant tumor excision, the operating surgeon must make the decision regarding immediate versus delayed reconstruction based on the medical information at hand. One common reason for delaying reconstruction is uncertainty about the possibility of local tumor recurrence. Many surgeons elect to take the conservative approach and wait approximately 1 year following the completion of surgery or radiation therapy. If recurrent cancer is diagnosed during this period, it is much easier to stage and treat without having disturbed the tissues by a reconstructive attempt. As a general rule, if there is any doubt about the frozen section diagnosis, or if the pathologist must wait for decalcification to give a judgment on the presence or absence of bone invasion, then the reconstruction attempts should be withheld until the diagnosis is final. Under those conditions, it is probably wise to delay reconstruction until adequate healing of the intraoral defect has occurred. One of the most important areas to look at histopathologically is the mandibular nerve, and a frozen section should always be considered before deciding on reconstruction.

Some consideration can also be given to selecting delayed versus immediate reconstruction based on the location of the mandibular defect. All things being equal, if the anterior symphyseal segment is absent, more consideration can be given to reconstructing the anterior arch in order to prevent the need for a long-dwelling tracheostomy and the associated speech and swallowing difficulties. Defects of the body and ramus of the mandible, such as those produced after composite tongue and tonsillar cancer resections, are much better tolerated by the patient in this regard. However, the final decision in all categories dealing with malignancies must be whether there remains a risk for recurrent or residual cancer at the mandibular site.

SPECIFIC TECHNIQUES OF RECONSTRUCTION

Autogenous Bone Grafts

The mainstay of mandibular reconstruction rests with the replacement of the missing mandibular segment by autogenous bone grafts. The two most commonly used graft materials are corticocancellous bone grafts obtained from the thoracic rib and iliac crest. As previously stated, the ribs in older patients are composed primarily of cortical bone with only a small amount of marrow or cancellous bone present. However, if the rib is split and placed in the mandibular compartment to serve as a spacing device, the trough it forms can be filled with iliac crest cancellous bone for its osteoneogenetic potential.[1] The best rib for excision is the fifth rib, but the sixth or seventh may also be used. If the patient requires a fairly curved segment of rib for mandibular replacement, then the rib may be obtained from the most lateral segment in the midaxillary line, in order to take advantage of the natural curvature at that point, However, it is usually easier for the head and neck surgeon to harvest the rib graft while the patient remains in the supine position, rather than the awkward lateral decubitus position. With an incision along the curvature of the rib margin as it approaches the xiphoid, the area of the fifth and sixth ribs are exposed and hemostasis achieved. The periosteum is incised on the superior and inferior margins of the fifth rib and by gentle dissection with a blunt elevator the rib is separated from its underlying periosteum and pleura. It is wise to leave periosteum on one cortical surface of the rib in an attempt to encourage revascularization of the bone. While a power saw can be used to sever the ends of the rib *in situ,* the safest technique is to use a mastoid drill to carefully produce a cleavage at the point of desired severance. If a small rent in the pleura is created, it may be sutured with Prolene suture and the patient observed for persistent leakage. However, for larger iatrogenic tears, a chest tube should be inserted in the second interspace in the usual fashion and the rent repaired.

The rib may be utilized in one of two ways for mandibular reconstruction. As previously mentioned, the rib may be split in half by drilling with the mastoid drill and wiring it on either side of the remaining mandibular fragments to form a trough (Figs. 177 to 181). The trough may be filled with cancellous bone chips. On the other hand, the inner table or the concave surface of the rib may be wedged in order to produce a controlled bending

Reconstruction of the Mandible 153

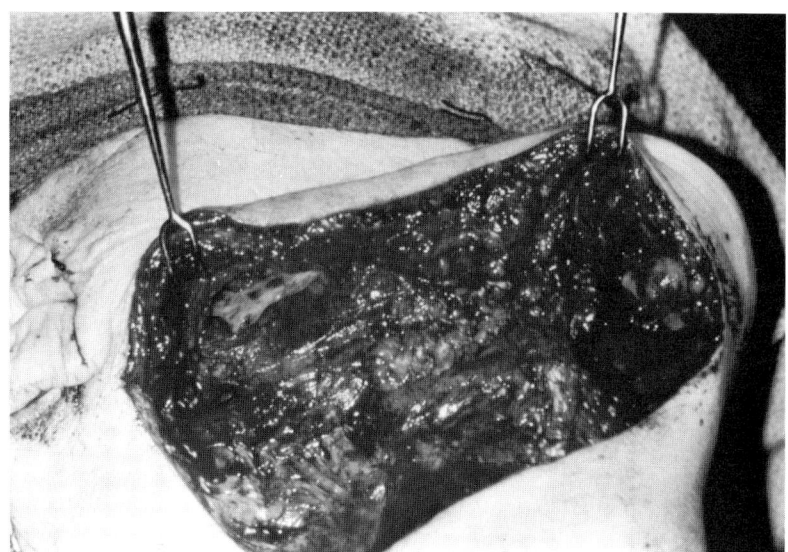

Figure 177. Patient 1 year after right partial mandibulectomy for alveolar squamous cell carcinoma. At reconstruction only a small fragment of ascending ramus is seen in the left center of the wound.

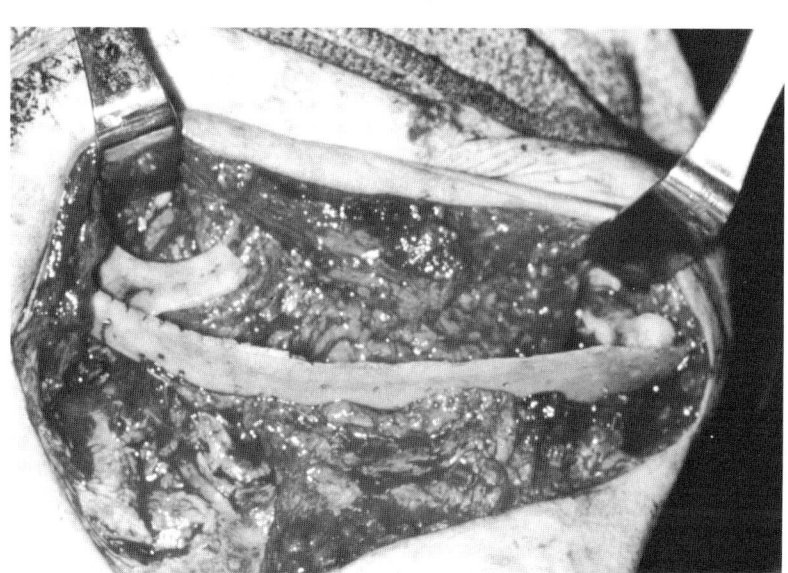

Figure 178. Split rib is utilized to form the new outline for the mandibular reconstruction.

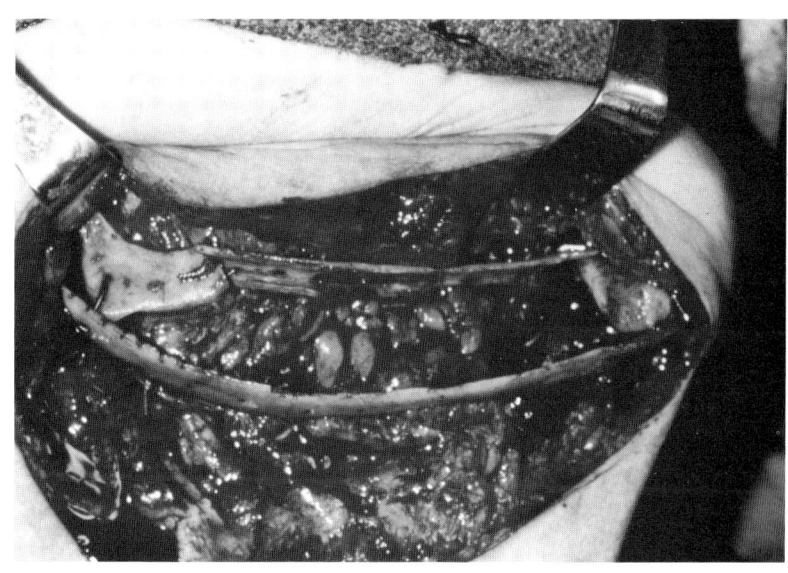

Figure 179. Both the superior and inferior borders have been reconstructed with split rib and wired into place at the ramus stump and the parasymphyseal region.

154 Surgery of the Mandible

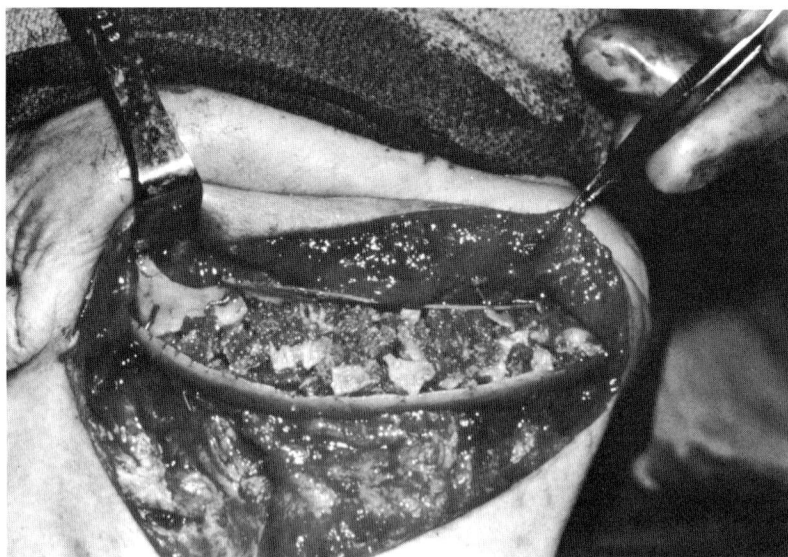

Figure 180. Autogenous iliac crest bone has been fragmented and placed into the split rib conformer.

of the rib to a more curved configuration to better simulate the mandibular requirements. Here the convex cortical surface, which has its attached periosteum, will actually be fractured in a "greenstick" manner, reducing its stability but also allowing it to conform better to the mandibular curvature.

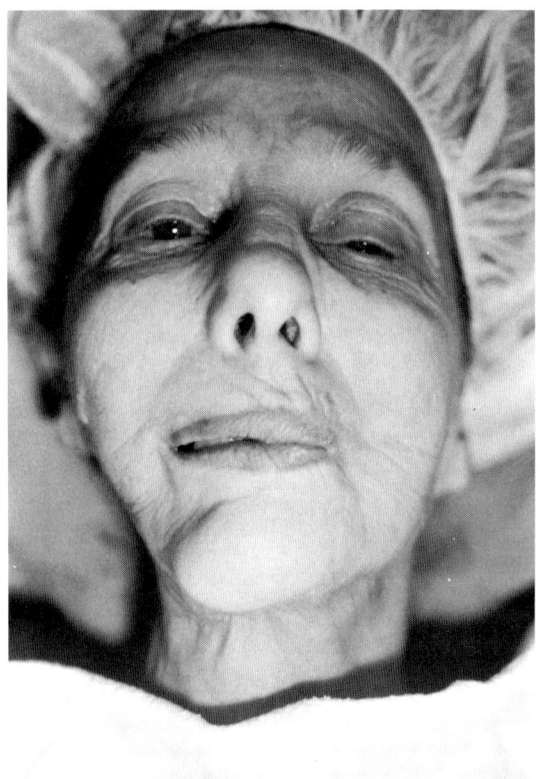

Figure 181. Patient 5 months after split rib-iliac crest bone reconstruction. Note right facial paresis seen as a complication of inadvertent pressure on the facial nerve trunk by the proximal portion of the split rib (see Chapter 14).

The rib is wired in place with intraosseous stainless steel wires in the usual fracture fashion.

The mainstay of the reconstruction of the mandible is the iliac crest corticocancellous bone graft. Because of the presence of cellular material that has the potential to differentiate into osteoblasts and osteoclasts, the entire process of bone resorption and osteogenesis occurs when the cancellous bone graft is utilized. Obviously, neovascularization has to occur to bring in the oxygen and nutrition that are required for bone growth. It is felt that the original matrix of the cancellous bone graft is absorbed to a certain degree but does maintain a certain amount of bulk intact. As will be mentioned in Chapter 14, there is a moderate amount of disability associated with obtaining an iliac crest graft which persists for several weeks after the actual surgical procedure. Grillon and associates have reported a technique for obtaining a cancellous bone graft from the ilium that appears to decrease the postoperative morbidity.[2] By raising an osteoperiosteal flap from the crest of the ilium and removing a medial corticocancellous bone block, the graft site morbidity is minimized. After the standard exposure via a curvilinear incision over the superior portion of the iliac crest only minimal dissection over the crest is performed. With an osteotome the bony-muscular "cap" is removed from the crest and relected superiorly. The periosteum is reflected off the medial surface of the crest and the inner cortical table is exposed. The corticocancellous plug is taken with a chisel or osteotome according to the reconstructive needs. The previously reflected bony-muscular cap is replaced and fixed in place using intraosseous wiring. The graft is stored in cold isotonic saline for later utilization. Postoperative drains are not used unless hemostasis is a problem. If a graft is required in a pediatric patient, the authors recommend use of the lateral iliac crest due to a possible disturbance in the growth of the cartilaginous portion of the iliac crest.

In certain benign conditions of the mandible, it is possible to replace the excised mandibular segment after removal of the abnormal pathology. An ideal case for this replacement is the excision of an arteriovenous malformation of the mandible.[3,4] Following removal of the vascular tumor by curetting and drilling out the cancellous portion of the mandibular segment, it can be replaced in the patient using intraosseous wiring, reconstruction plates, or a metallic mesh for attachment to the remaining segments (Figs. 182 to 195). The replaced segment of mandible is essentially an autogenous bone trough which can be filled with cancellous bone from the iliac crest. The indications are few for utilizing the mandibular segment in this manner and there is always a slight risk that the arteriovenouus malformation might reestablish itself in small channels not completely eradicated.

Leipzig and Cummings have recently reported their final comments following several years of animal and patient studies on the use of autogenous frozen mandibular grafts for reconstruction.[5] They

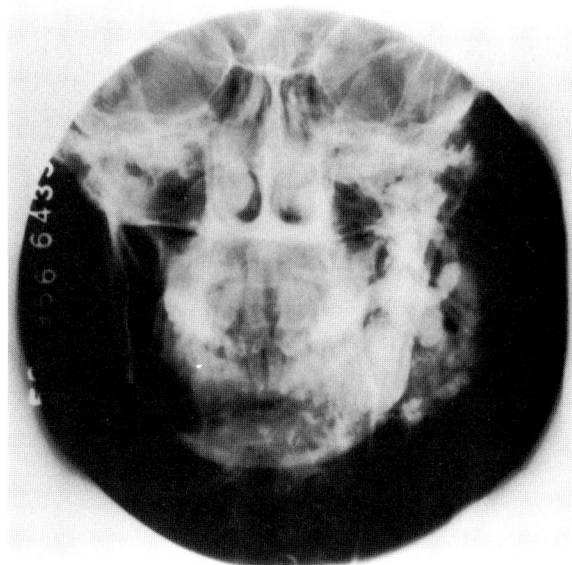

Figure 183. Arteriogram of patient with extensive arteriovenous malformation of left mandible.

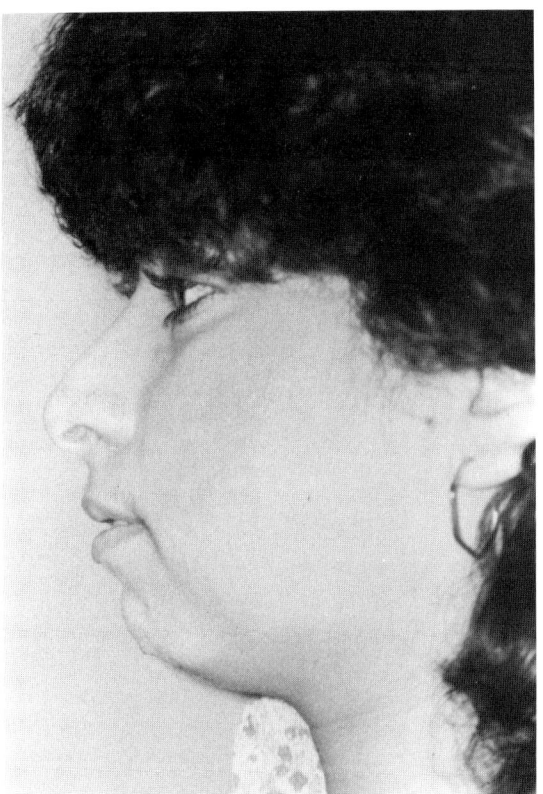

Figure 182. Patient with extensive bony and soft tissue involvement in left mandibular region with arteriovenous malformation.

originally felt that the functional and cosmetic debility surrounding mandibular resection was significant enough to warrant an attempt to replace the patient's own mandible following cancer surgery. They stated that "use of the patient's own mandible should ideally adapt perfectly to provide a solution that satisfies both functional and cosmetic demands." Freezing kills the bone, however, and it serves merely as a cortical stent that should be filled with marrow to allow restitution of osteoblastic activity. Previous animal studies had shown that the frozen, grafted mandibular segment demonstrated evidence of osteoneogenesis.[6,7] In the Leipzig and Cummings report, they utilized frozen autogenous mandible to reconstruct patients after excision of clinical stage 4 cancer of the floor of the mouth. In all six patients the regrafted mandibular site failed to heal and the authors have abandoned the procedure at the present time as a form of immediate reconstruction of the mandible. It is important to note that these grafts failed even in the presence of a soft tissue flap used to reconstruct the floor of the mouth and provide adequately vascularized tissue around the graft. The causes of failure included contamination from intraoral complications and tumor recurrence in adjacent soft tissues.

On the other hand, Hamaker and colleagues have reported a 66% success rate when using irradiated mandibular autografts for reconstruction of mandibular defects after cancer surgery.[8] Following removal of the specimen for total extirpation of the tumor, the mandibular segment is dissected free of the specimen and the bone is centrally drilled,

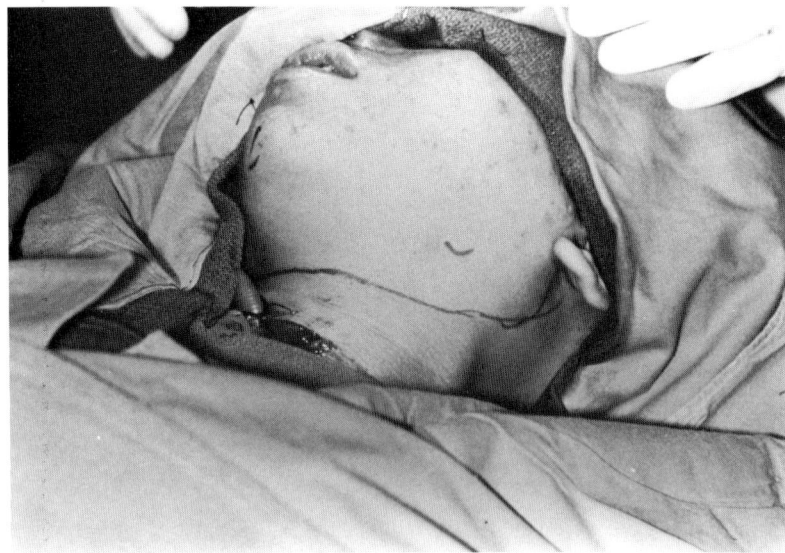

Figure 184. Following elective tracheostomy the arteriovenous malformation was exposed via a horizontal upper neck incision.

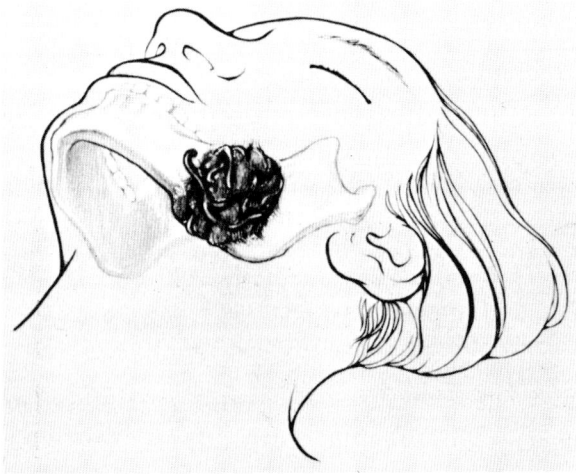

Figure 185. Artist's conception of extent of involvement of patient's mandible with arteriovenous malformation.

removing all material, including nerve, except for the cortical shell. This segment is then placed in a bag with saline and 100% oxygen introduced by catheter. The bag is then transported to the radiation therapy suite where it is subjected to 10,000 rad of external beam radiation. This usually takes 30 to 40 min, allowing time for closure of the intraoral defect or the placement of a regional flap. The mandibular segment is then wired back into position and the wound dead space is closed. If the mandibular condyle has been removed with the bone, it is replaced into the glenoid fossa. Hamaker and associates report ten successes in 15 patients. However, there was no evidence at the time of publication of osteoneogenesis. One difficulty noted was the poor success in closing the usually inadequate mucosa at the region of the anterior mandible,

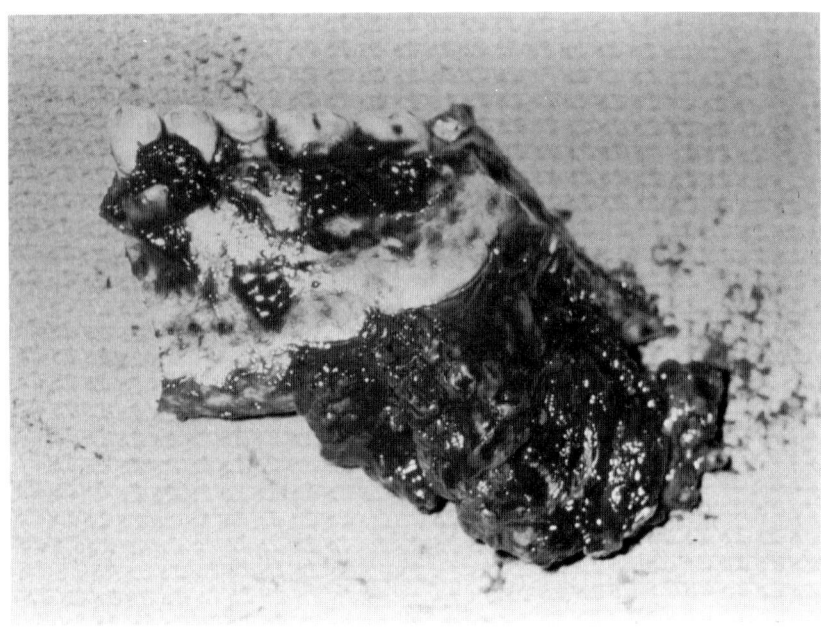

Figure 186. Gross pathologic specimen of arteriovenous malformation involving mid-body of left mandible and adjacent soft tissues.

Reconstruction of the Mandible 157

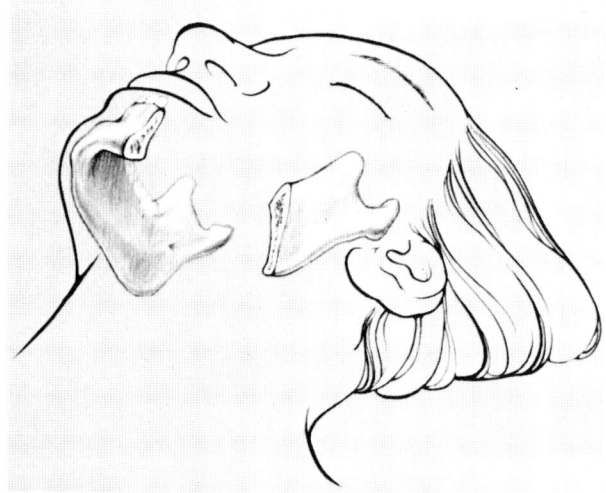

Figure 187. Extent of resection of mandibular body to excise arteriovenous malformation.

the "attached gingiva." The authors stressed that this procedure was not indicated in a mandible that had preoperative osteoradionecrosis.

Alloplastic Materials

A large number of alloplastic materials are available and have been used for mandibular reconstruction; Parel and associates have summarized the literature and historical aspects of their use.[9] Metallic implants have been widely utilized and include aluminum, gold, stainless steel, vitallium, tantalum, and titanium. While these metallic devices are relatively free from tissue graft rejection phenomena, certain inherent properties of these metallic devices make them difficult to maintain in the tissues for extended periods of time. The main

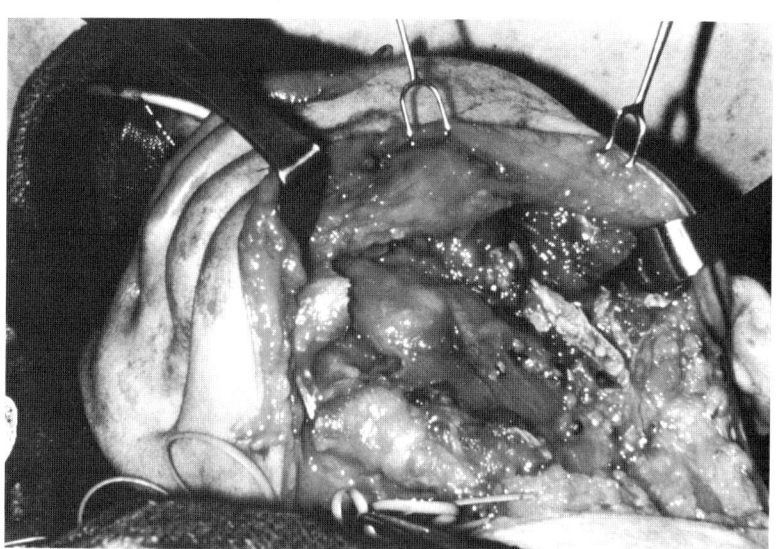

Figure 188. Operative view of defect in mandible after excising arteriovenous malformation.

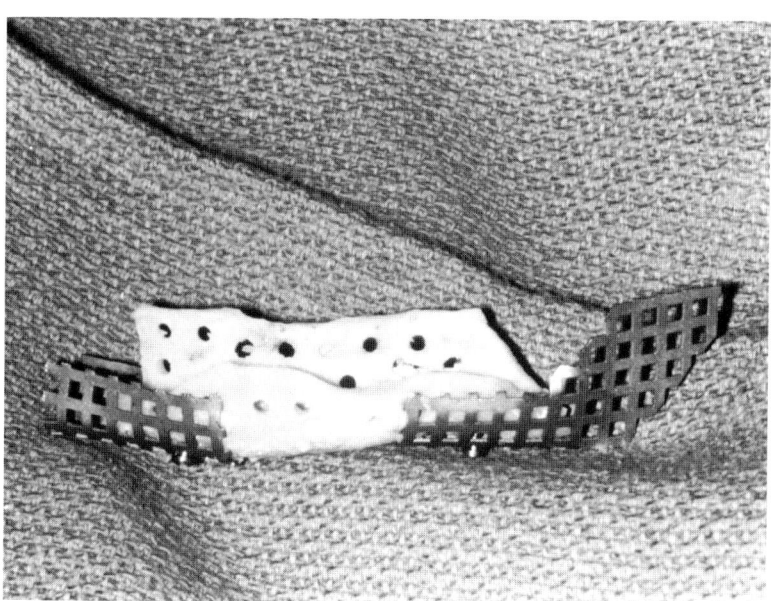

Figure 189. After drilling the arteriovenous malformation out of the mandible, a cortical trough was produced, which when wired to the mandibular defect would provide a tray for autogenous bone chips.

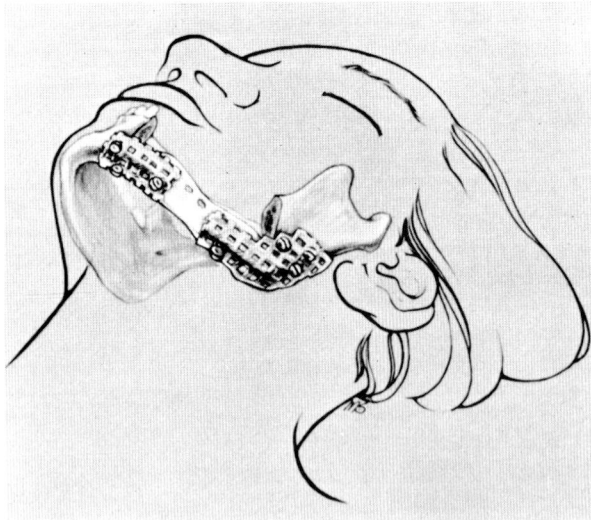

Figure 190. Artist's conception of drilled mandibular segment repositioned in situ and held in place with a tantalum mesh tray.

difficulty centers around their relative rigidity in the tissues so that if there is less than abundant overlying soft tissue, the metallic device has a tendency to become exposed through erosion. Another property of their rigidity is their tendency to produce uncomfortable or painful areas adjacent or overlying the actual implant. This is the indication for the removal of most metallic implants that have achieved a position of homeostasis with the recipient site. Because of these two major problems, most metallic prosthetic devices are removed electively to prevent complications. Additionally, it is felt that the relatively early removal of the devices that are utilized with an autogenous bone graft allows the acceptance of forces by the autogenous graft and provides for the dynamic remodeling of the new bone. Most metallic devices are utilized currently mainly to provide internal fixation to the mandible or to the graft material when utilized with

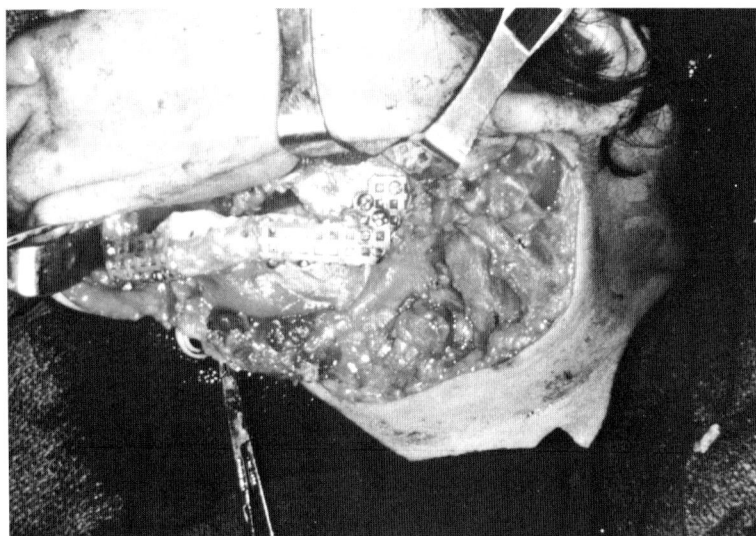

Figure 191. Operative view of reconstructed mandible in place.

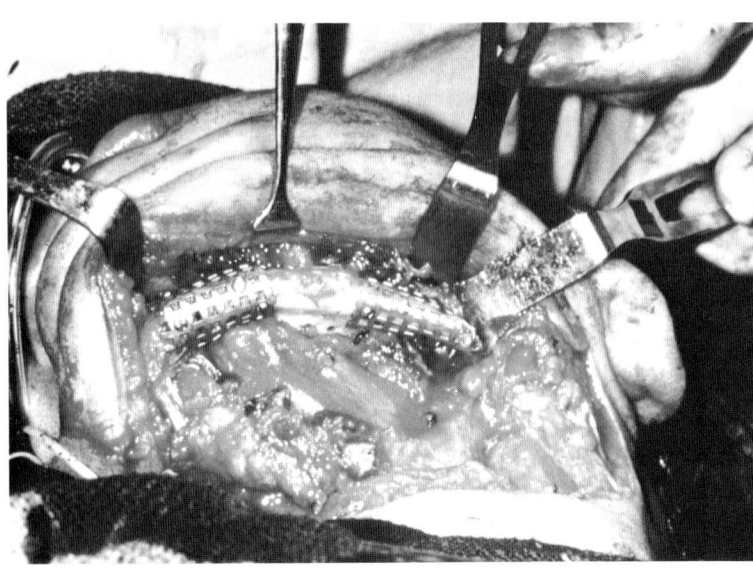

Figure 192. More inferior view of mandible showing mesh trays holding carved mandibular segment in place.

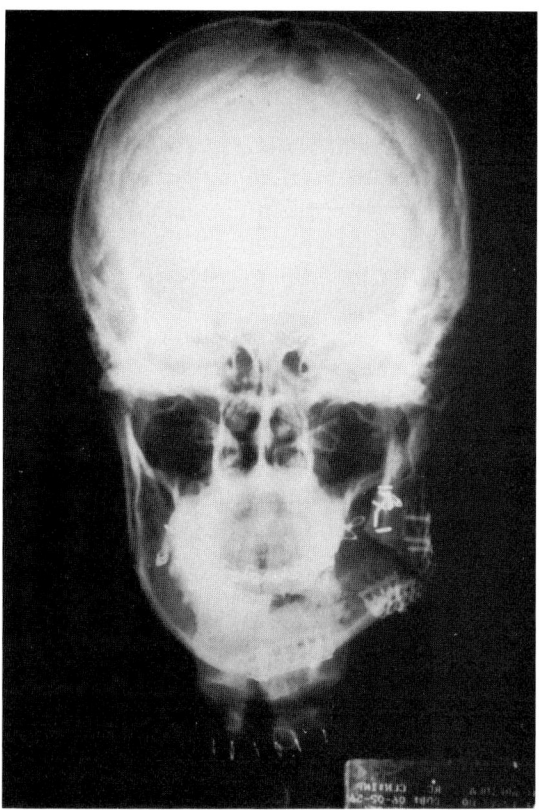

Figure 193. Postoperative radiograph showing mandibular-maxillary fixation in place and the screws fixing the tray to the mandibular segments. Also note the vascular clips in the region of the internal maxillary artery.

bone grafting. This will be discussed in Mandibular Reconstruction Plates and Trays, below.

Organic or naturally occurring materials such as calcium aluminate, calcium apatite, and calcium sulfate have been used with limited success in mandibular reconstruction. Calcium sulfate (plaster of paris) has been reported by McKee and Bailey as satisfactorily replacing lost mandible in canine studies.[10] They implanted the material both with and without the overlying periosteal covering. While the presence of infection limited the success of the graft, in those animals without infection, successful replacement of the calcium sulfate by normal bone occurred both with and without the presence of periosteum. It was these investigators' conclusion that calcium sulfate has osteogenic properties if in contact with bone and/or periosteum and that its action may be due to the fact that it stimulates pleuripotential cells to differentiate into osteoblasts with subsequent ossification. McKee and Bailey felt that since periosteum was not required, this technique could be used in patients where bone and periosteum have been lost secondary to trauma or sacrificed secondary or neoplasia or infection.

Synthetic materials have been developed largely as a by-product of the manufacturing industry and include methylmethacrylate, Proplast, and Teflon (from the space technology industry). One important material used widely in surgery is medical-

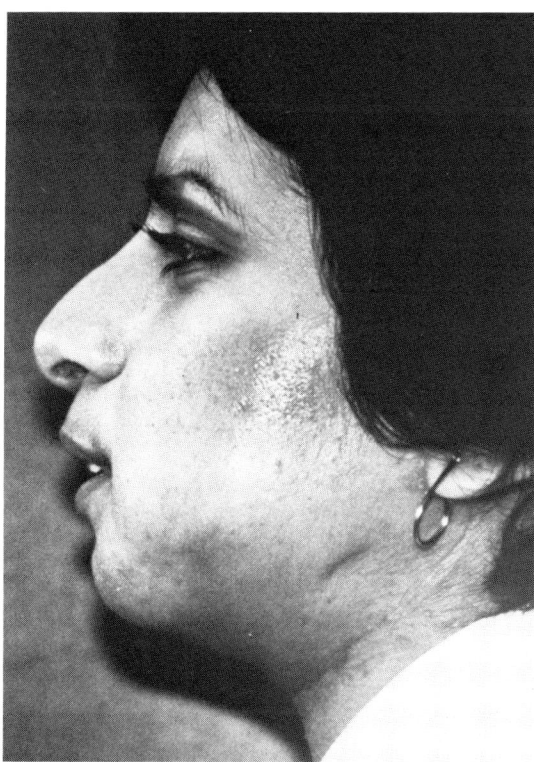

Figure 194. Postoperative view of patient 6 months after mandibular reconstruction. Note soft tissue defects over mandibular region.

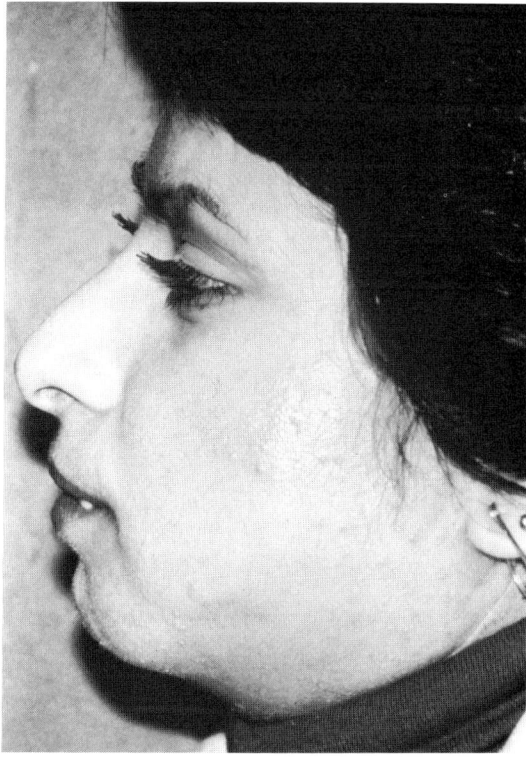

Figure 195. Same patient 3 months after soft tissue augmentation over left mandibular region with a dermis-fat graft.

grade silicone rubber, which was developed in 1953. It proved to be biocompatible but when considering its use in mandibular reconstruction, it was not felt to be strong enough to provide its own internal fixation. As an alternative, Dacron felt was bonded to the silicone rubber to permit tissue ingrowth and to improve the stability of the graft. McKenzie recently reported a case where such a device was utilized to completely replace the mandible and found it to be successfully functioning in a patient 15 years after its placement.[11] Since the use of silicone rubber for mandibular replacement has not been widely successful, the author proposed that its success in this patient was due to his novel eating habits, to the fact that the patient did not attempt to wear dentures, and that he had experienced no external trauma in the region of the mandible since its reconstruction.

In 1984, Schwartz reported the use of a Dacron-urethane prosthesis in conjunction with autogenic cancellous bone to reconstruct the mandible in 32 patients.[12] The Dacron cloth mesh is stiffened by impregnation with urethane and formed into a trough having roughly the same shape as the mandible. Fresh autogenic bone from the iliac crest was placed into the trough as it allowed the transplantation of large numbers of viable osteoblasts which would then form new bone for the mandible. These patients had a wide variety of etiologies to their defects including benign and malignant osseous lesions, and trauma secondary to gunshot wounds and following osteoradionecrosis. In 14 patients, mandibles were reconstructed primarily with this technique, and in 18 patients the technique was used secondarily for reconstruction. There was only one failure and that was in a patient who developed a B-hemolytic streptococcus infection. These prostheses were never electively removed, but if part of the graft became exposed, the prosthesis was debrided and a flap was used to obtain adequate soft tissue coverage over it. The prosthesis was internally secured with stainless steel wires. The author recommends this synthetic prosthesis over metallic devices because it is stated that no galvanic current current will be set up between dissimilar metals and because radiation therapy can be used postperatively without the beam-scattering effect of the metals. Because such synthetic prostheses are not entirely rigid, the elasticity present may absorb some mild shocks to the mandibular region without incurring injury to the prosthesis.

While the synthetic materials used in reconstruction of the mandible are for the most part biocompatible and nonbiodegradable, there still exists the possibility that rejection or untoward reactions still exist and larger studies will be required before their use becomes widespread.

Mandibular Reconstruction Plates and Trays

Since it is widely accepted that successful mandibular reconstruction depends, in part, on rigid fixation of the reconstruction materials, considerable experience has been gathered in the use of metallic reconstruction plates and trays. Traditionally, the earliest fixation devices were composed of stainless steel and were simply interosseous wires. The use of K-wires to "skewer" the bony fragments to a bone graft were not very successful. Newer techniques now include the use of stainless steel or rare metal bone plates and trays. The bone plates are of two types: compression plates or noncompression plates. The advantage of the compression plate centers around its rigid fixation and ability to produce osteoneogenesis at the bone fragment interface (Fig. 196). The same type of

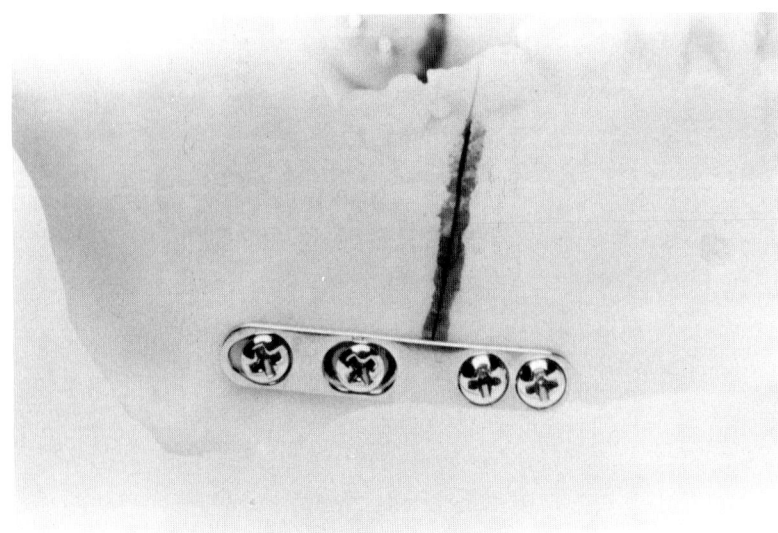

Figure 196. Mandibular model showing compression plate fixation of unfavorable body fracture. Note eccentric screw holes on posterior part of plate which create the compression at the fracture site when tightened against the regular screw holes anteriorly.

bony union does not occur in noncompression plate fixation. Strelzow has reported good success with the use of the Synthes Maxillofacial Bone Plating System for reconstruction of segmental jaw defects.[13] Several different types of materials were used for reconstruction including Proplast, freeze-dried mandibular autografts, fresh iliac crest bone, and irradiated mandibular autografts. The reconstruction plates were utilized to secure these grafts into place. Two of the ten grafts failed, both due to exposure of the graft through an intraoral dehiscence. The author relates that these plates can be bent to fit the defect and the size of the graft material, and are secured in place either with osseous screw or stainless steel wire; they can be used in the compression or noncompression style (Figs. 197–205). Their drawback is that the large bulk of metal may potentially serve as a foreign body, and requires very good overlying soft tissue coverage. Strelzow feels it is very important to properly stabilize the nonvascularized bone graft and to allow maximal revascularization and long-term viability. If the plates hinder subsequent new bone remodeling, they can be removed.

Raveh and associates found that when using conventional screws for reconstruction plates, the narrow layer of fibrous tissue that developed between the bone and metal eventually loosened the plate. In dog studies where some of the animals' mandibles had been irradiated, these investigators utilized titanium plates and screws for reconstruction and reported good stabilization and good bone-to-metal contact.[14] Later, Roweh and colleagues reported the use of these titanium screws in patients and found that bone grew into the hollow screws, affording a tight interface between bone and screw, which was increased with increasing duration of

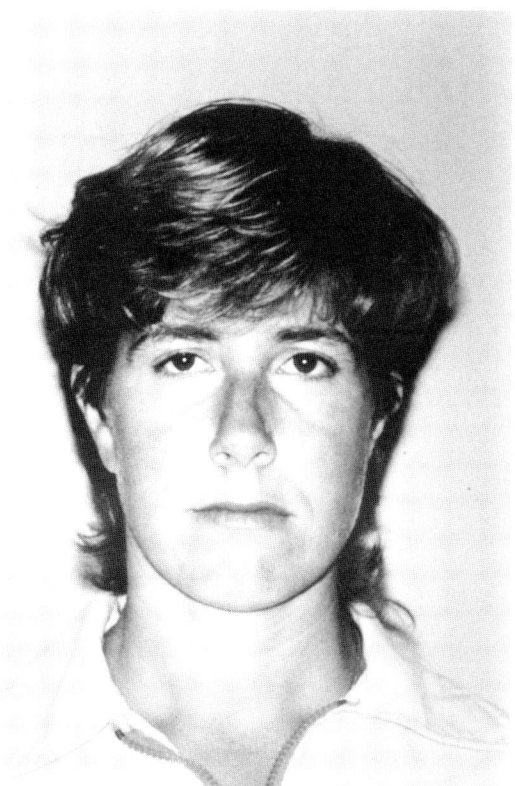

Figure 197. Patient with asymptomatic (unrecognized) ameloblastoma of left mid-body of the mandible.

implantation.[15] They also developed a special reconstruction plate which allowed attachment of an adjustable temporomandibular joint (TMJ) condyle prosthesis which could be adjusted to permit precise restoration of articular guidance to the reconstructed side while preventing incorrect loading of the opposite joint.

It is very important when using reconstruction

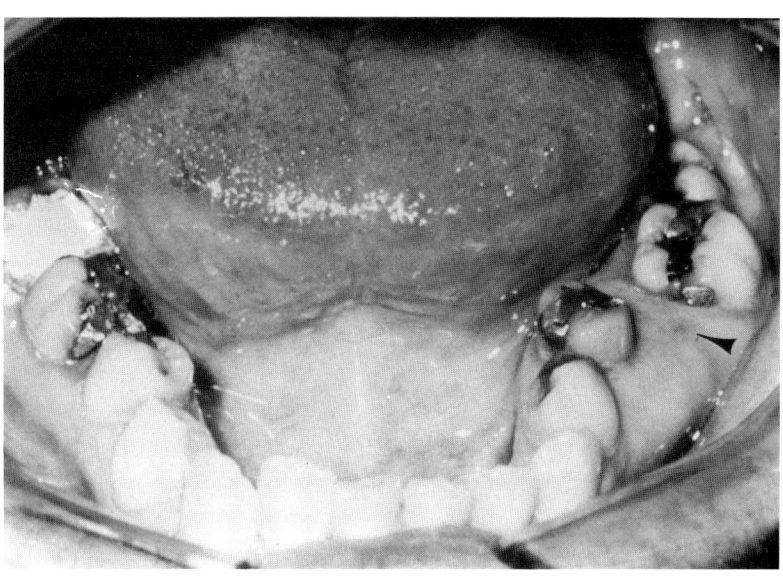

Figure 198. Intraoral view of ameloblastoma of left mandibular alveolus (arrow).

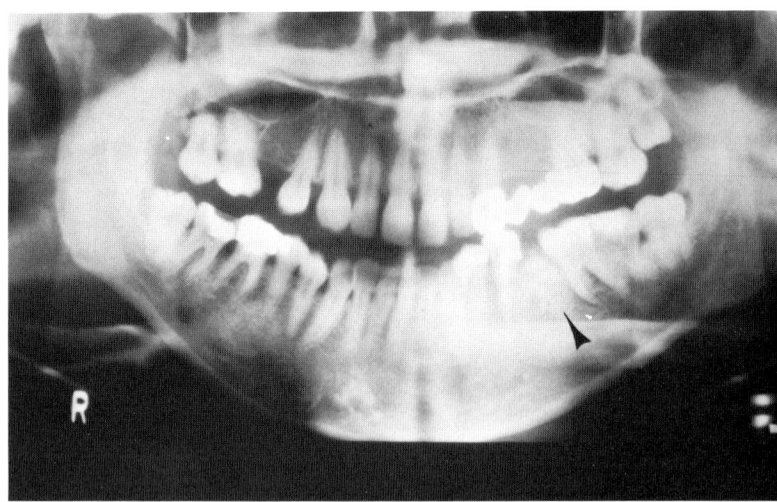

Figure 199. Panorex showing left mid-body alveolar ameloblastoma (arrow).

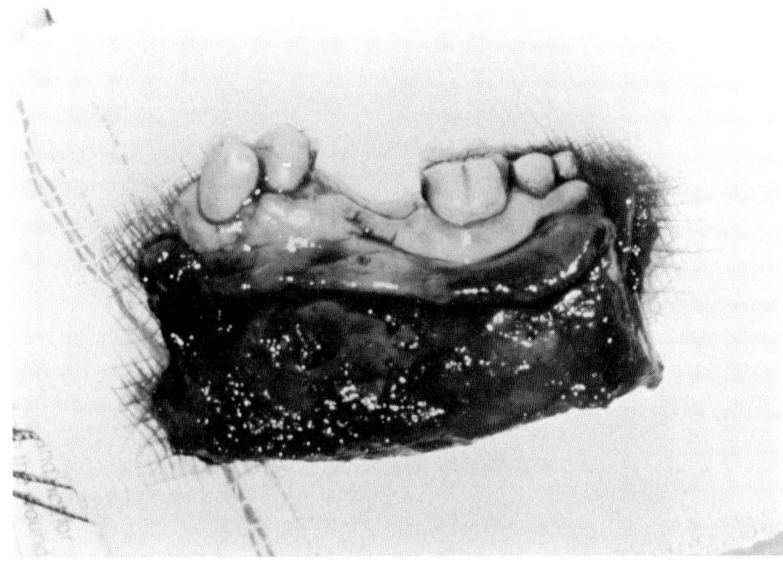

Figure 200. Surgical specimen showing extent of resection to include two teeth anterior and posterior to the bony tumor.

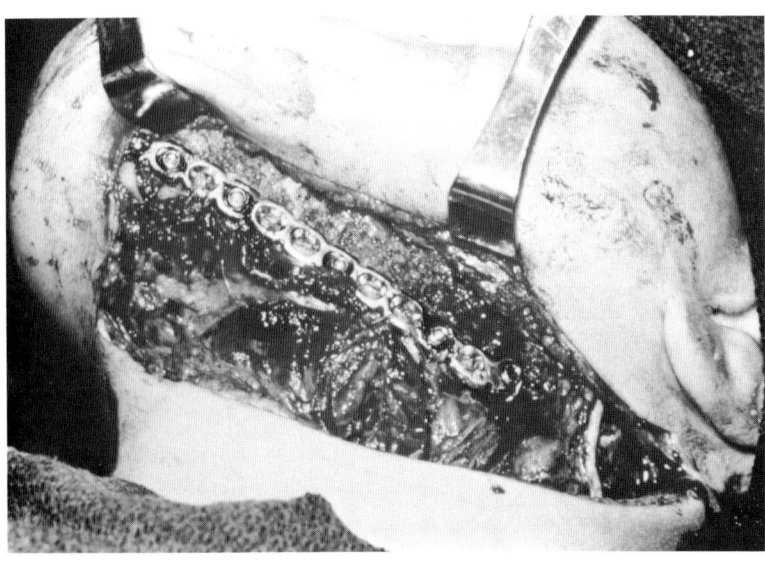

Figure 201. Reconstruction of surgical resection of mid-body left mandible using noncompression reconstruction bar screwed into proximal and distal mandibular segments.

Figure 202. Inferior view of operative field showing iliac crest autogenous bone graft secured to reconstruction plate to serve as primary source of osteoneogenesis.

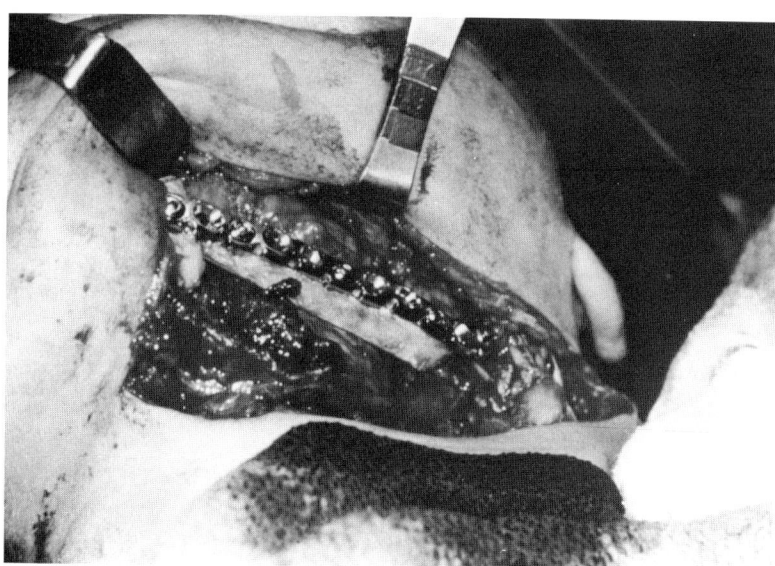

Figure 203. Panorex demonstrating maxillary-mandibular fiation and position of bone graft and reconstruction plate.

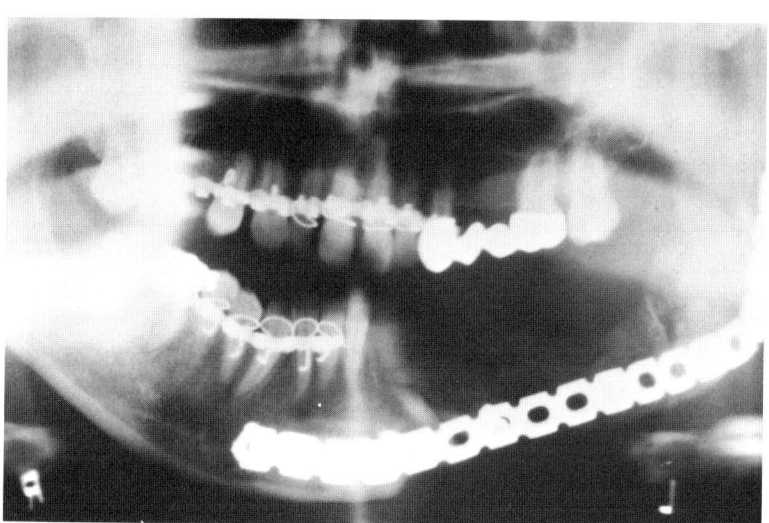

Figure 204. Intraoral view of patient after removal of reconstruction plate and solid healing of iliac bone graft.

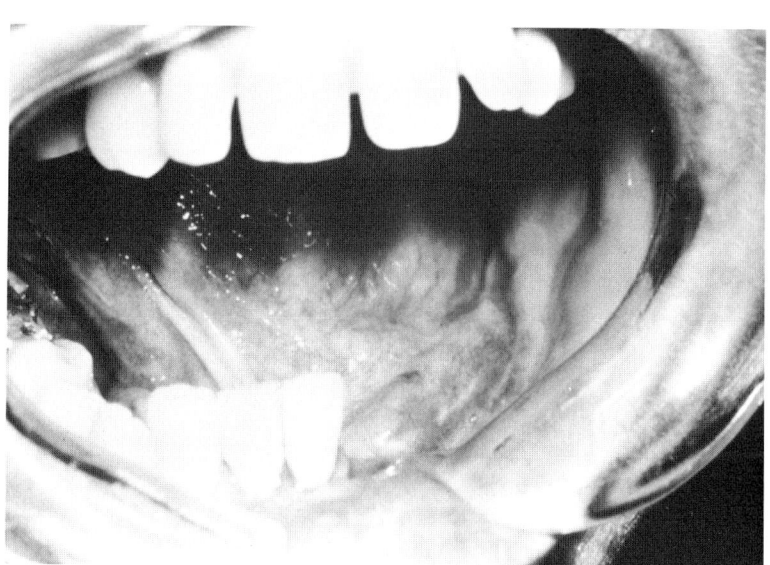

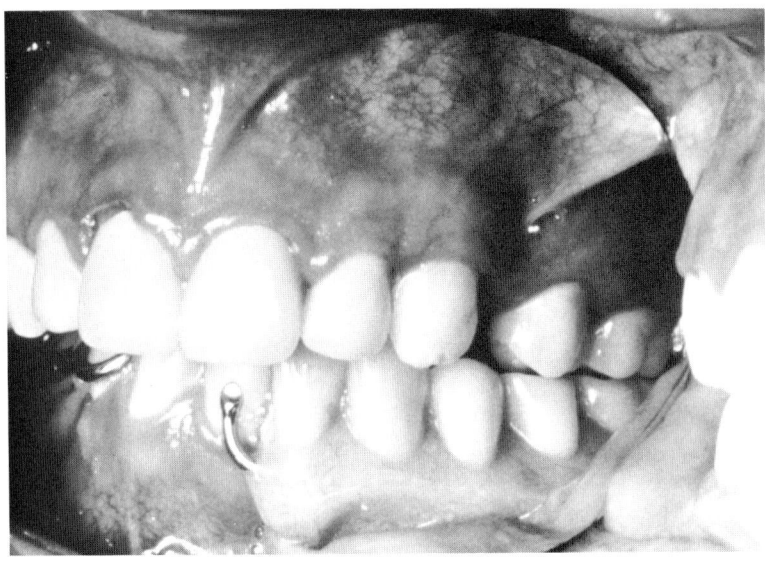

Figure 205. Same patient as in Figure 204 with partial denture in place to rehabilitate dental-alveolar defect in left mandible.

plates to have adequate soft tissue in the area, both intra- and extraorally. Additionally, the dead space around a reconstruction plate should be completely obliterated, both by sutures and closed space drainage to prevent fluid accumulation and its subsequent infection. Without adequate overlying soft tissue, reconstruction plates tend to cause soft tissue thinning, pain over the plate, and eventual exposure of the plate itself. In most patients the reconstruction plate is removed electively after 3 to 4 months to allow remodeling of the mandible under the functional stress of weight and tension loading.[16] If a pseudoarthrosis occurs at the fracture site after removal of the reconstruction plate, Kruger and Krumholz recommend that a second bone graft should be inserted, along with another compression-type reconstruction plate, approximately 6 months after the first operation.[17] In their series of bone plate mandibular reconstruction, there was 80% success with 30% pseudoarthrosis in patients where the oral mucosa was open, and 97% success with only 15% pseudoarthrosis when the approach was extraoral.

A mesh tray utilized for mandibular reconstruction is generally used as a crib to contain autogeneous bone fragments (Figs. 206–212). In most patients its strength is sufficient to support the mandible without mandibular-maxillary fixation with minimum loading. According to Lawson, its failure rate is about 10%.[18] These crib graft trays are composed of many different materials including stainless steel, titanium, and vitallium. The trays are of a meshwork design to allow ingrowth of blood vessels and osteoneogenesis. These trays can

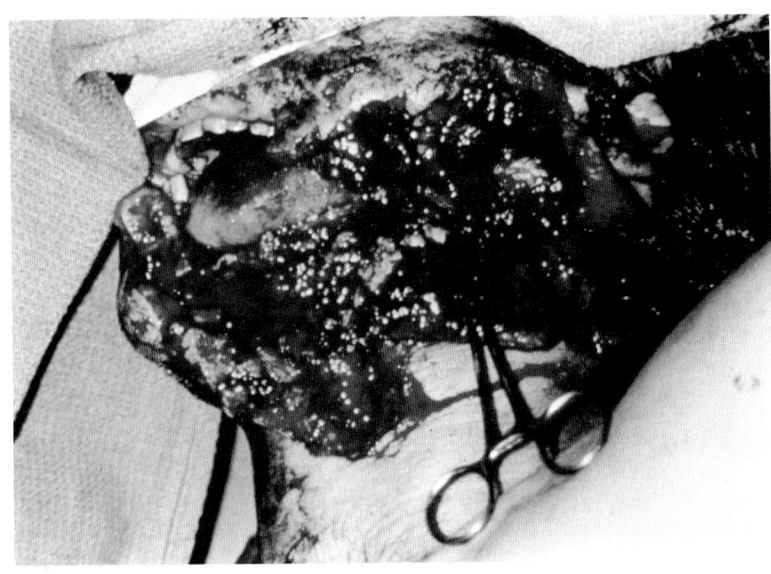

Figure 206. Patient with severe gunshot wound to left mandible with loss of entire left body and angle of mandible.

be secured in place with screws or with wire fixation and can be cut and shaped to fit the defect. While the trays are manufactured to common sizes of full, half, or partial mandibular replacement, the metal is soft and can be trimmed easily or bent with pliers to more readily conform to the individual patient requirements. Although trays can be used as a spacer device, the reconstruction plates are better utilized in that capacity, reserving the tray for actual secondary reconstruction. The main advantage of the mandibular tray is that it allows the autogenous cancellous bone graft to remodel in the resemblance of the mandibular form while giving strength to the mandibular segment immediately.

In most patients the mandibular tray is removed approximately 6 months after insertion or when there is good radiographic evidence of osteoneogenesis. The author prefers to make this decision based upon both a computed tomography (CT) scan and, if equivocable, a radionuclide bone scan. At the time of removal of the tray, great care should be exercised not to allow intraoral contamination to occur and not to accidentally fracture the new mandibular segment while removing the tray. Normally the tray can be removed by gentle prying and separation from the underlying bone with a flat bone elevator. If the new mandibular segment is somewhat atrophic (and it usually is) and the overlying soft tissues are thin, then augmentation of the defect can be accomplished using either a free dermal-fat graft or a pedicled soft tissue flap, such as one based upon the sternocleidomastoid (SCM) muscle. In most patients the SCM muscle will undergo significant atrophy if the overlying dermis is not transferred to the soft tissue defect site along with the muscle (see Chapter 14).

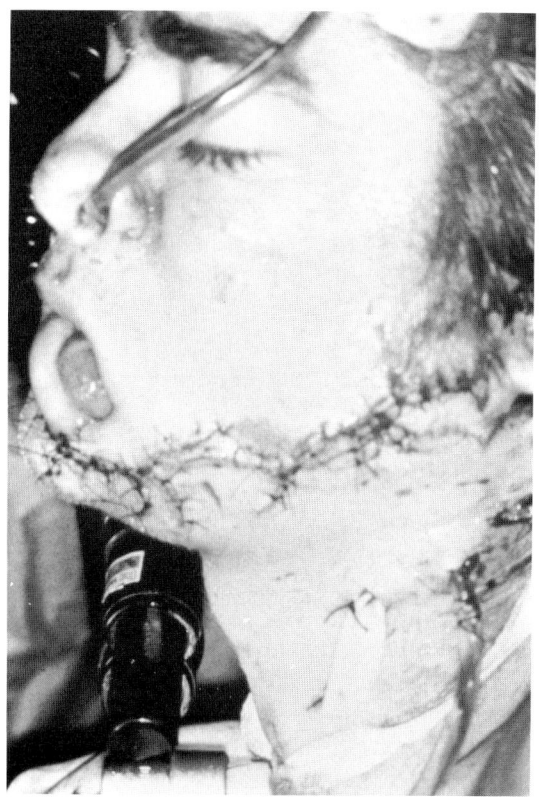

Figure 207. Primary repair including closure of intraoral defect, debridement of tissues, and closure of skin defect.

Free Composite Bone Flaps

In some patients, where there has been an incontinuity resection of the mandible and intraoral soft tissues, consideration can be given to utilization of a free composite bone graft to reconstruct the bone and soft tissue defect in a one-stage procedure. Obviously, this technique is limited to

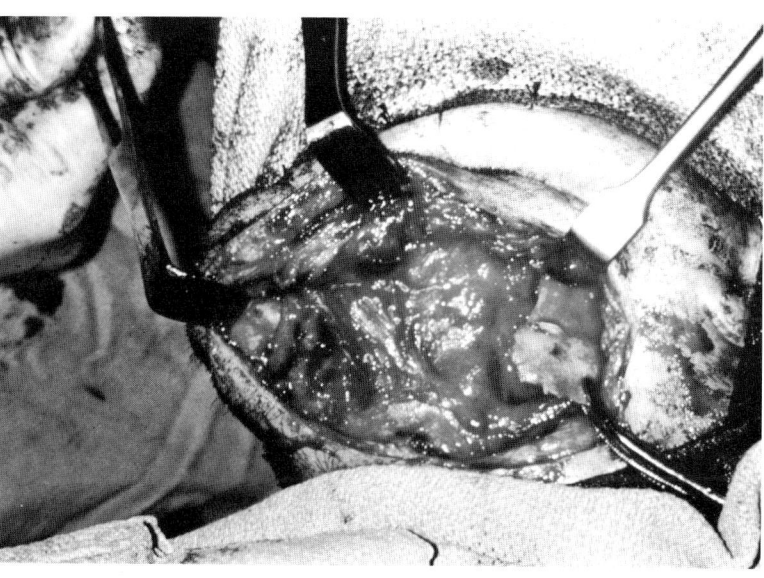

Figure 208. Approximately nine months after healing of primary closure, patient underwent secondary reconstruction of mandible, beginning with exposure of remaining mandibular segments.

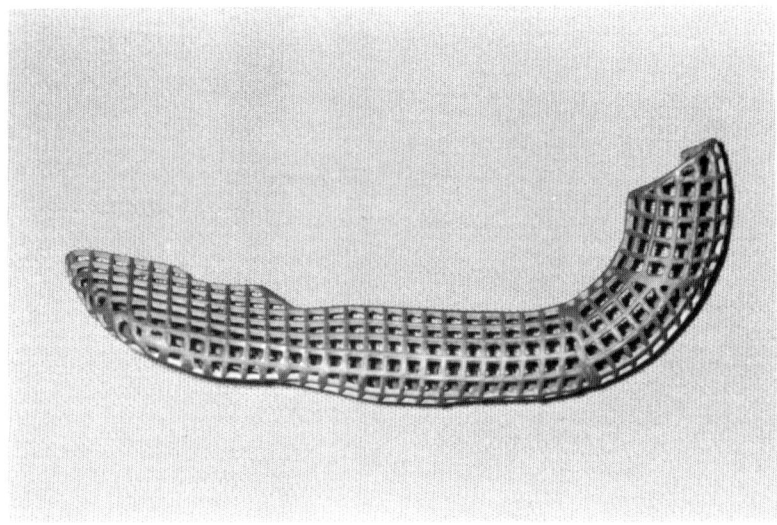

Figure 209. Vitallium crib (mesh) tray used to reconstruct missing mandibular segment and to serve as a trough for autogenous iliac crest bone.

those surgeons who have special expertise in microvascular reconstruction. In some patients, a two-team approach can be utilized, where one team performs the resection while the second team harvests the graft from the donor site and transplants the flap to the mandibular region. Several perimandibular vessels can be utilized as the recipient vessels, including the facial artery and vein, the superficial temporal system, and the superior thyroid vessels. However, if the entire external carotid artery system has been removed with the cancer ablation procedure, this type of reconstruction is not favorable.

Bitter and colleagues described the use of an iliac bone or osteocutaneous transplant pedicled to the deep circumflex iliac artery for mandibular replacement.[18] Approximately a 15 to 20-cm-sized free flap can be harvested with the iliac crest attached to the flap. Because the iliac bone crest is relatively flat, if it is required so that the anterior mandible may be replaced, it can be cut along its antevascular side with wedges of cancellous bone inserted in the cuts to keep the crest in a curved shape. Additional support from major myocutaneous flap (MMF) or reconstruction plates is used to strengthen the mandible during healing. Postoperative technetium scintography can be utilized to evaluate the effectiveness of the pedicled blood supply. Possible complications include those associated with iliac crest and groin incisions and the transient numbness that can occur if the lateral femoral cutaneous nerve was stretched but left intact. Taylor described the techniques for harvesting the free iliac crest graft, and mentioned that one can alter the bone taken from the hip to fit the mandibular defect since the entire iliac crest is nourished by the deep circumflex iliac system.[19]

MacLeod and Robinson prefer the free osteocutaneous flaps derived from the foot for immediate or delayed one-stage mandibular reconstruction.[20]

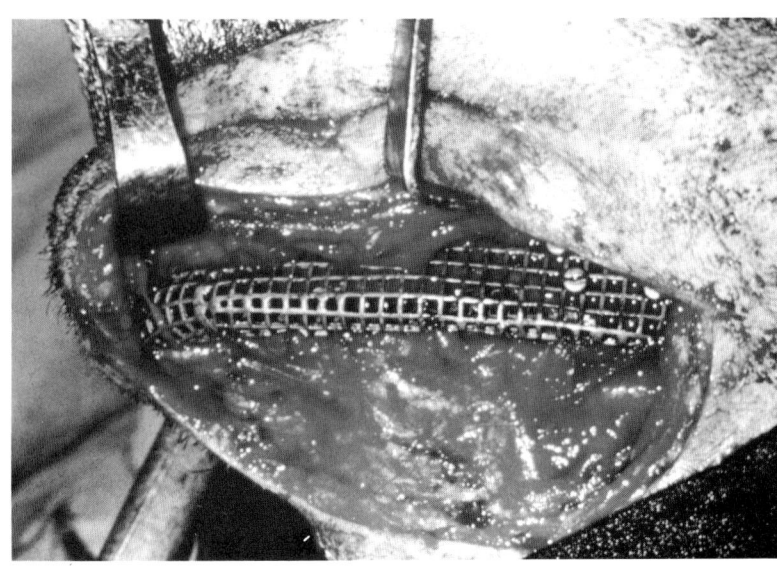

Figure 210. Operative view showing crib tray in place, secured to the remaining mandibular segments and ready to receive the particles of iliac crest corticocancellous bone.

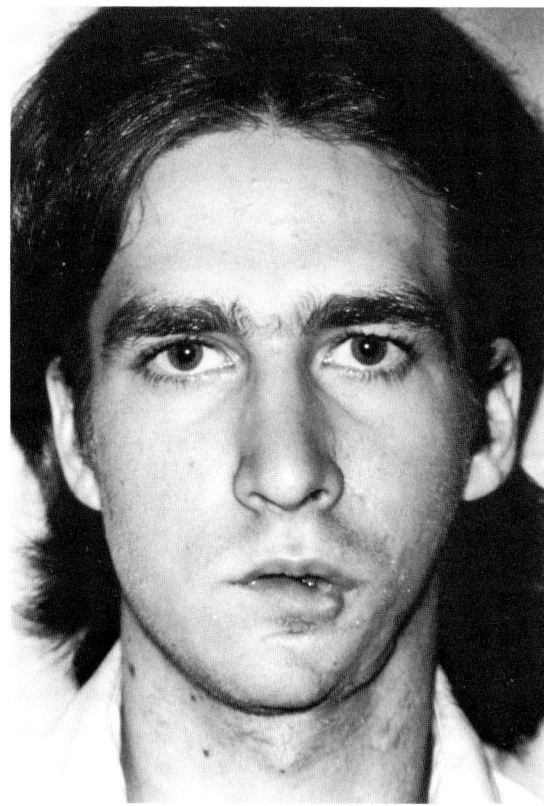 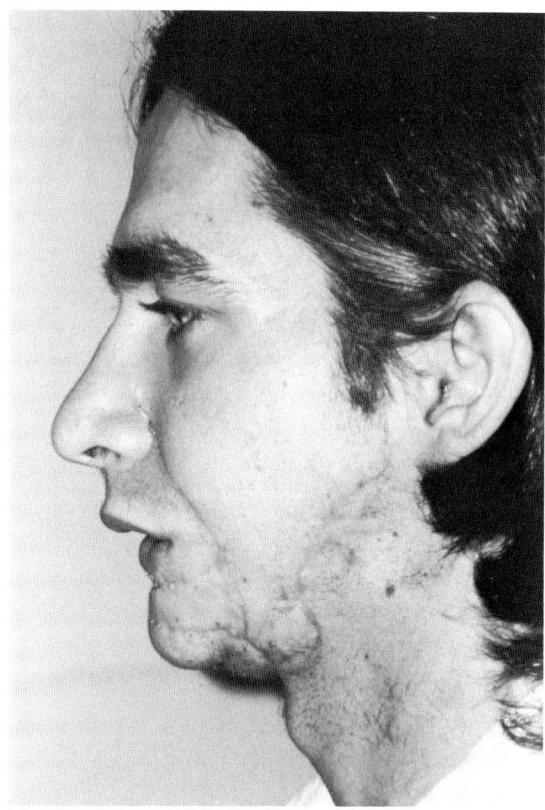

Figure 211. (A) Left, frontal view; and right, (B) left lateral view approximately 9 months after reconstruction of the mandible with crib tray-bone graft technique.

The curvature of the mandible can be mimicked by the bones of the mid-foot, and the hairless thin flap provides adequate tissue to form a new buccal and lingual sulcus. A long vascular pedicle can be obtained from the anterior tibial and long saphenous systems. Of 12 patients in these authors' series, failure occurred in only 1, and this was due to venous obstruction. MacLeod and Robinson recommend bony fixation by interosseous wire with the metatarsal placed at the lower border of the mandibular defect to give more room for the flap to fit in above it.

When the mandible is reconstructed using a latissimus dorsi free flap, the skin portion is designed over the seventh, eighth, and ninth ribs. The thoracodorsal artery is located and the perforators are

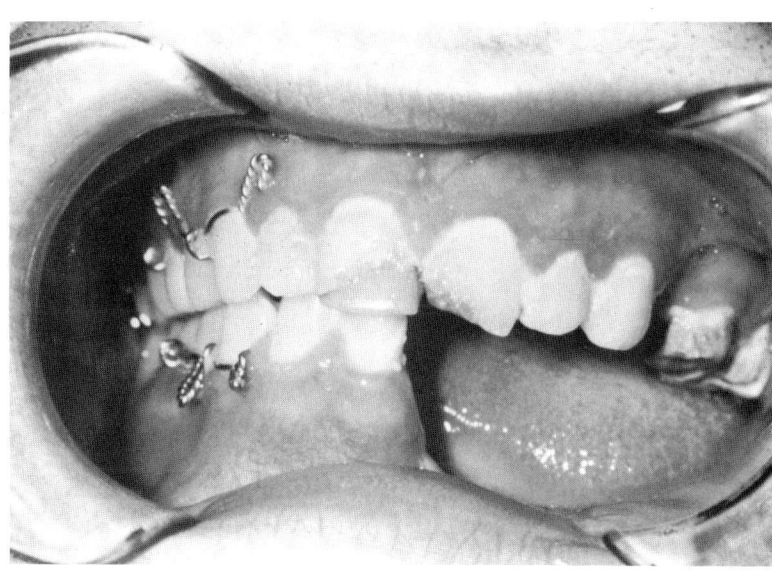

Figure 212. Intraoral dental-alveolar defect remaining after healing of reconstructed mandible.

preserved. It is apparently wise to include the intercostal vessels on the inferior margin of the rib to enhance the chance for collateralization of the blood supply.[21] This leaves the latissimus dorsi muscle and its overlying skin island and underlying rib attached by the vascular insertion and the thoracodorsal artery in the axilla. Suitable recipient vessels include the facial and superfacial temporal systems. The long vascular pedicle allows the anastomosis to be performed low or high in the neck or on the contralateral side.

These free bone flaps are effective in the repair of mandibular bone grafts only when utilized by experienced microvascular surgeons. Because these skills are not commonly held by most head and neck surgeons, one-stage reconstruction may best be accomplished by the development of osseomyocutaneous flaps whose use is more universally applied.

Osseomyocutaneous Pedicle Flaps

Failure of mandibular reconstruction in the irradiated patient often occurs when prosthetic devices or free bone grafts are utilized, primarily because of inadequate soft tissue coverage and insufficient vascularity to sustain a free graft. In one of the earliest articles dealing with osteocutaneous flaps for reconstruction of the head and neck, Conley described the use of a rib graft and its connecting periosteum and muscle for intraoral reconstruction.[22] The most commonly used osteomyocutaneous flaps at this time include the pectoralis major myocutaneous flap with the attached fifth rib, the SCM flap with attached clavicle, and the trapezius myocutaneous flap with the scapular spine.[23] In most patients the pedicle can be brought up to the mandible either externally or internally.

In 1980, Cuono and Ariyan first reported a case of a pectoralis major composite reconstruction of the mandible, including within that flap the portion of the underlying fifth rib from beyond the border of the ectoralis muscle to the sternum—the flap subsequently survived.[24] They emphasized the need to raise the cartilage with the rib because the costal origins of the pectoralis major muscle arise from the cartilaginous portions of ribs 2 to 6. It thus becomes a chondroosseomyocutaneous flap. If used, a pectoralis minor muscle component from the fourth to fifth ribs periosteum can serve the role as a nutrient bridge between the thoracoacromial supply of the pectoralis major free border and the lateral bony fifth rib, probably from the arborized bed of the lateral thoracic artery with the pectoral branch of the thoracoacromial artery and the intercostal arteries. The plane of dissection is between the periosteum and perichondrium and the pleura of the chest wall. Little and associates state that if the rib is used to reconstruct a straight segment of mandible, then less rib length will be required than if a curved segment is needed.[25] They burr off the rib cortex and insert only the cancellous bone into the corresponding cancellous bone of the mandibular stumps. For horizontal body and ramus portion, overlapping mortised joints can be fashioned and wired into place. Since rib is very soft, most authors report the concomitant use of an external fixation device for stabilization in the postoperative period.

Potential complications of the Pectoralis major composite flap include pleural tears, which can either be sewn or used to insert a chest tube for closed drainage, and a chest deformity at the rib excision site. The defect can be strengthened by reflecting superiorly a rectus abdominus flap. Since there is a 9 to 15 degree range of movement at the costal cartilage-rib junction, this motion can be deleterious if the pectoralis major composite flap is used for reconstructing a straight mandibular segment; however, that same motion may be used to a positive advantage when reconstructing the TMJ.[26]

Panje recommends the use of the trapezius osteomusculocutaneous flap, particularly for anterior arch defects or following osteordionecrosis of the mandible.[27] When this flap is used for primary reconstruction, Panje reports an 87% overall success rate. This is a composite island flap consisting of skin, trapezius muscle, and the medial scapular spine based on the transverse cervical artery and vein. Panje cautions that one should include three to four paraspinous perforators within the flap's muscle. By leaving the scapular spine attached to the trapezius muscle, adequate vascular perfusion of the bone's periosteum and marrow is possible. Only the posterior-medial scapular spine can be taken with the flap so as to leave the acromion. Panje also uses an external fixation device to stabilize the graft and to prevent migration; however, the vascularized bone graft can tolerate weight-bearing more like the original bone than a free bone graft. The healing of vascularized bone grafts appears to take much less time than with a nonvascularized free graft.

A disadvantage of the trapezius composite flap is the possible loss of shoulder muscle function with loss of a length of trapezius muscle and denervation of the remainder. Panje recommends suturing the chin to the shoulder temporarily to prevent excessive tension on the vascular pedicle and its subsequent injury.

PROSTHETIC REHABILITATION OF THE RECONSTRUCTED MANDIBLE

One of the most difficult tasks of a maxillofacial prosthodontist is to fabricate functionally useful dentures in a patient who has undergone successful bony reconstruction of a mandible. Most prosthodontists will not allow that patient the use of dentures for 6 to 12 months after the successful reconstruction. Perhaps the major difficulties center around the intraoral soft tissue status which is often either too thin or too thick. The surgeon can assist the prosthodontist by attempting to only insert enough soft tissue as is required to cover and nourish the graft and to bring the height of the mandible to the level of the adjacent attached gingiva. Most prosthodontists simply recommend that the patient not be fitted with dentures, and restrict the patient to a soft diet, or will fabricate the dentures so that most of the loading forces will be absorbed by the normal mandible. Other problems include the disruption of the normal paired muscle activity, the occasional loss of ipsilateral tongue bulk and function, and difficulty in swallowing due to the unilateral activity of the elevator muscles on the unaffected side causing the mandible to rotate and deviate with respect to the maxilla.[28]

Other goals of the successful prosthetic rehabilitation of the reconstructed mandible include the restoration of normal facial appearance, the permitting of bilateral mandibular articulation, and the facilitation of speech. It is often necessary to secondarily reconstruct buccal and lingual sulci by inserting skin grafts after incising the soft tissues on either side of the new mandibular segment. Once a denture is fabricated, cinefluoroscopy may be used to check the relationship of the denture to the mandible during swallowing. Much work may be required by the prosthodontist in fabricating a conventional denture that comfortably promotes speech and swallowing.

However, a new method of securing prosthetic devices to the reconstructed mandible has been developed by Branemark and colleagues at the Institute for Applied Biotechnology in Gothenburg, Sweden. Originally, these investigators utilized a pure titanium mold which was inserted into the iliac crest surface to outline the required segment of bone to reconstruct the mandible.[29] They found that this "cookie cutter" technique allowed for the harvesting of a segmen of corticocancellous bone which very closely fit the shape of the previously resected or lost segment of mandible. Then, using their principle of osseointegration whereby special titanium screws are inserted into bone and induce osteoneogenesis around them, Branemark and co-workers preinserted the screw fixtures into the outlined mandibular segment while it was still within the iliac crest. Following a 4 to 5-month period to allow the fixtures to become integrated within the bone, the unit was transferred to the defect in the mandible. The fixtures then served two purposes: first, some of the screws were used to secure the bone graft in place; second, other screws, placed vertically, were used as a foundation on which to build a supporting structure for a denture.[30]

However, currently the most successful use of titanium fixtures is to insert them directly into the reconstructed mandibular segment after remodeling and healing has occurred (Figs. 213–217). Fixtures can also be inserted into the unviolated mandibular portion if the patient is edentulous, as well as into the maxilla to completely restore the dentition. This

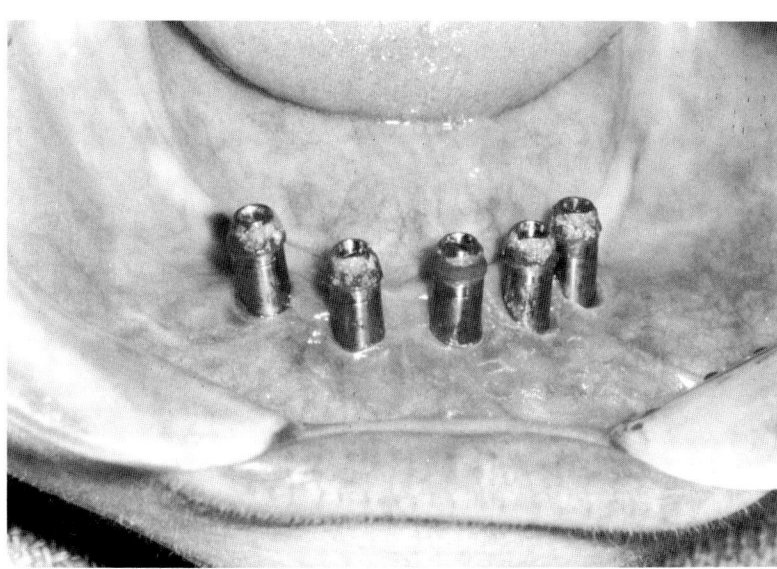

Figure 213. Rehabilitation of reconstructed mandible using osseointegrated titanium fixtures. Here, the fixtures have penetrated the skin and are attached to titanium abutments.

170 Surgery of the Mandible

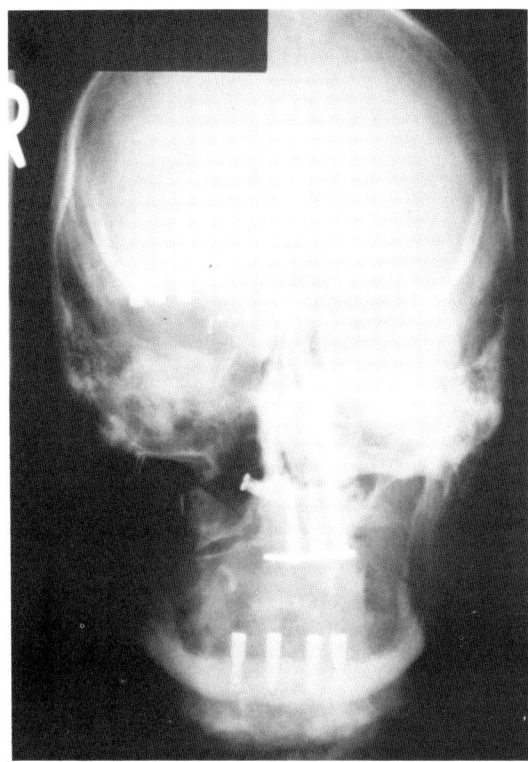

Figure 214. Typical radiographic appearance of osseointegrated fixtures in the mandible, maxilla, and right superior orbital rim to rehabilitate a patient following orbital exenteration and bone resorption of the jaws.

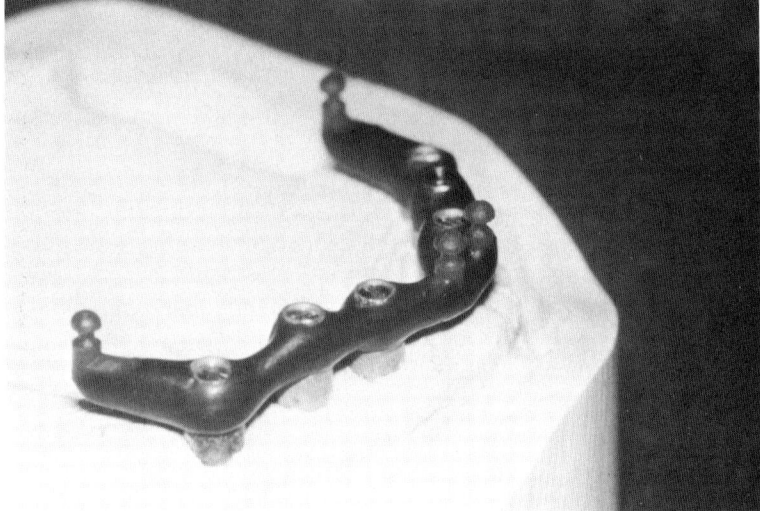

Figure 215. Dental model showing method of fabricating bridgework between abutments and the attachments of "knobs" that will hold the denture in place.

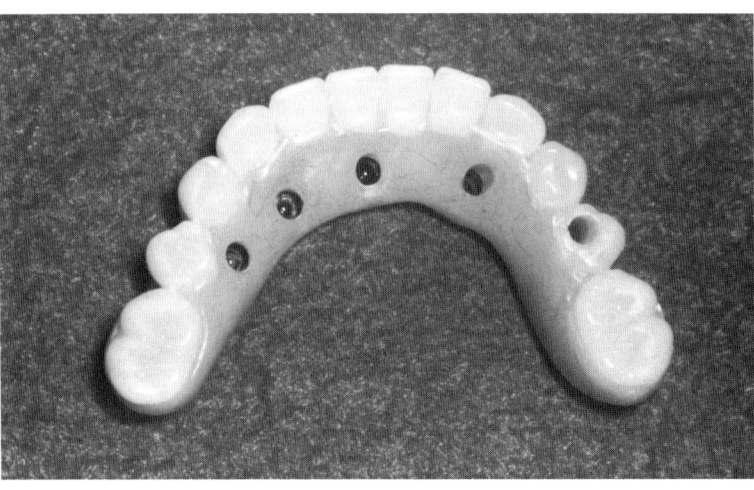

Figure 216. Mandibular denture showing position of receptacles for mating of denture to abutments.

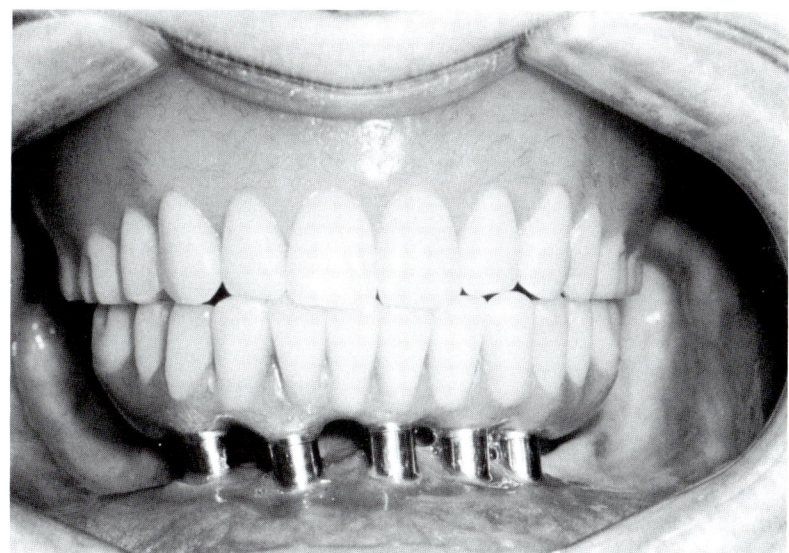

Figure 217. Final denture in place on abutments. Denture and fixtures are capable of sustaining normal tension-loading during chewing.

technique of using osseointegrated fixtures to rehabilitate the mandible has been followed for nearly 20 years with nearly 95% clinical success.[31] The future of restoration of difficult cases of mandibular reconstruction likely lies within the work being performed on the osseointegration techniques.

REFERENCES

1. Tingchun W. Zhe C, Fengchen T, et al.: Ameloblastoma of the mandible treated by resection, preservation of the inferior alveolar nerve, and bone grating. J Oral Maxillofac Surg 42:93–96, 1984
2. Grillon GL, Gunther SF, Connole PW: A new technique for obtaining iliac bone grafts. J Oral Maxillofac Surg 42:172–176, 1984
3. Babin RW, Osbon DB, Khangure MS: Arteriovenous malformations of the mandible. Otolaryngol Head Neck Surg 91:366–371, 1983
4. Holt GR, Tinsley PP Jr, Aufdemorte TB, et al.: Arteriovenous malformation of the mandible. Otolaryngol Head Neck Surg 91:573–578, 1983
5. Leipzig B, Cummings CW: The current status of mandibular reconstruction using autogenous frozen mandibular grafts. Head Neck Surg 6:992–997, 1984
6. Hamaker R: Irradiated autogenous mandibular grafts in primary reconstruction. Laryngoscope 9:1031–1051, 1981
7. Dougherty TP, Rafetto LK, Edwards RC, et al.: Reimplantation of freeze-treated bone in immediate reconstruction of the mandible. J Surg 144:463–465, 1982
8. Hamaker RC, Singer MI, Shockley WW, et al.: Irradiated mandibular autografts. Cancer 52:1017–1021, 1983
8. Parel SM, Drane JB, Williams EO: Mandibular replacements; a review of the literature. J Am Dent Assoc 94:120–125, 1977
10. McKee JC, Bailey BJ: Calcium sulfate as a mandibular implant. Otolaryngol Head Neck Surg 92:277–286, 1984
11. McKenzie ML: Mandibular reconstruction using silicone: Fifteen year followup. Plast Reconstr Surg 74:531–534, 1984
12. Schwartz HC: Mandibular reconstruction using the Dacron-urethane prosthesis and autogenic cancellous bone: A review of 32 cases. Plast Reconstr Surg 73:387–392, 1984
13. Strelzow VV: Mandibular reconstruction using implantable stabilization plates. Arch Otolaryngol 109:333–337, 1983
14. Raveh Y, Stich H, Sutter F, et al.: New concepts in the reconstruction of mandibular defects following tumor resection. J Oral Maxillofac Surg 41:3–16, 1983
15. Raveh J. Stich H, Sutter F, et al.: Use of the titanium-coated hollow screw and reconstruction plate system in bridging of lower jaw defects. J Oral Maxillofac Surg 42:281–194, 1984
16. Kruger E: Reconstruction of bone and soft tissue in extensive facial defects. J Oral Maxillofac Surg 40:714–720, 1982
17. Kruger E, Krumholz K: Results of bone grafting after rigid fixation. J Oral Maxillofacial Surg 42:491–496, 1984
18. Bitter K, Schlesinger S, Westerman U: The iliac bone or osteocutaneous transplant pedicled to the deep circumflex iliac artery. J Maxillofac Surg 11:241–247, 1983
19. Taylor GI: Reconstruction of the mandible with free composite iliac bone grafts. Ann Plast Surg 9:361–377, 1982
20. MacLeod AM, Robinson DW: Reconstruction of defects involving the mandible and floor of mouth by free osteocutaneous flaps derived from the foot. Br J Plast Surg 35:239–246, 1982
21. Schmidt DR, Robson MC: One-stage composite reconstruction using the latissimus myoosteocutaneous free flap. Am J Surg 144:470–472, 1982
22. Conley J: Use of composite flaps containing bone for major regions in the head and neck. Plast Reconstr Surg 49:522–526, 1972
23. Pearlman NW, Albin RE, O'Donnell RS: Mandibular reconstruction in irradiated patients utilizing myoosseocutaneous flaps. Am J Surg 146:474–477, 1983
24. Cuono CB, Ariyan S: Immediate reconstruction of a composite mandibular defect with a regional osteomusculocutaneous flap. Plast Reconstr Surg 65:477–482, 1980
25. Little JW III, McCulloch DT, Lyons JR: The lateral pectoral composite flap in one-stage reconstruction of the irradiated mandible. Plast Reconstr Surg 71:326–335, 1983
26. Jones NF, Sommerland BC: Reconstruction of the zygoma, TMJ and mandible using a compound pectoralis major osteomuscular flap. Br J Plast Surg 36:491–497, 1983
27. Panje WR: Mandible reconstruction with the trapezius osteomusculocutaneous flap. Arch Otolaryngol 111:223–229, 1985
28. Watson RM, Welfare RD, Islami A: The difficulties of prosthetic management of edentulous cases with hemimandibulectomy following cancer treatment. J Oral Rehab 11:201–214, 1984
29. Branemark PI, Breine U, Hallen O, et al.: Repair of defects in mandible. Scand J Plast Surg 4:100–106, 1970
30. Lindstrom J, Branemark PI, Albrektsson T: Mandibular reconstruction using the preformed, autologous bone graft. Scand J Plast Surg 15:29–35, 1981
31. Odell R, Lekholm U, Rochler B, et al.: Osseointegrated titanium fixtures in the treatment of edentulousness: A 15 year followup study. Int J Oral Surg 10:387–393, 1981

13 Principles and Preferences in Mandibular Reconstruction

Byron J. Bailey, M.D.

The field of mandibular reconstruction has advanced rapidly during the past decade. New and better reconstructive flaps and more durable and versatile metallic and alloplastic materials have provided strong stimuli for the numerous investigations that have been undertaken. A critical period of transition must elapse between the introduction of new concepts for reconstruction and the time when it is possible to say with certainty that one procedure is "the best." We are currently moving ahead in that transition from surgical innovation to clinical application in the field of mandibular reconstruction.

The goals of the surgeon have changed little during the past 50 years and can be listed as follows:

1. To restore mandibular form and function.
2. To minimize malocclusion and mandibular drift.
3. To accomplish simultaneously skeletal reconstitution and soft tissue coverage.
4. To reconstruct the mandible primarily when possible.
5. To reconstruct the mandible using a single-stage procedure whenever possible.
6. To minimize the operative and postoperative morbidity at the donor and recipient sites.
7. To utilize techniques that are compatible with preoperative and postoperative radiation therapy.

In this chapter, we would like to share some personal preferences of this author and those of other head and neck surgeons engaged in mandibular reconstruction.

OPTIONS FOR MANDIBULAR RECONSTRUCTION

The leading authorities in surgical reconstruction of the mandible have progressed through a cyclical pattern during the past 20 years. During the 1960s, simple spacing devices such as the Kirschner wire and similar pins and plates were used most commonly in mandibular reconstruction. During the 1970s, more elaborate, complex, and expensive procedural options were introduced and promoted. Some of these options experienced initial popularity, followed by numerous reports of complications and other problems so that in their rate of utilization subsequently declined. A definite attitude of restraint and conservatism characterizes most surgeons at present. While the reasons for this state of affairs are understandable, the need remains pressing for continuing, aggressive investigation into all of the possible opportunities to improve the postoperative condition of patients who lose segments of mandible from trauma or surgical resection.

The surgeon may select a reconstructive approach from various options. Each of the following techniques has been the subject of numerous published reports and presentations at recent scientific meetings:

1. *Soft tissue closure without skeletal reconstruction*. This technique has been recommended particularly for short, lateral segmental defects of the mandible. Occasionally, it may yield acceptable results for anterior defects (Figs. 218 and 219).

2. *Kirschner wire and other simple spacing devices followed by a period of observation* (Figs. 220–223). This approach leaves open assorted options for secondary reconstruction and is advised when of malignant lesions are likely to recur locally or in the neck. Several authors have reported their preference for this approach because of the relatively low success rate of primary repair, largely due to difficulties with postoperative infection. Various secondary reconstructive procedures can be accomplished with much higher success rates.

3. *Dynamic bendable defect bridging plates*. These plates have become popular with some surgeons because of their versatility and reliability. They are heavier and more durable than the Kirschner wire but introduce a much smaller amount of metallic foreign material than do the larger metallic cribs.

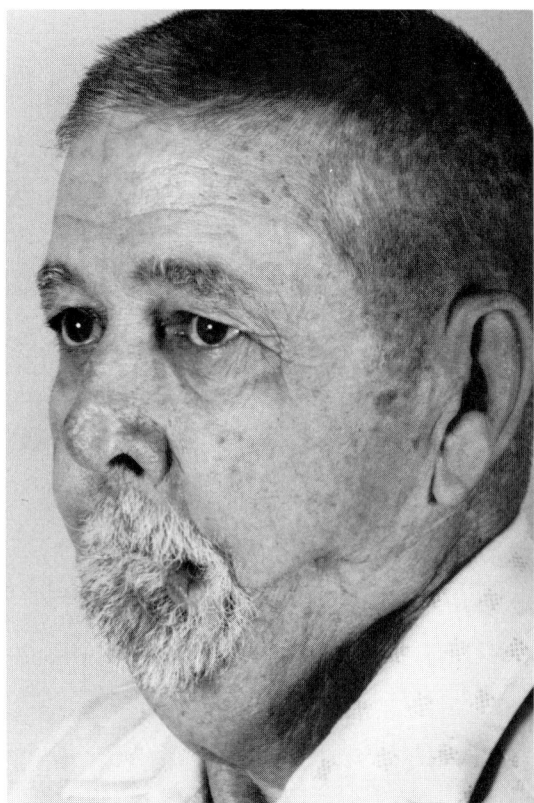

Figure 218. Resection of symphysis and anterior body bilaterally for carcinoma of anterior floor of mouth. Kirschner wire was used temporarily as a spacer, but was removed at 8 months postoperatively when it became displaced. Patient does not desire further reconstruction.

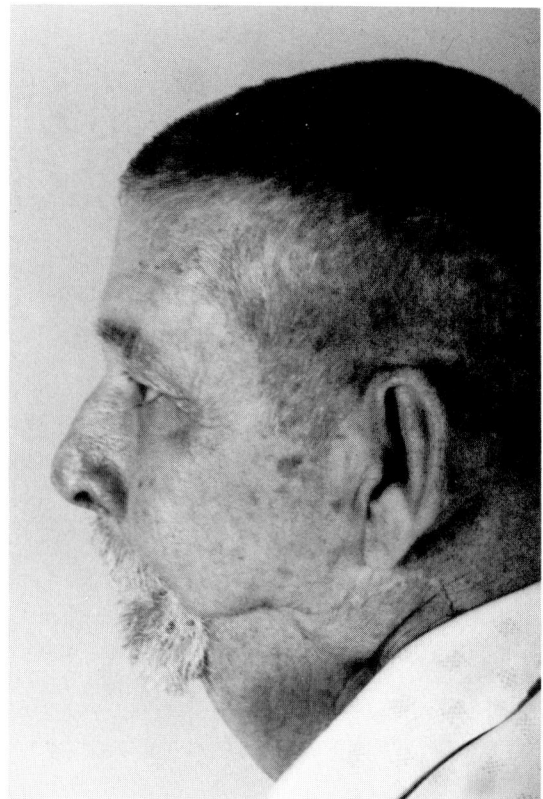

Figure 219. Same patient viewed from laterally. Speech articulation and deglutition are satisfactory and there is salivary continence.

Surgeons at the University of Minnesota have reported their experience with mandibular reconstruction using A-O plates.[1] Their use of these bendable plates in 11 patients with mandibular defects achieved a solid mandibular arch in every case (Figs. 224–226).

Strelzow has described the use of implantable stabilization plates to control the position and relationship of the mandibular segments after partial resection.[2] He illustrates the technique with examples of defect management at the angle (Figs. 227 and 228) and at the symphysis (Figs. 229–231).

4. *Myocutaneous flaps without osseous components.* These flaps are proposed for the muscle bulk that is introduced to maintain special relationships.[3] Furthermore, they are useful for increasing blood supply (Figs. 232–234).

5. *Myocutaneous flaps with bone segments.* Four flaps are included in this group: the sternocleidomastoid-clavicular flap, the trapezius flap along with the spine of the scapula, the pectoralis major myocutaneous (PMM) flap that incorporates a segment of the fifth rib, and the more recently described PMM flap that incorporates a bone graft implanted beneath the flap at a previous procedure.

The trapezius osteomyocutaneous island flap for mandibular reconstruction was introduced into the American literature by Panje and Cutting in 1980. Subsequently, they published a report of their results with 24 patients in whom they used this composite flap to repair mandibular defects. They achieved a success rate of 87% and the procedure appears to be particularly useful for immediate reconstruction.[4] The anatomic features of the blood supply and the incision are shown in Figures 236 and 237.

Maisel and Adams[5] recently summarized their observations regarding mandibular reconstruction with a pectoralis major osteomycutaneous flap that incorporates a segment of the fifth rib (Figs. 238–240). They emphasized the financial savings that can be realized when immediate reconstruction is successful. When secondary repair is either chosen electively or forced by events, the patient may require from 24 to 47 additional hospital days rather than a 1- to 2-year period.

6. *Free rib grafts.* Wersall and co-workers[6] had

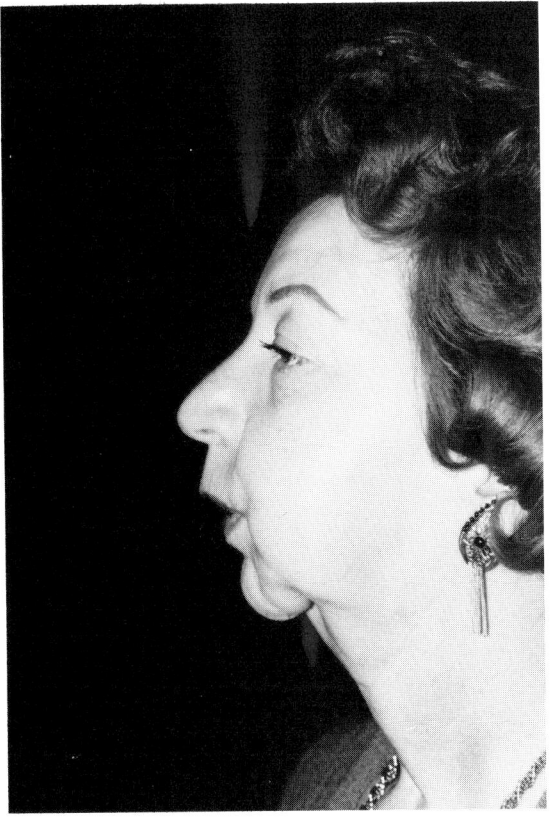

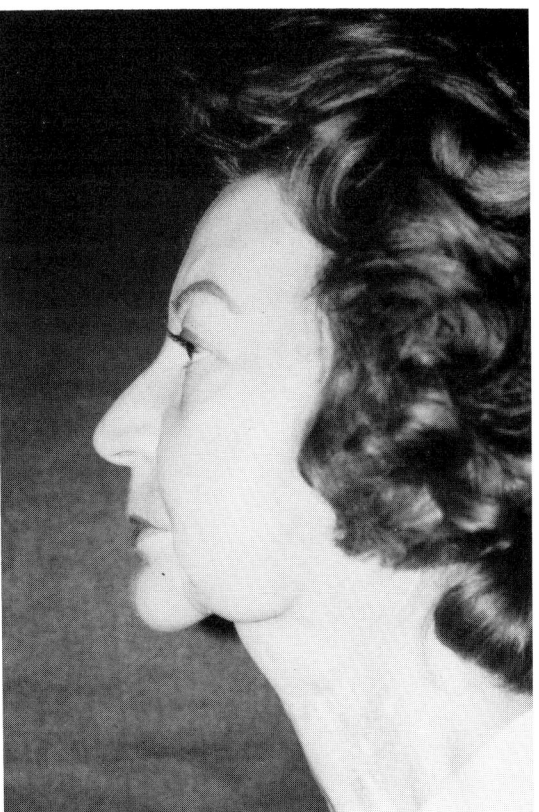

Figure 220. Resection of anterior mandibular arch (symphysis and anterior body bilaterally) in continuity with anterior floor of mouth and tongue. Kirschner wire was used temporarily as a spacer to bridge defect and maintain mandibular relationships during healing. Lateral (profile) views shows chin deformity at 3 months postoperatively.

Figure 221. Same patient 6 months later after a more curved Kirschner wire with a Silastic outer layer was implanted to provide chin advancement. Although speech articulation is moderately impaired, there is salivary continence and deglutition is satisfactory.

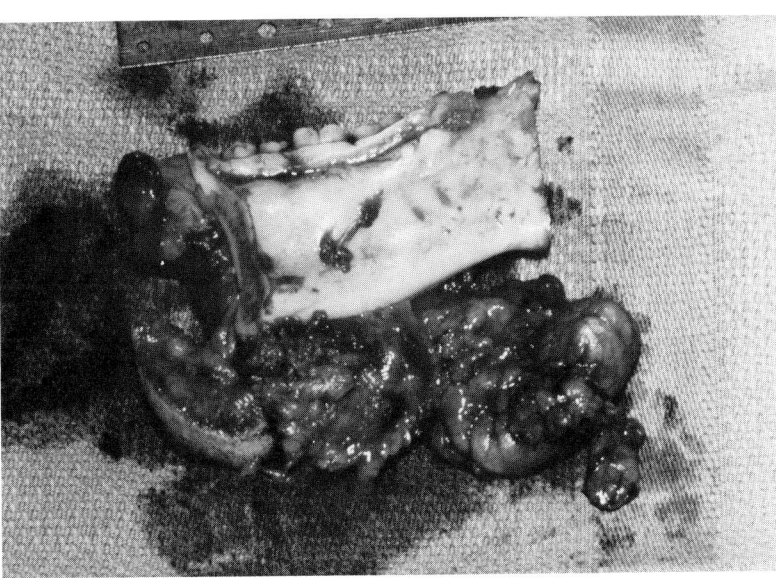

Figure 222. Hemimandibulectomy and neck dissection specimen. Mandibular symphysis resected as well because of direct extension from lip cancer plus perineural tumor spread along inferior alveolar nerve.

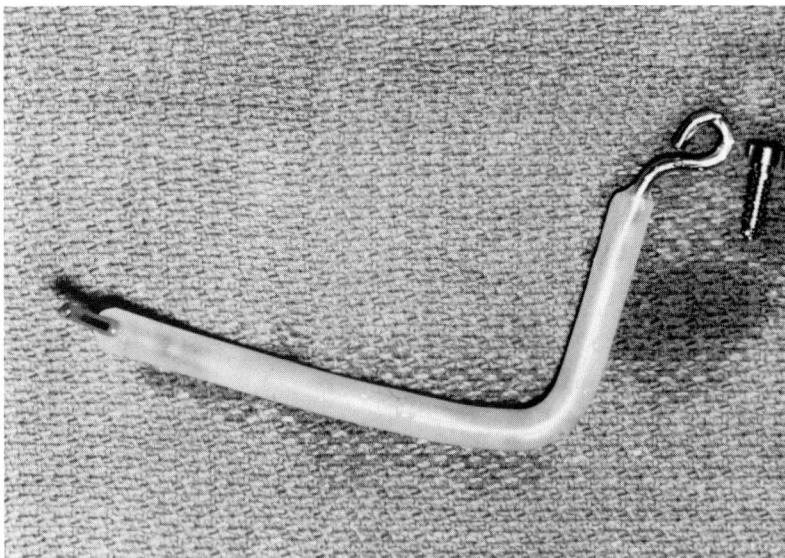

Figure 223. Kirschner wire plus Silastic spacing prosthesis with eyelet fashioned to permit attachment by screw to proximal segment of mandibular ramus.

good success with split-rib free grafts for mandibular reconstruction in a group of 23 patients. We have recently used similar treatment for some of our patients. First, the defect is prepared to receive the graft, the external biphasic appliance is put in place, and adequate hemostasis is achieved (Fig. 241). The rib is split longitudinally and the two halves are wired together with the marrow surfaces outward and the cortical surfaces touching each other. This bone graft unit is then wired into position in the defect (Figure 242). and the wound is closed.

7. *Iliac crest and other bone grafts without microvascular anastomosis.* The use of bone grafts without microvascular anastomosis has been widely reported and reviewed. Lawson and Biller[7] have studied a series of 60 patients who underwent mandibular reconstruction; many of these patients were managed by block bone grafts. These surgeons emphasizes that oral contamination of the graft site is the major factor involved in the failure of this approach when it is employed as a primary technique at the time of tumor resection. Block bone grafts removed from the iliac crest or ribs are extremely reliable in reconstituting the continuity of the mandibular arch when the following three conditions are met:

1. An extraoral surgical approach is employed.
2. Adequate immobilization of the graft is achieved.
3. The technique is employed as a *delayed* (secondary) approach after of the original surgical wound has healed completely.

When these principles are followed, this technique can be used successfully, even in patients who have undergone high-dose radiation therapy.

8. *Iliac crest grafts with microvascular anastomosis.* The successful use of a free feusor fascia lata osteomyocutaneous flap in the reconstruction of mandibular defects has been reported by Baker.[8] This approach requires the special technical expertise of microvascular anastomosis. Its advantages include more rapid healing in poorly vascularized areas, less risk of bone graft absorption, and greater resistance to infection and extrusion. Figures 243—247 illustrate this technique and the results.

Panje[9] has described his short-term success with a free compound groin flap (containing a segment of iliac crest) in the repair of extensive anterior mandibular defects (Figs. 248–250). The bone grafts have survived despite their placement in an irradiated field in the presence of salivary contamination.

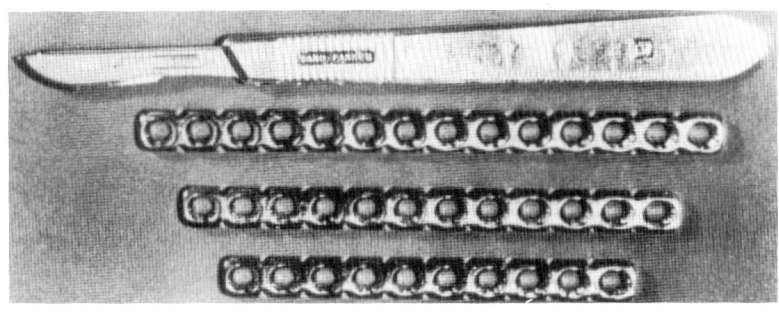

Figure 224. Three of several different reconstructive plates that are commercially available. (From Hilger PA and Adams GL: Arch Otolaryngol 111:470, 1985. With permission.)

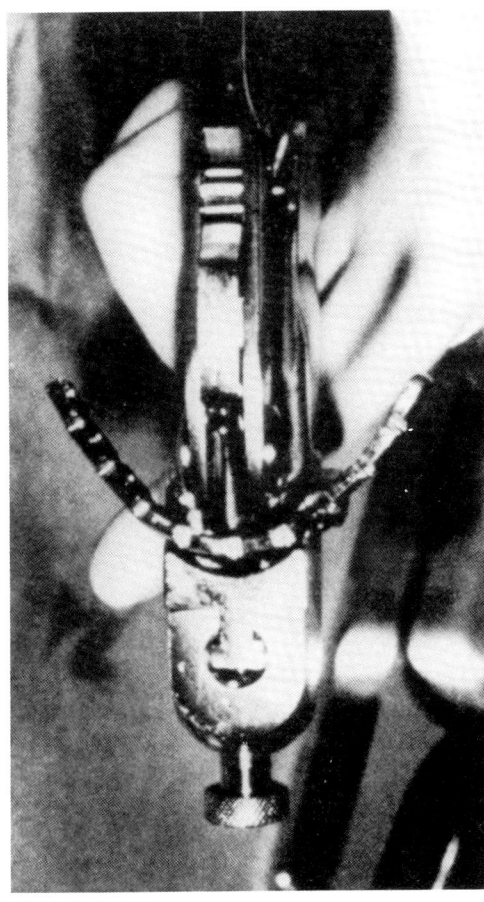

Figure 225. Shaping the reconstructive plate is accomplished using the orthopedic plate bender. (From Hilger PA and Adams GL: Arch Otolaryngol 111:470, 1985. With permission.)

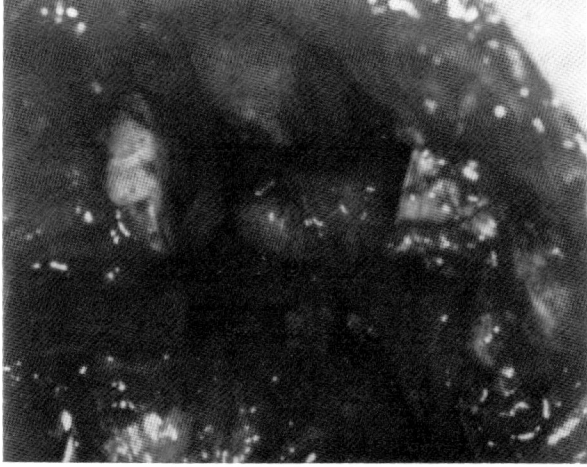
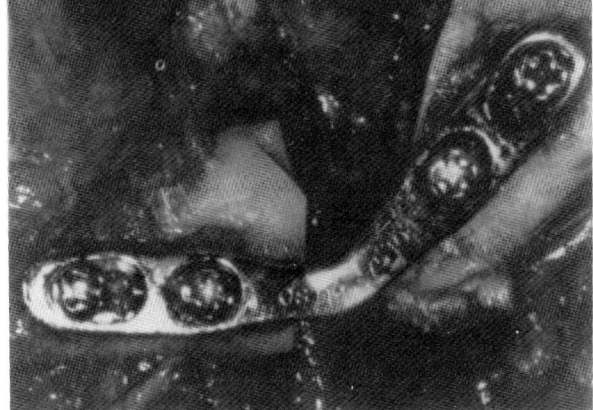
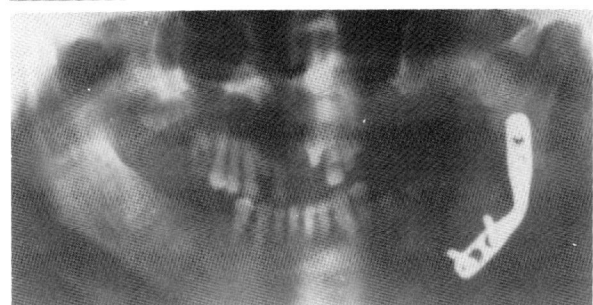

Figure 227. Top: mandibular defect (5.5 cm) after composite resection. Center: advanced bone segments with 62-mm "spanner" plate. Bottom: postoperative roentgenogram showing left spanner plate. (From Strelzow VV: Arch Otolaryngol 109:334, 1983. With permission.)

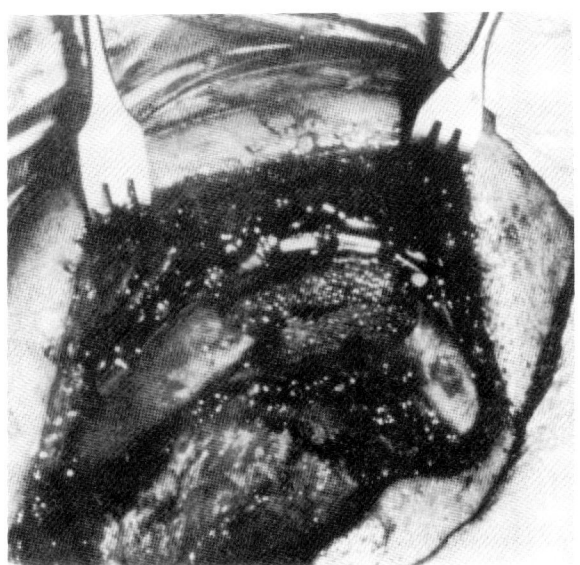

Figure 226. Reconstructive plate in place with cortical and cancellous bone filling the defect. (From Hilger PA and Adams GL: Arch Otolaryngol 111:470, 1985. With permission.)

Continued bone viability was documented by technetium^{99m} (Tc^{99m}) pyrophosphate scanning and other techniques.

Harrison and Quillen[10] report the same technique from a slightly different perspective. They note the usefulness of the free osteocutaneous groin flap in the repair of extensive lateral and posterior defects (Figs. 251 and 252).

9. *Bone banks or autogenous frozen or irradiated homograft replacements for the mandible.* These approaches to mandibular reconstruction have been proposed by deFries[11] and by Cummings and

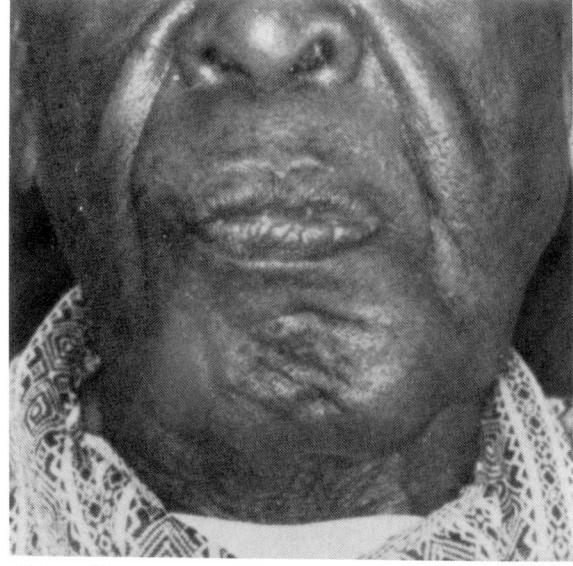

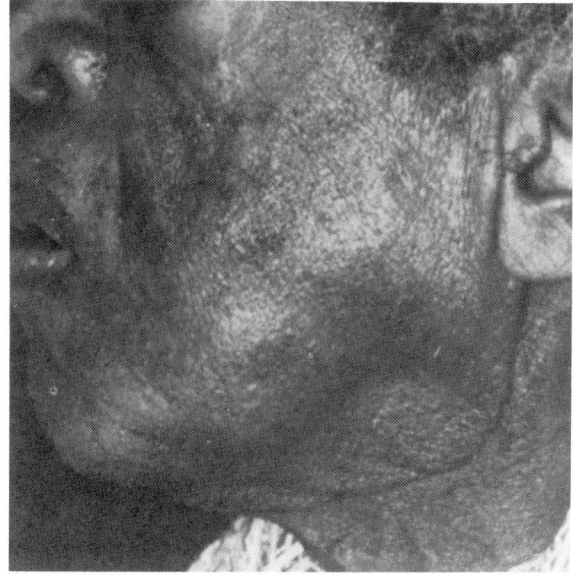

Figure 228. Top: Frontal view. Bottom: Laterial view, 6 months postoperative. (From Strelzow VV: Arch Otolaryngol 109:335, 1983. With permission.)

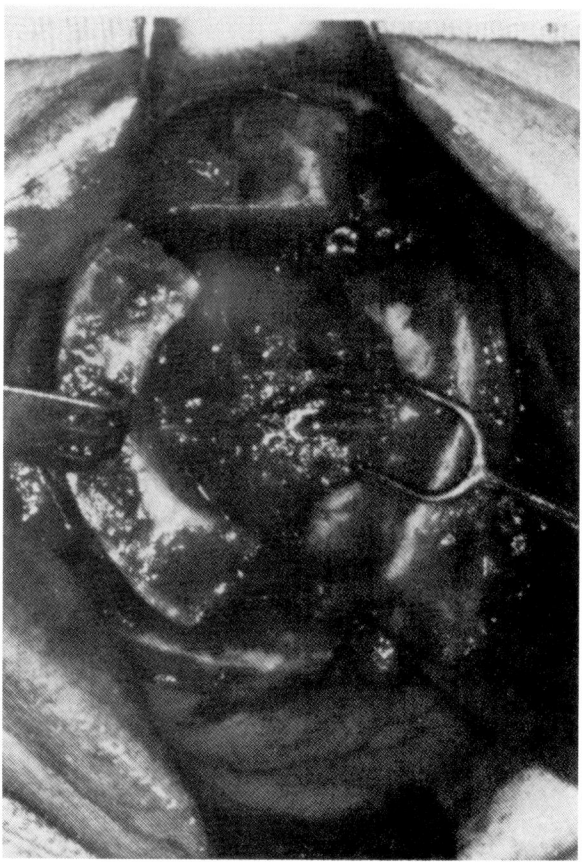

Figure 229. Anterior mandibular arch defect. (From Strelzow VV: Arch Otolaryngol 109:335, 1983. With permission.)

Leipzig.[12] They may have a broader clinical usefulness in the future than they currently enjoy for successful reconstruction after cancer surgery. It does seem that deFries has had good success (12 of 14 patients) when the repair is used for traumatic mandibular loss or when the patient has not undergone irradiation therapy (Table 13–1).

10. Metal cage/crib prostheses without autoge-

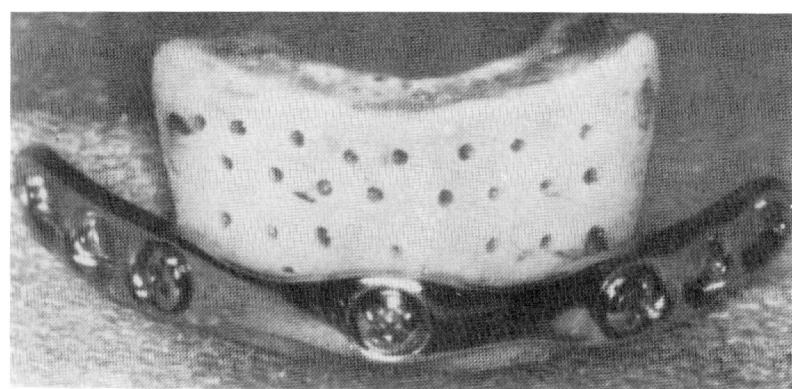

Figure 230. Stabilization plate, 92 mm, with freeze-treated bone graft. (From Strelzow VV: Arch Otolaryngol 109:335, 1983. With permission.)

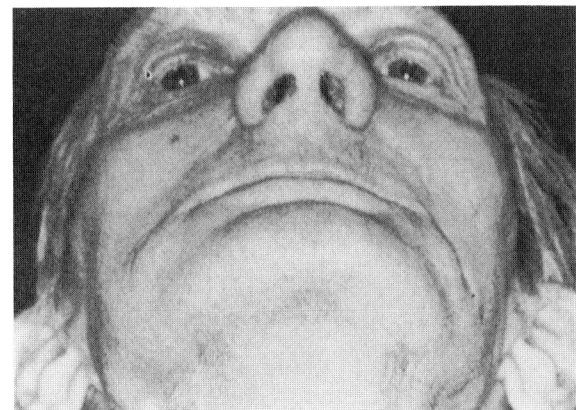
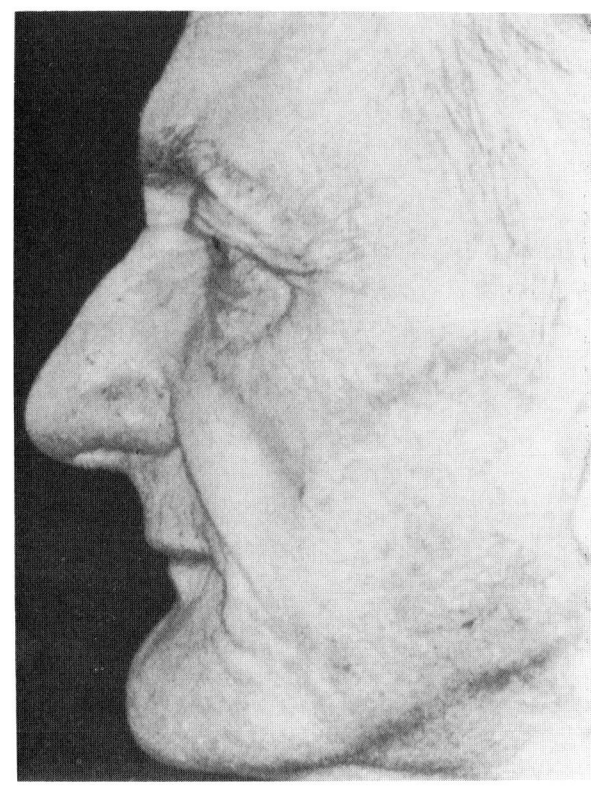

Figure 231. (A) Frontal—submental view. (B) Lateral view, 12 months postoperative. (From Strelzow VV: Arch Otolaryngol 109:335, 1983. With permission.)

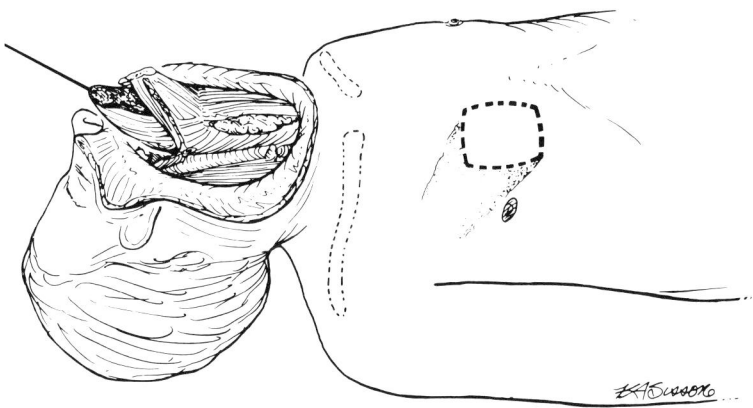

Figure 232. Flap outlined on chest. (From Berktold RE et al.: Otolaryngol Head Neck Surg 94:181, 1986. With permission.)

nous particulate cancellous bone graft material. Schuller and co workers[13] reported the successful use of titanium tray mandibular reconstruction without using cancellous bone fragments in the trays. The technique (Figs. 253–255) was effective in patients with mandibular loss following gunshot wounds. The objectives of this type of repair are to restore the integrity of the mandibular arch and to improve appearance and function, using a reliable single-stage technique. The limitations of masticatory function and the risk of late extrusion must be weighed carefully in the surgeon's decision.

11. *Metal cage/crib prostheses with autogenous particulate cancellous bone.* These prostheses were advocated for repair of posttraumatic mandibular defects by Boyne[14] in 1969. This technique has been employed successfully for the delayed repair of defects resulting from oncologic surgery but has

Table 13–1. Combined Mandibular Homograft-Autograft (1970–1978)

	No. of Patients	Success (No. of Patients)	Failure (No. of Patients)
Trauma	12	10	2
Cancer resection			
Without prior radiation	2	2	0
With prior radiation	12	2	10

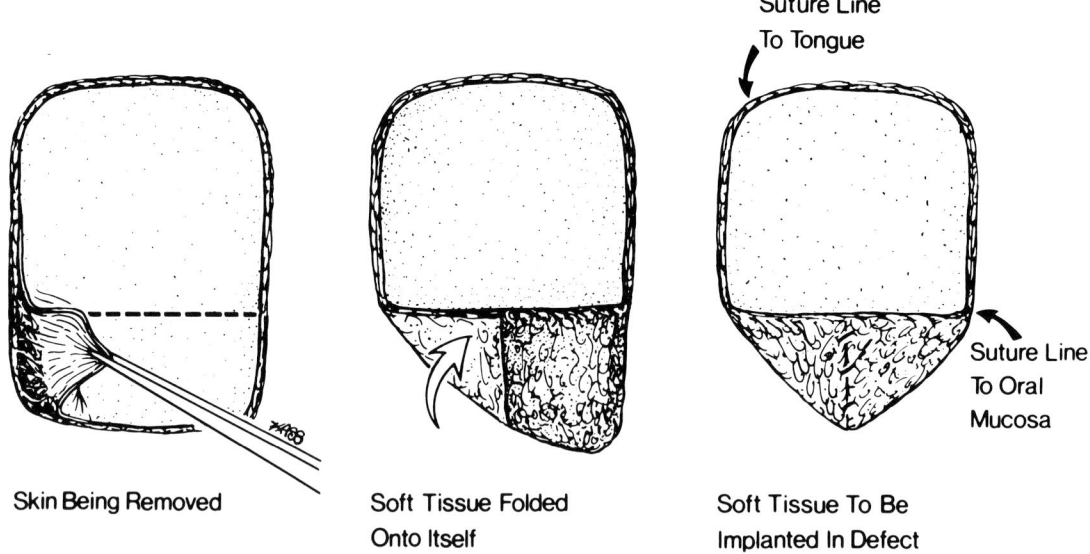

Figure 233. Details of flap modification. (From Berktold RE et al.: Otolaryngol Head Neck Surg 94:182, 1986. With permission.)

been problematic as a primary reconstructive technique. A recent report by Shrewsbury[15] reviews this technique (Figs. 256 and 257) and related options for repairing complicated mandibular defects. These include dynamic compression plates and reconstructive plates attached to custom-fitted cortical-cancellous bone plugs.

12. *Alloplastic prostheses without autogenous particulate cancellous bone (e.g., Silastic or Proplast)*. Numerous attempts have been made to utilize alloplastic materials as permanent, functional replacements for missing mandibular segments. Despite occasional success, most surgeons find that greater problems with late infection and extrusion with this technique than they are with other reconstructive options. This approach may prove ultimately to be successful, but more research and development are needed.

13. *Alloplastic prostheses with autogenous particulate cancellous bone (Dacron mesh tray)*. The

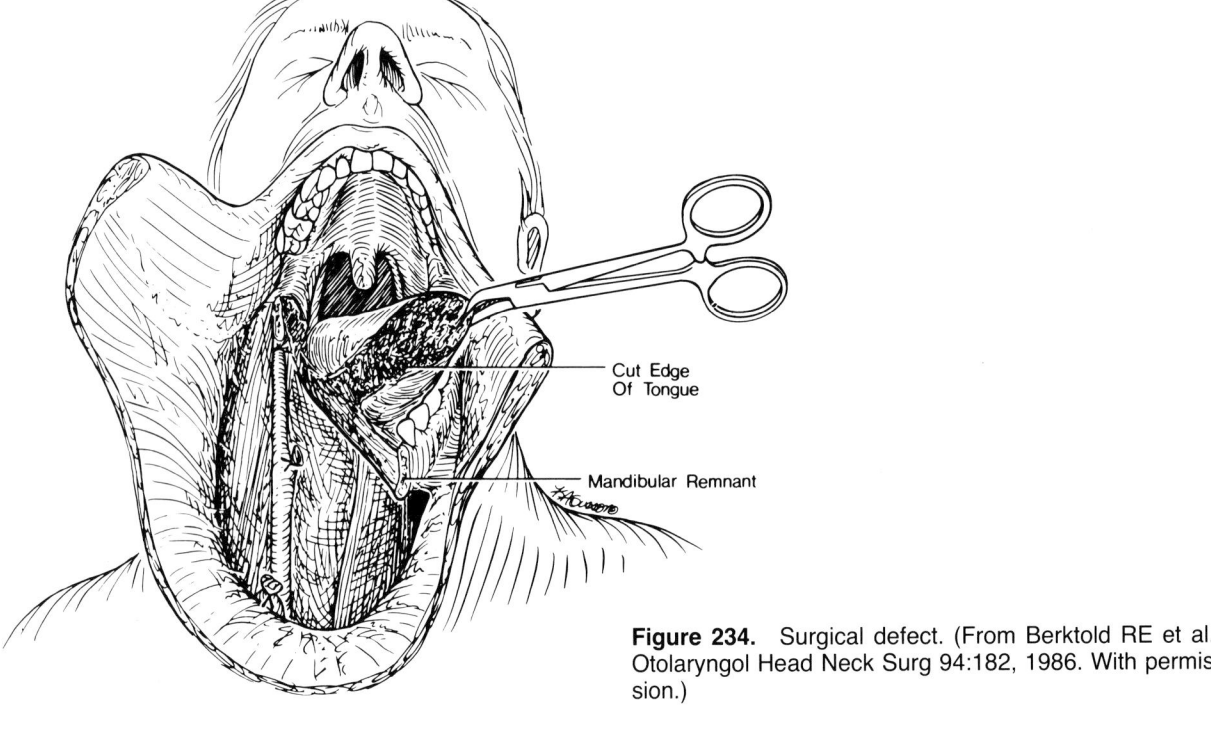

Figure 234. Surgical defect. (From Berktold RE et al.: Otolaryngol Head Neck Surg 94:182, 1986. With permission.)

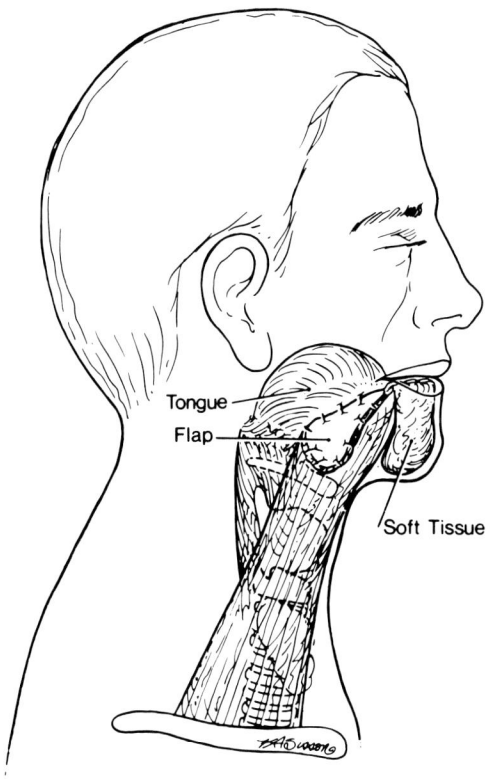

Figure 235. Finished result shows soft tissue part of flap replacing chin. (From Berktold RE et al.: Otolaryngol Head Neck Surg 94:183, 1986. With permission.)

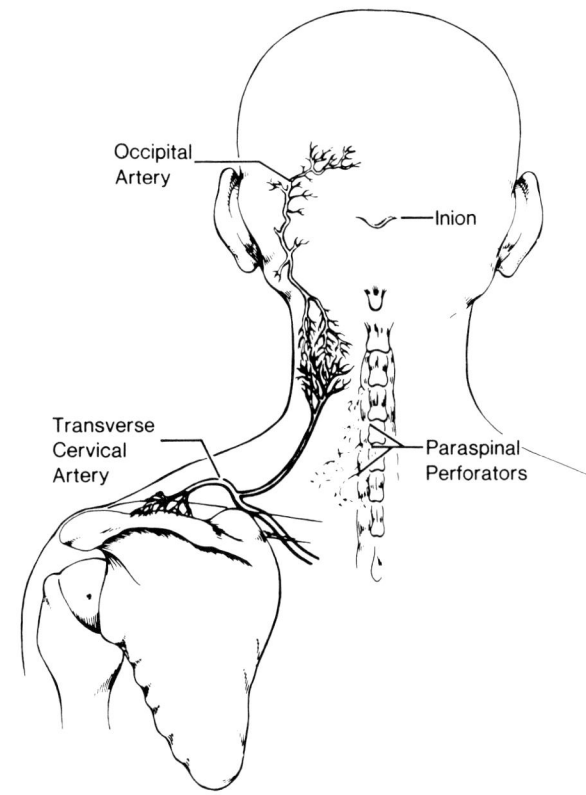

Figure 236. Tripartite blood supply to upper half of the trapezius muscle. Osteomyocutaneous flap can survive on either transverse cervical vasculature alone or paraspinous perforators with or without occipital vasculature. (From Panje WR: Arch Otolaryngol 111:224, 1985. With permission.)

apparent exception to the problems of alloplastic prosthetic mandibular replacement is the Dacron mesh tray, originally described by Leake.[16] Recently, Albert and colleagues[17] reported successful achievement of solid functional mandibles in a group of patients with posttraumatic and postoperative mandibular defects.

This reconstructive procedure (Figs. 258–260)

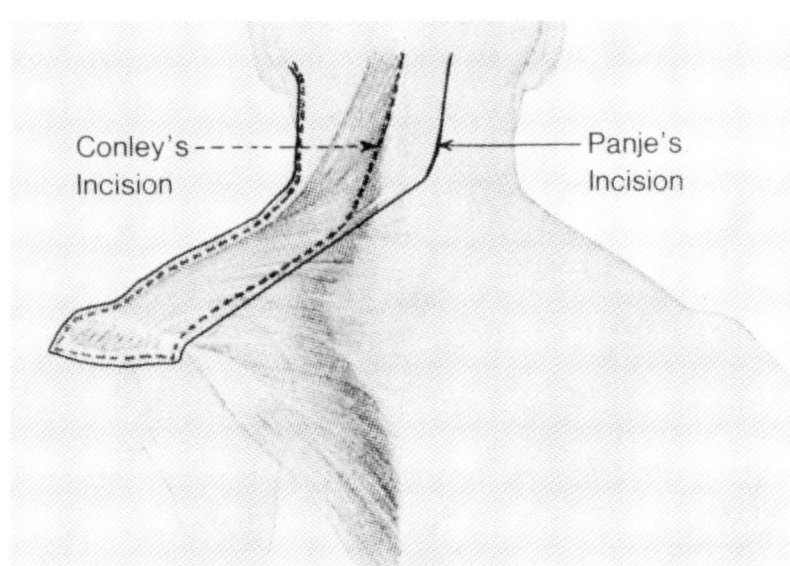

Figure 237. Broken line indicates incision used by Conley for trapezius composite flap. This flap is dependent on occipital vasculature. Solid line indicates incision to allow inclusion of paraspinous vasculature with pedicled trapezius osteomyocutaneous flap. (From Panje WR: Arch Otolaryngol 111:224, 1985. With permission.)

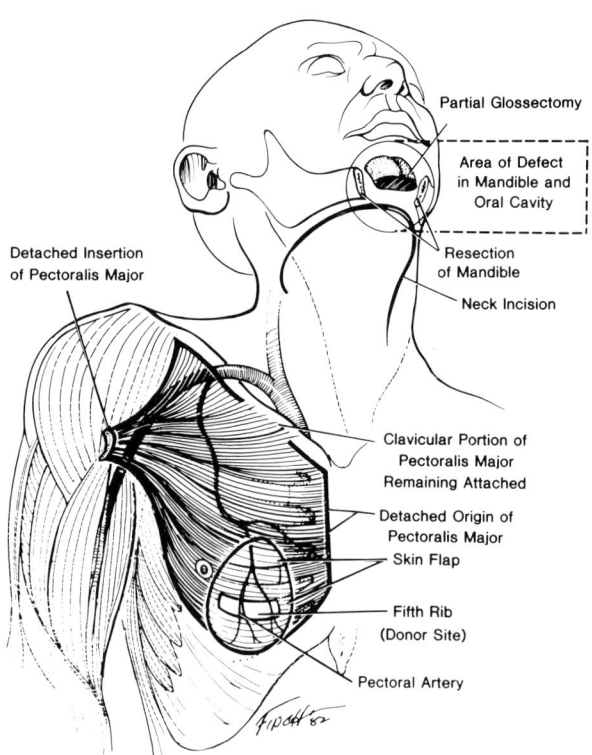

Figure 238. Harvesting of osteomyocutaneous flap. Pectoralis muscle is drawn in situ. (From Maisel RH and Adams GL: Arch Otolaryngol 109:732, 1983. With permission.)

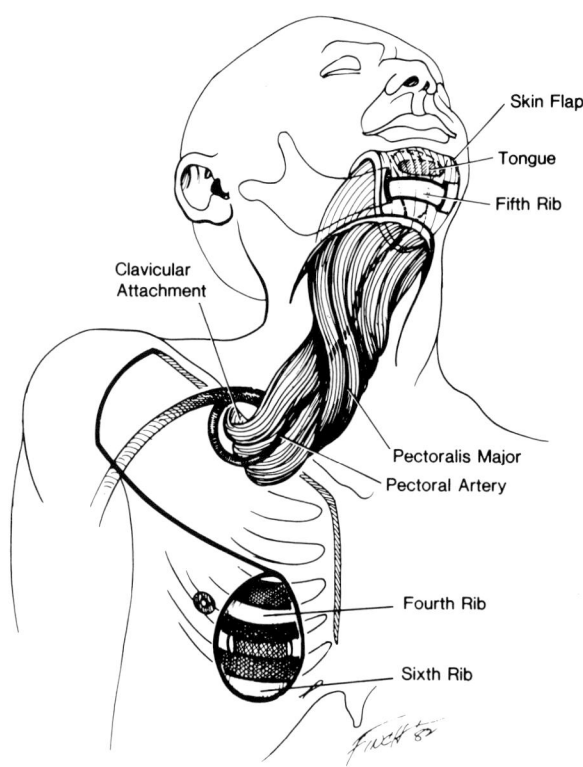

Figure 240. Lateral view. Flap is rotated to ensure preservation of artery. Skin of flap is sutured to soft tissues of tongue and lip. Bulk of muscle further protects bone from intraoral exposure. (From Maisel RH and Adams GL: Arch Otolaryngol 109:732, 1983. With permission.)

requires careful attention to surgical technique and to the authors' recommended guidelines, including the following:

—Delayed reconstruction.
—Adequate soft tissue coverage, externally and intraorally.
—Immobilization of the mandible.
—Avoidance of salivary contamination.
—Preoperative and postoperative use of hyperbaric oxygen therapy in those patients with prior radiation therapy or osteoradionecrosis.

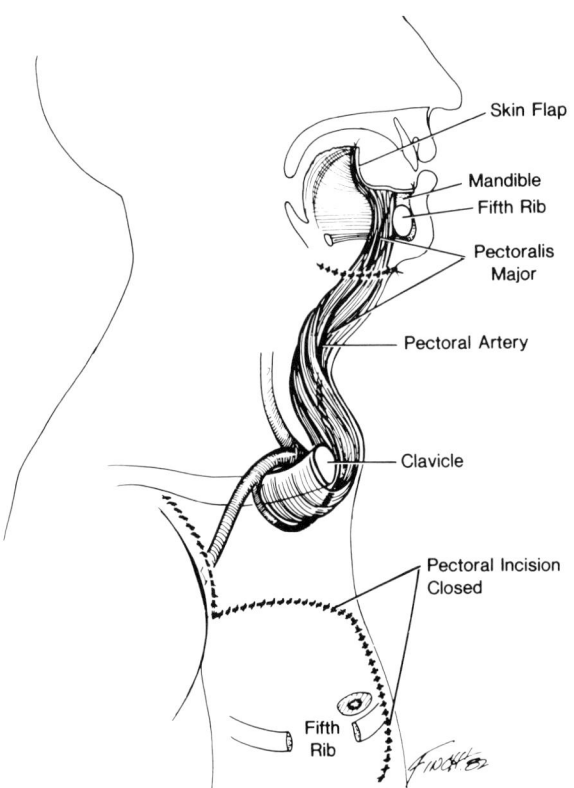

Figure 239. Osteomyocutaneous flap is elevated over clavicle and deep to skin of neck until it is in position at anterior mandible. (From Maisel RH and Adams GL: Arch Otolaryngol 109:732, 1983. With permission.)

14. *Hydroxyapatite calcium sulfate and free periosteal grafts as bone repair materials.* Mandibular reconstruction may require the replacement of lost bone substance, without the need for immediate restoration of full mandibular strength. Numerous materials including assorted metals, several alloplastic materials, and different types of organic substances have been used with varying propotions of success and problems. McKee and Bailey[18] have investigated the use of calcium sulfate as a bone implant for the repair of surgically created mandibular defects in dogs (Fig. 261). We observed that

Principles and Preferences in Mandibular Reconstruction 183

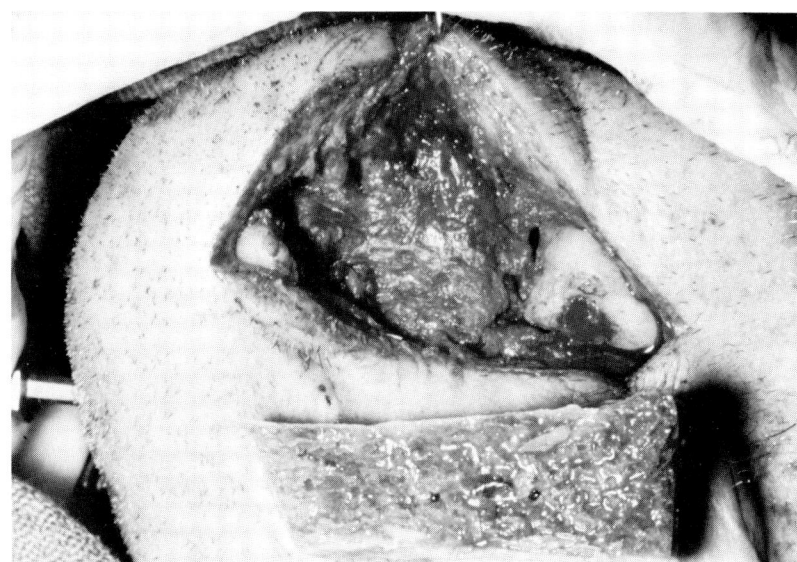

Figure 241. Defect of left parasymphyseal area after surgical resection and radiation therapy. Free split-rib graft prepared and shaped after external biphase appliance has secured segments.

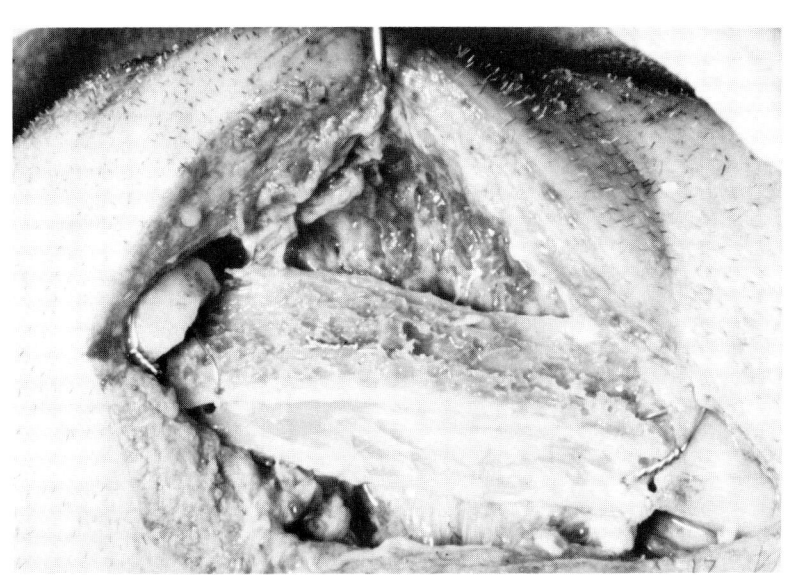

Figure 242. Split-rib graft is secured in defect using interosseous wire fixation.

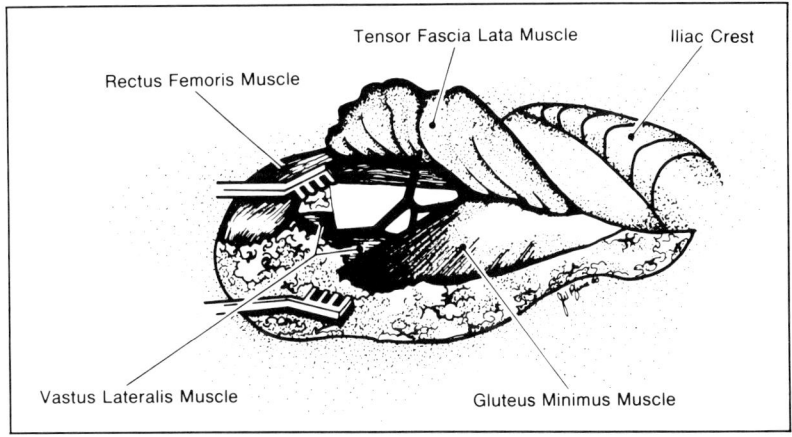

Figure 243. Cadaver dissection demonstrating branching of lateral femoral circumflex artery. Artery supplies branches to vastus lateralis and gluteus minimus muscles before continuing as transverse branch to tensor fascia late muscle. (From Baker SR: Arch Otolaryngol 107:417, 1981. With permission.)

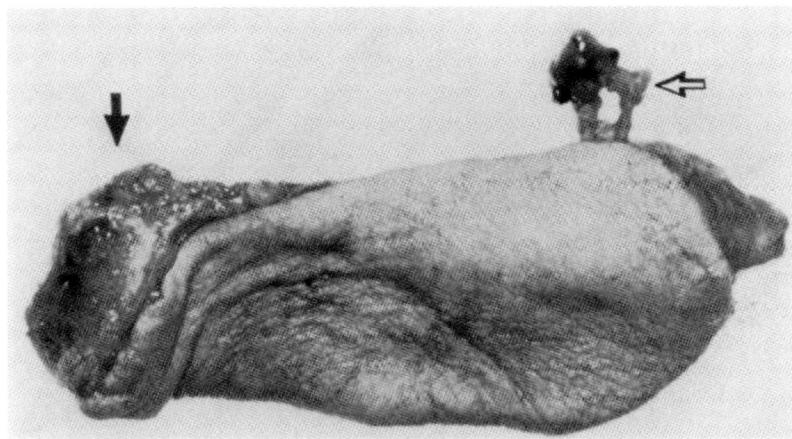

Figure 244. Tensor fascia lata osteomyocutaneous flap has been harvested and is ready for transfer to oral cavity. Vascular pedicle (outlined arrow) and attached segment of iliac crest bone (arrow) are noted. (From Baker SR: Arch Otolaryngol 107:416, 1981. With permission.)

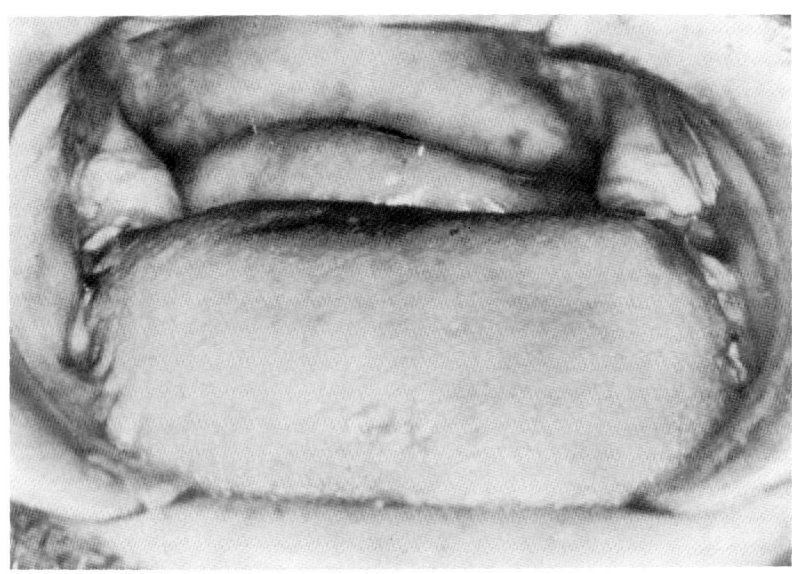

Figure 245. Tensor fascia lata osteomyocutaneous flap, 10 days postoperatively. (From Baker SR: Arch Otolaryngol 107:416, 1981. With permission.)

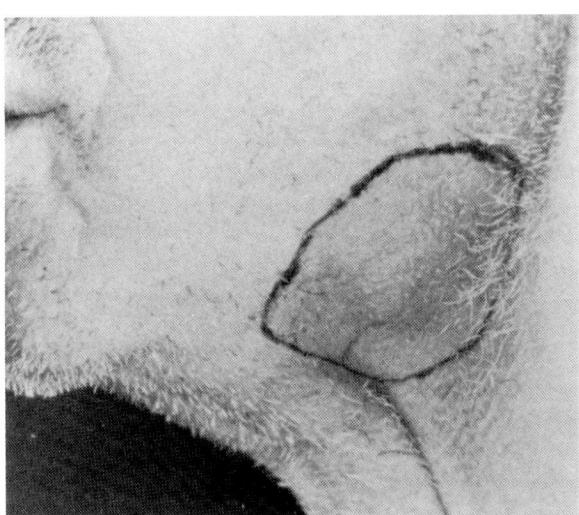

Figure 246. Metastatic squamous cell carcinoma to submandibular lymph nodes with attachment to body of mandible and overlying skin. (From Baker SR: Arch Otolaryngol 107:416, 1981. With permission.)

calcium sulfate can overcome problems of rejection, late infection, and failure to establish bony fusion with the adjacent mandible. The calcium sulfate appears to be a stimulus for osteoneogenesis, with new bone forming through and around the calcium sulfate, even when the periosteum has been excised with the underlying bone.

Stanley and Rice[19] accomplished a similar result using autoclaved, reimplanted bone grafts in association with free periosteal grafts. They removed 1.0 × 3.0-cm segments of bone from the lower border of the mandible in dogs (Fig. 262) and found that the bone grafts were solidly healed 8 weeks later.

15. *Adjunctive prosthetic devices to enhance function.* In conceptualizing mandibular reconstructive options, we must remind ourselves that function is the key in determining postoperative success. In dealing with the complex act of deglutition it helps to think of the oral cavity structures as a

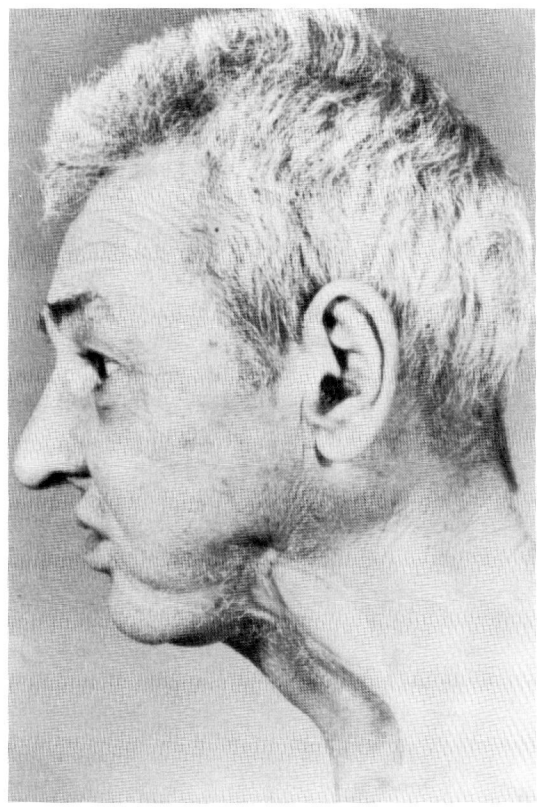

Figure 247. Tensor fascia lata osteomyocutaneous flap, 8 months postoperatively.(From Baker SR: Arch Otolaryngol 107:416, 1981. With permission.)

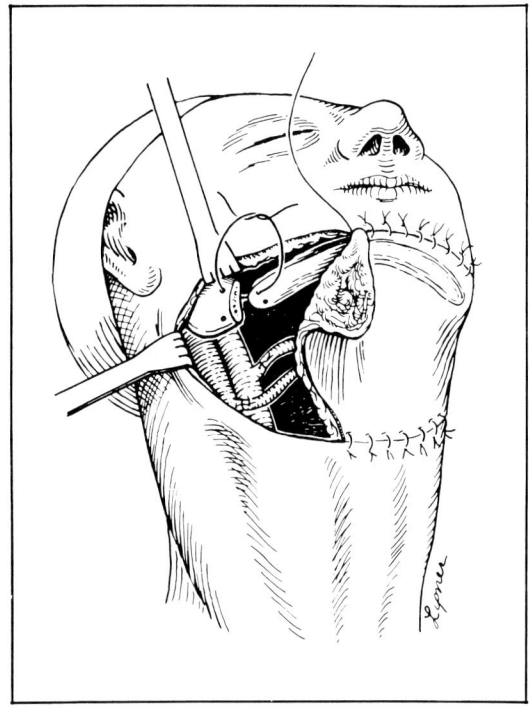

Figure 249. Illustration of compound flap being placed into recipient site. (From Panje WR: Arch Otolaryngol 107:19, 1981. With permission.)

series of four valves (lips, tongue, hard and soft palate, and velopharyngeal port).[20] A mandibular resection may have a marked effect on the first three of these valves, and patients will often benefit greatly from a prosthesis designed to enhance their ability to propel a food bolus into the pharynx. The compensatory prosthetic augmentation (Figs. 263 and 264) will provide enough improvement in many patients to permit a much more rapid return to near-normal nutritional patterns.

The availability and promotion of such a varied set of options carries the same implication in this field of surgery as in all other surgical fields. They indicate that no single approach works reliably in a sufficient number of settings to be designated at this time as "the best method."

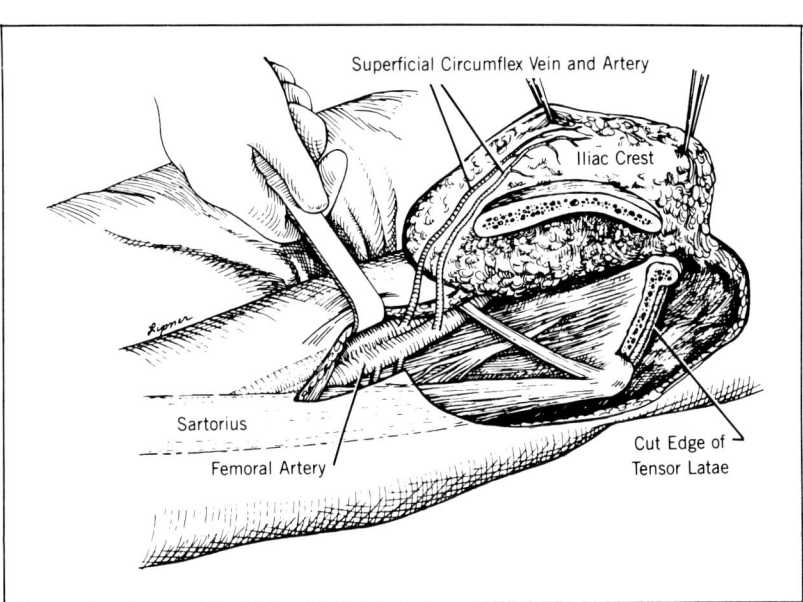

Figure 248. Illustration of compound groin flap reflected from ilium. (From Panje WR: Arch Otolaryngol 107:18, 1981. With permission.)

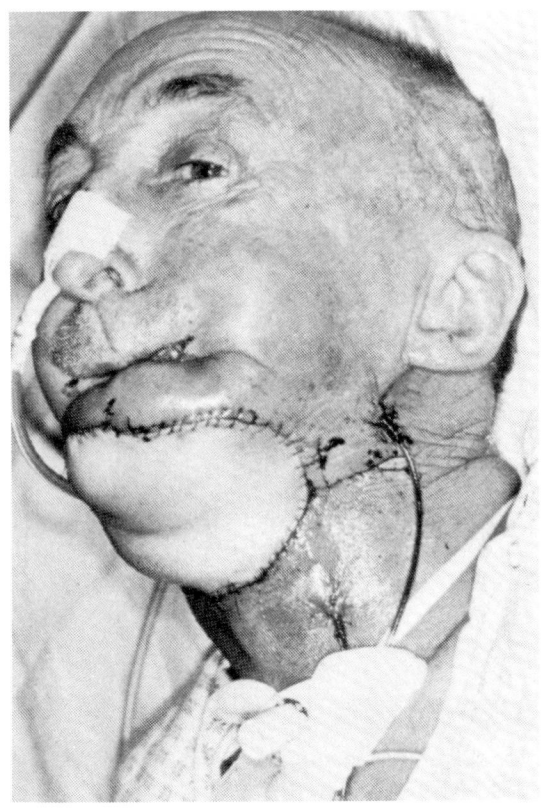

Figure 250. Early postoperative period. (From Panje WR: Arch Otolaryngol 107:19, 1981. With permission.)

The mature surgeon always keeps in mind that the performance of a reconstructive procedure carries no assurance that a positive step has been taken toward the goals stated in the first section of this chapter. An unsuccessful reconstructive effort may result in a patient who has lost more mandibular form and function than would have been lost with a simple soft tissue closure. We must be certain that neither our primary resection nor our reconstructive intervention is responsible for creating an "oral cripple."

On a more positive note, advances in the field of mandibular reconstruction have brought us to a period when previously "unresectable" tumors can now be resected, and previously "unreconstructable" defects can now be reconstructed. Patients in whom the risks of loss of function and extensive postoperative deformity would have been too great to permit the adequate surgical excision of an oral cavity primary are now becoming infrequent.

SUMMARY OF MANDIBULAR RECONSTRUCTIVE PRINCIPLES

The plan for surgical management of oral neoplasms and trauma involving the mandible is a challenging mix of immediate concern for managing the surgical procedure in the most appropriate way and a long-term projection of the patient's status months and years in the future. In dealing with the interaction of surgical resection and surgical reconstruction, the surgeon must consider numerous conditions that deal with both the positive factors of healing and repair and the most common mechanisms of surgical failure.

Some of the issues that must be considered include the following:

—The oral cavity soft tissue closure and the external skin closure over the mandible must be complete and watertight. Salivary contamination of a skeletal repair or reconstruction will almost always lead to infection despite perioperative antibiotic therapy.
—Techniques employed in tumor resection and mandibular reconstruction must preserve an adequate blood supply for the prevention of various postoperative complications.
—Reconstruction of the soft tissues in the surgical defect of the oral cavity should be durable enough to tolerate a moderate degree of trauma. The soft tissue repair should be performed in a manner that retains maximum tongue mobility, which is so crucial for articulation and swallowing.
—Mandibular reconstructive techniques must be followed by a period of complete immobilization.
—Mandibular reconstructive techniques must result in a sufficient degree of postoperative strength and durability to permit relatively normal activities.
—The reconstructive techniques selected should be compatible with preoperative and postoperative radiation therapy. Preoperative radiation therapy results in scarring and a degree of vascular compromise that often cause problems for the introduction of prosthetic materials and free bone grafts. The ability to deliver radiation therapy precisely is diminished by the introduction of large metallic prostheses.
—The training and experience of the surgeon must be compatible with the surgical objectives.
—The desires and general medical status of the patient may eliminate some options. Malnutrition, severe cardiovascular disease, and diminished pulmonary function are factors that limit the techniques that are feasible.

Principles and Preferences in Mandibular Reconstruction 187

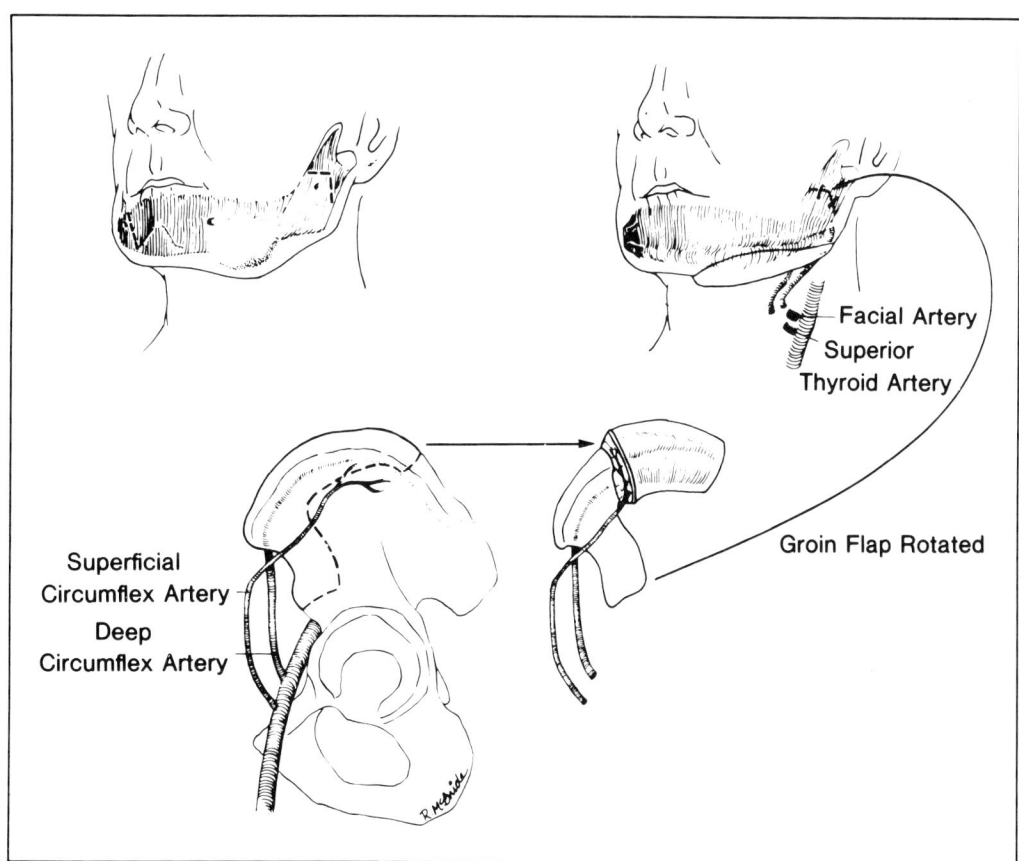

Figure 251. Schema of entire free osteocutaneous groin flap procedure. Top left: View of carcinomatous mass and area of mandible to be excised. Dotted lines indicate limits of mandibular resection. Bottom left: harvesting of groin flap and its transfer as mandible and facial replacement. Anatomic location of flap with dotted lines indicate limits to iliac resection. Bottom right: schematic drawing of composite groin flap. Both arteriovenous systems, superficial circumflex iliac, and deep circumflex iliac are used in our groin flap to promote better survival. Top right: Final reconstruction showing position of bony and cutaneous portions of graft and arterial anastomoses. (From Harrison TJ and Quillen CG: Arch Otolaryngol 109:486, 1983. With permission.)

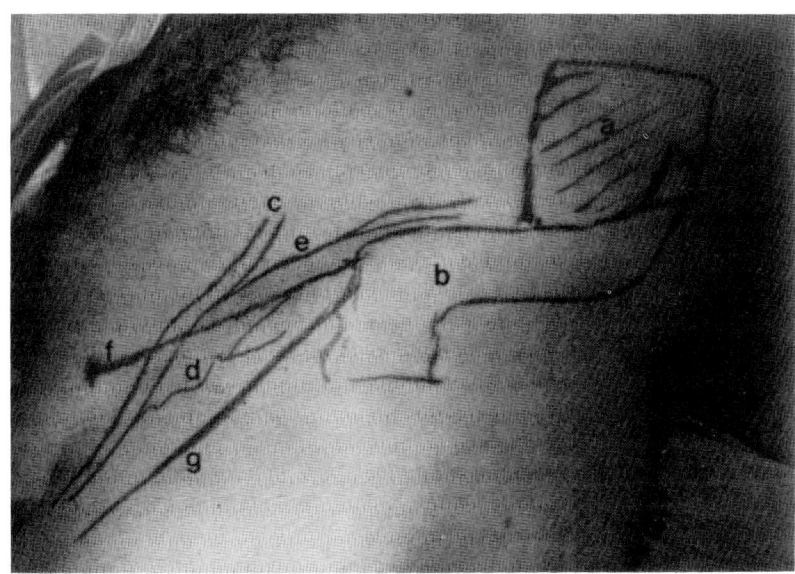

Figure 252. (a) Design of osteocutaneous groin flap. Anatomy shown consists of groin skin to be transplanted. (b) Iliac crest bone to be transplanted. (c) Femoral artery. (d) Superficial circumflex iliac artery. (e) Deep circumflex iliac artery. (f) Inguinal ligament. (g) Border of sartorius muscle. (From Harrison TJ and Guillen CG: Arch Otolaryngol 109:486, 1983. With permission.)

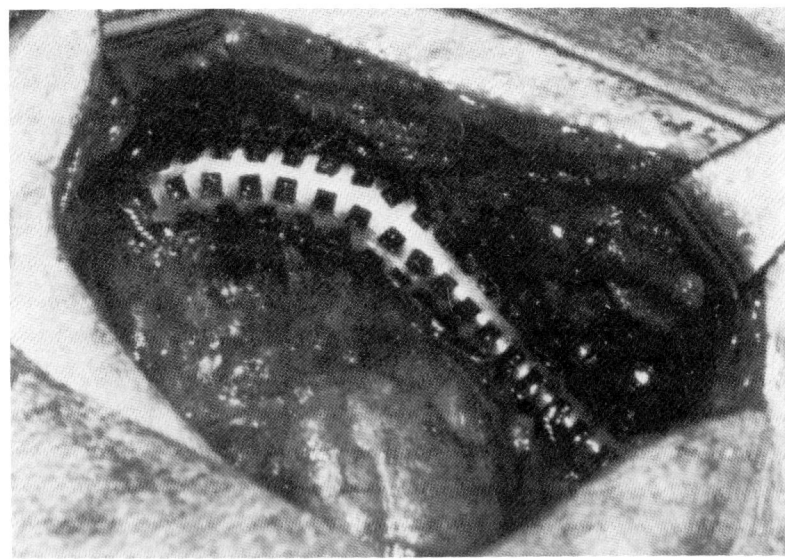

Figure 253. Titanium tray secured in position and packed with particulate cancellous marrow grafts from iliac crest.

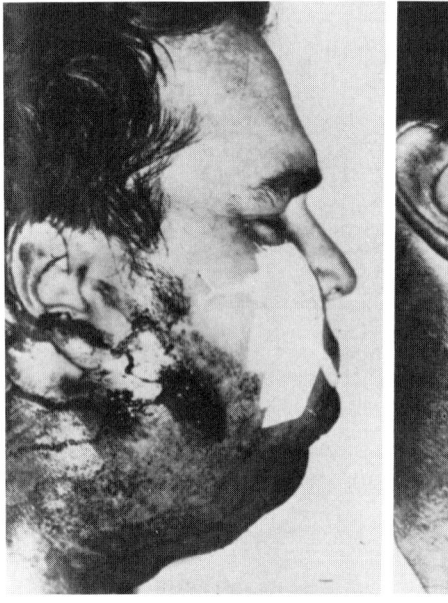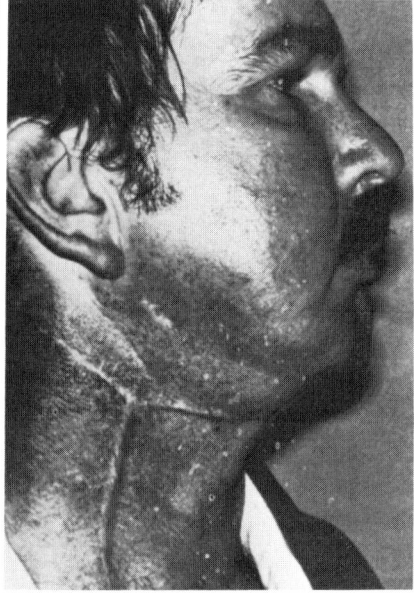

Figure 254. Left: patient who sustained facial gunshot wound that destroyed mandibular body and avulsed facial skin and soft tissue. Right: exploration of this wound was performed through inferior neck incision to provide access for eventual mandibular reconstruction without placing incision directly over future site of titanium tray. (From Schuller DE et al.: Arch Otolaryngol 108:175, 1982. With permission.)

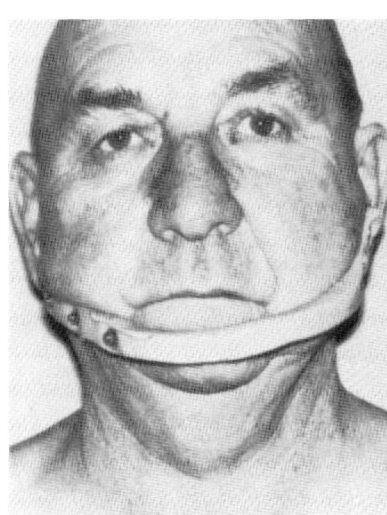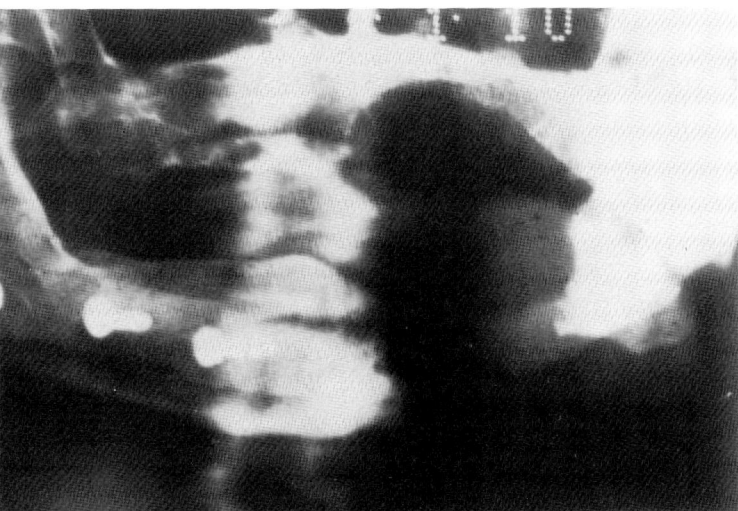

Figure 255. Left: Biphase external mandibular splint maintains proper position of mandibular fragments after mandibular resection, as seen in roentgenogram (right). (From Schuller DE et al.: Arch Otolaryngol 108:176, 1982. With permission.)

Figure 256. Cancellous bone within cobalt-chromium alloy (Vitallium basket). (From Shrewsbury DW et al.: Arch Otolaryngol 108:164, 1982. With permission.)

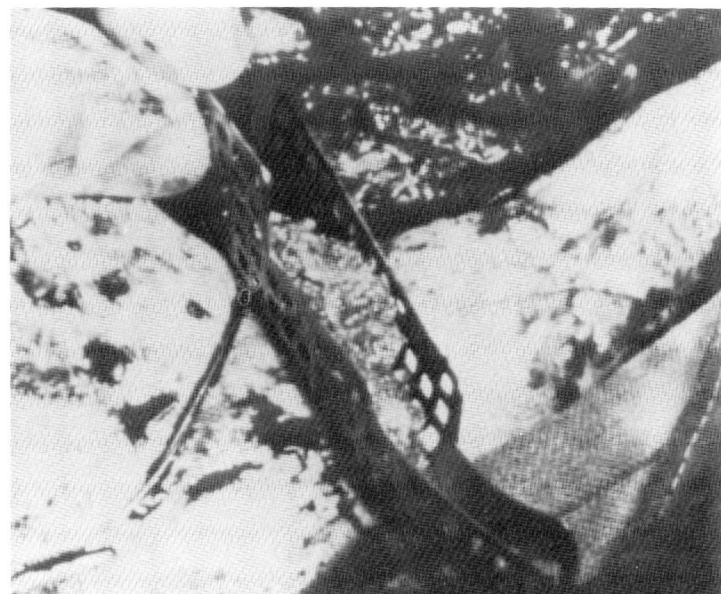

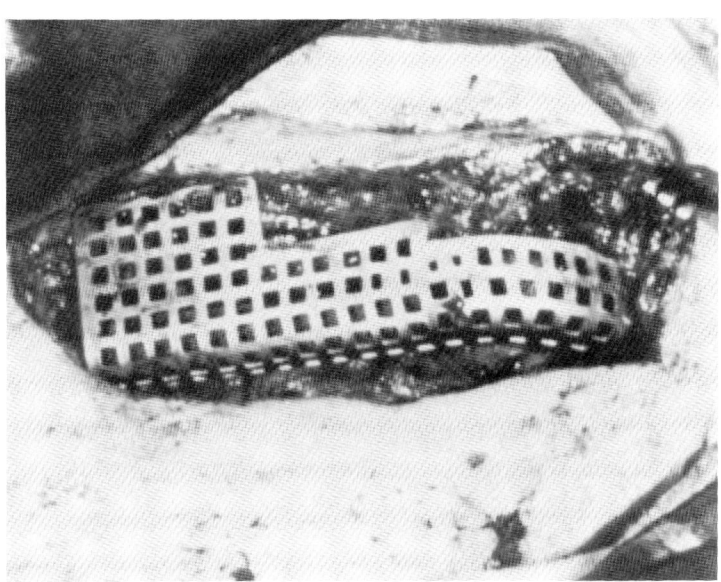

Figure 257. Basket is secured to mandibular stumps. (From Shrewsbury DW et al.: Arch Otolaryngol 108:164, 1982. With permission.)

Figure 258. Dacron-urethane mesh tray, male size. (From Albert TW et al.: Arch Otolaryngol Head Neck Surg 112:53, 1986. With permission.)

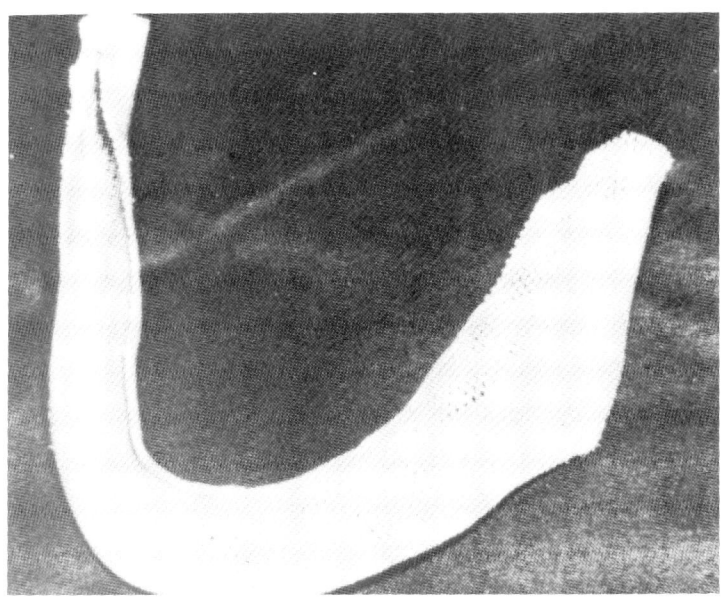

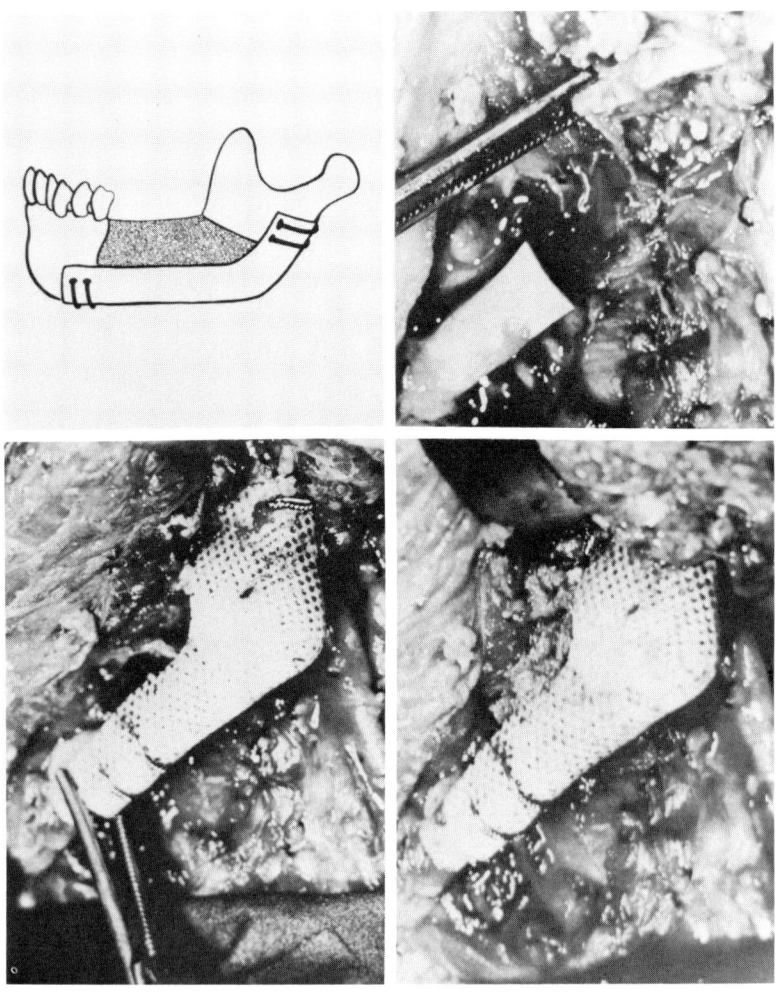

Figure 259. Top left: diagram of Dacron-urethane mesh tray bridging mandibular defect. Top right: mandibular defect in patient. Bottom left: mandibular defect bridged by Dacron-urethane mesh tray. Bottom right: Dacron-urethane mesh tray filled with cancellous bone. (From Albert TW et al.: Arch Otolaryngol Head Neck Surg 112:53, 1986. With permission.)

—The time that will be required to complete the reconstruction and the cost to the patient must be considered.
—The patient's prognosis for cure.
—The size and location of the mandibular defect.
—The amount of donor site morbidity.

Many other variables of less significance may be thought of as "fine points" affecting the decision to favor one type of reconstruction versus another. These secondary issues include the following:

—Issues concerning the antigenicity of reconstructive material. Autogenous bone grafts

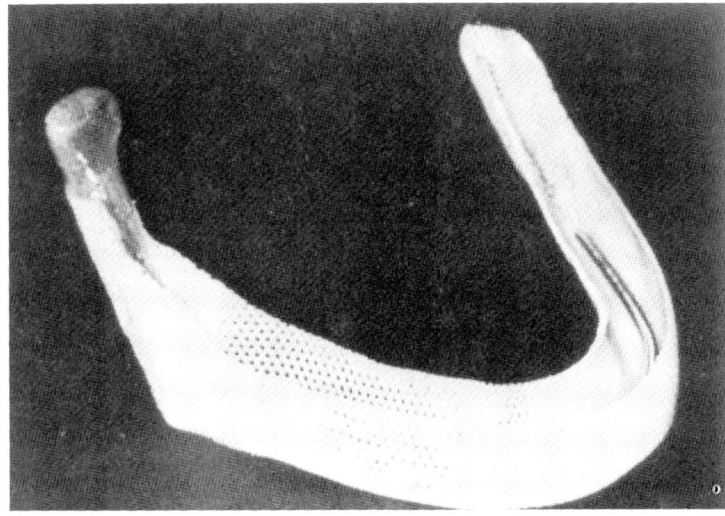

Figure 260. Special Dacron-urethane mesh tray with fabricated polyurethane condyle. (From Albert TW et al.: Arch Otolaryngol Head Neck Surg 112:55, 1986. With permission.)

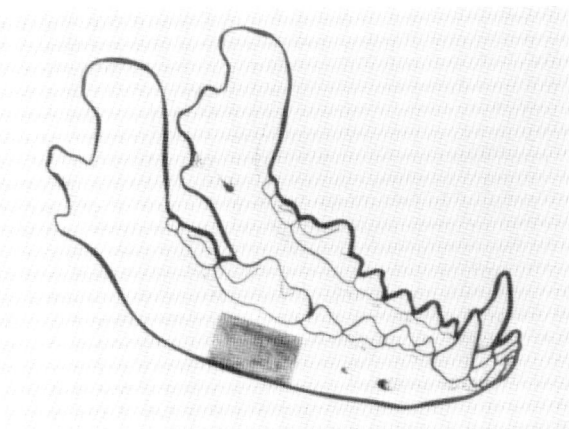 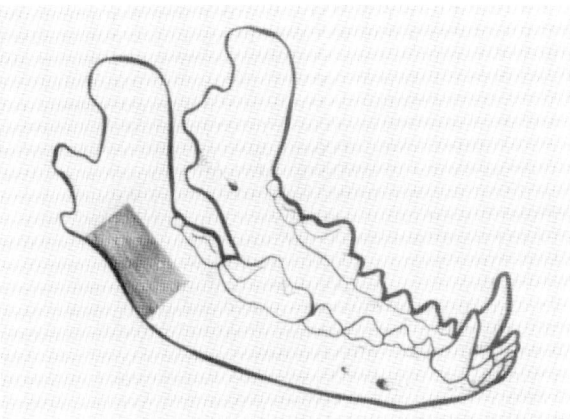

Figure 261. Depicts segments of the body and the ramus that were excised and repaired with calcium sulfate. (From McKee JC and Bailey BJ: Otolaryngol Head Neck Surg 92:278,1

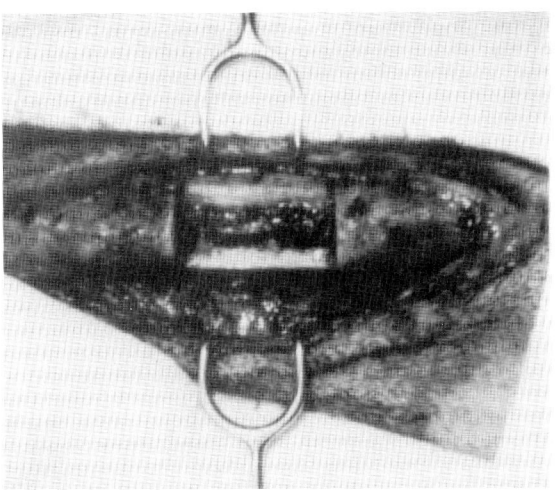 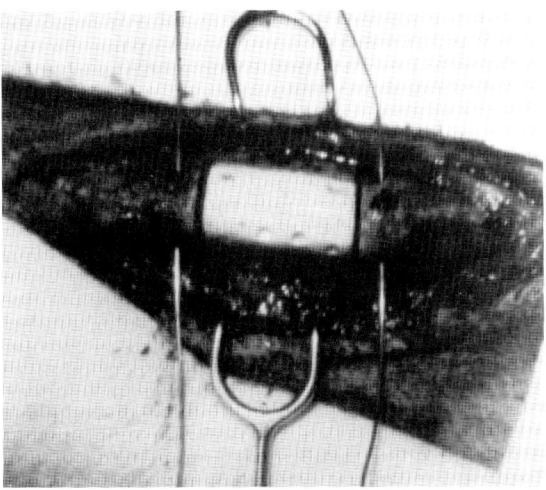

Figure 262. Left: lower border of mandibular body with 1 × 3-cm segment of bone removed. Right: autoclaved bone in position prior to wiring. (From Stanley RB and Rice DH: Otolaryngol Head Neck Surg 89:415, 1981. With permission.)

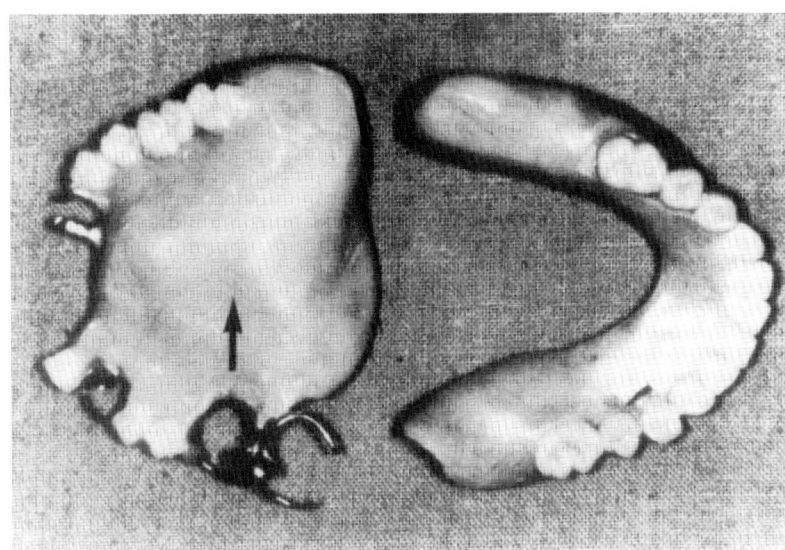

Figure 263. Palatal prosthesis with built-up area (arrow). (From Wurster CR et al.: Arch Otolaryngol 111:530, 1985. With permission.)

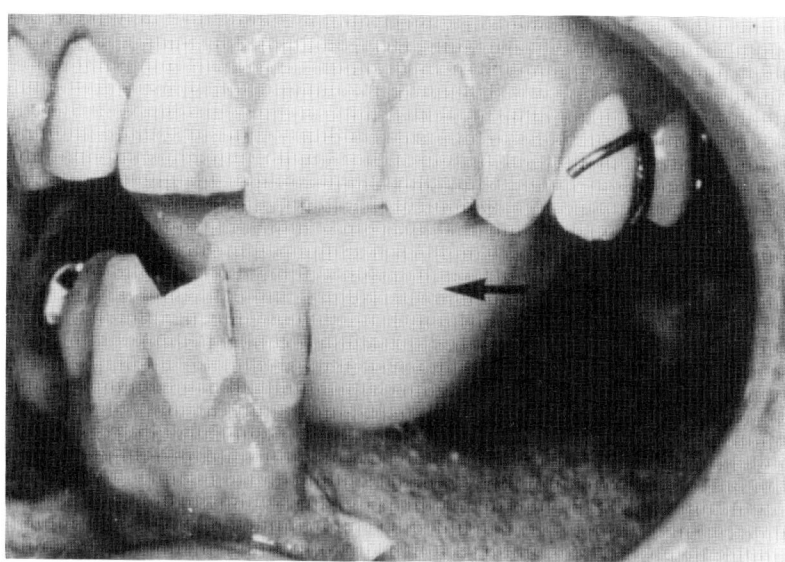

Figure 264. Palatal prosthesis augmentation in place (arrow). Two months after surgery. (From Wurster CR et al.: Arch Otolaryngol 111:531, 1985. With permission.)

are considered more desirable than homologous or bone bank specimens.

—Reconstructive techniques that can be accomplished with maximum preservation of mandibular periosteum are favored.

—Fresh autologous bone grafts are preferred to frozen autologous bone grafts as templates for new bone growth.

—The less foreign material implanted, the less the risk of postoperative infection.

—Techniques that require less time, less patient repositioning, and less complex interoperative activity are preferable if they can accomplish the same goals. Microvascular anastomosis and extensive drilling and shaping of bone fragments may or may not contribute significantly to the maximum postoperative result. Further experience by a larger number of reconstructive surgeons will be necessary to answer that question.

—Careful attention to fundamental principles of surgical technique is vital. The most meticulous reconstructive procedure can fall victim to the infected hematoma that results from inadequate hemostasis. Gentle handling of tissue and the elimination of "dead space" in the wound are very important.

In the present period of medical cost-consciousness, we must be able to justify the level of our surgical intervention in terms of mandibular reconstruction. Even though we lack a perfect understanding in this area, cost tissues cannot be avoided or dismissed lightly. Mandibular reconstruction requires individualization in every patient. For example, the cost-to-benefit ratio may be favorable for the reconstruction of defects in the region of the mandibular symphysis, but it may be unfavorable for short, lateral mandibular defects.

All in all, mandibular reconstruction entails one of the most controversial, difficult, complex decision processes that is faced by surgeons in any field.

INVESTIGATION AND STANDARDIZATION

The unanswered questions regarding mandibular reconstruction deserve a major program of coordinated research activity. Currently, there are reports in the medical literature that involve only small numbers of patients and short durations of follow-up. Consequently, the results and recommendations seem to be confusing, contradictory, and frequently based only on the personal preference of individual authors.

To arrive at a clearer understanding of "the best" method of mandibular reconstruction for specific types of defects, we must undertake either a large prospective clinical investigation or, at the very least, agree to standardize the reporting of results. The current economic reality for research funding reduces the probability that a major national prospective study will be undertaken in the area of mandibular reconstruction. Nevertheless, we must recognize the need for such a study and to encourage its consideration at every possible opportunity.

What we can do is agree to report our results in a standardized fashion. The following factors should be indicated clearly in every report that deals with mandibular reconstruction:

1. Duration of hospitalization associated with the proposed technique.
2. Cost of the procedure. This should include in a comprehensive manner all hospital costs, charges by surgeons and other physicians, cost of all outpatient services, and cost of the patient's loss of time from work.
3. Number of operative procedures required to accomplish all stages of the original procedure, any reoperations, and any surgical revision techniques that are necessary.
4. Degree of patient acceptance, compliance, and satisfaction.
5. Mastication (ability and limitations).
6. Ability to wear any type of denture.
7. Deglutition (types of food, oral transit time).
8. Speech articulation and intelligibility.
9. Compatibility of the procedure with preoperative radiation therapy.
10. Compatibility of the procedure with postoperative radiation therapy.
11. Facial appearance.
12. Donor site morbidity, including pain, appearance, and decreased function.

SURGICAL PREFERENCES AND CASE EXAMPLES

This section contains a review of some surgical options for various types of reconstructive mandibular surgery. They are presented in the format of illustrative case examples, selected to show how the operative principles discussed throughout this book are applied. We do not mean to suggest that any one technique has been proven superior to others that may be chosen. Some cases were provided by Roger Crumley, M.D., San Francisco, and Charles Cummings, M.D., Seattle; we appreciate their assistance in the preparation of this chapter.

Flap Reconstruction Without Mandibular Reconstruction

Case 1. This 63-year-old man noticed a lesion inside the right cheek approximately 1 month prior to consulting a physician. Physical examination disclosed a 3 cm × 3 cm fungating lesion in the right inferior gingivobuccal region. The lesion was contiguous with the mandible and a firm fullness was palpable in the submandibular region. A single 2 cm × 2 cm right jugulodigastric lymph node was mobile and nontender. Radiographic assessment of the mandible disclosed erosion and decalcification of the posterior mandibular body adjacent to the oral cavity tumor. Biopsy disclosed the presence of squamous cell carcinoma Grade 1. At the time he was admitted to the hospital, the patient had an abscess on the skin adjacent to the tumor and overlying the mandible. The abscess was drained and thorough evaluation revealed no evidence of distant metastasis. A treatment program of surgery, postoperative radiation therapy, and chemotherapy was designed.

Surgical management for this patient is illustrated in Figs. 265–270. The course of the thoracoacromial artery can be outlined by Doppler "tracking" from the skin surface. The margins of the deltopectoral flap are incised and the flap is elevated (even though it will not be used in the primary reconstruction).

After a wide excision of the tumor, overlying

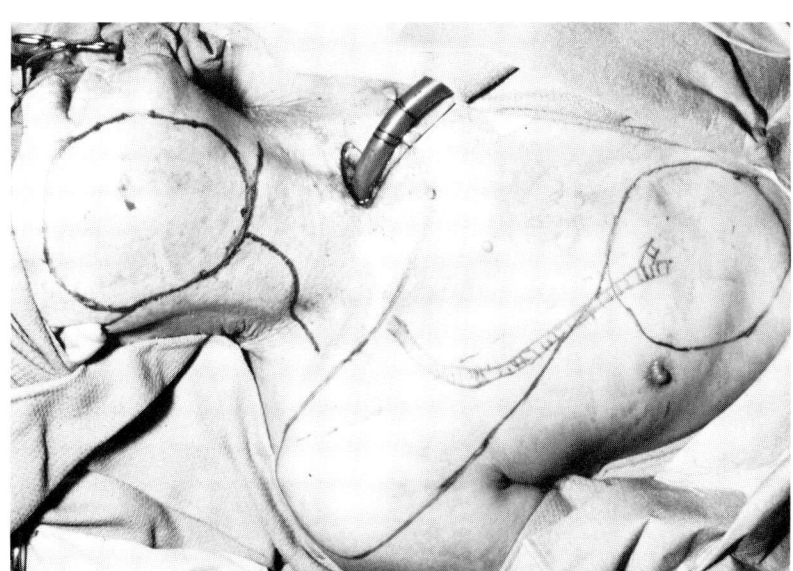

Figure 265. The patient is prepped for surgery. The skin overlying the area of gingivobuccal carcinoma and mandibular invasion will be excised, and the defect will be closed with a pectoralis major myocutaneous flap.

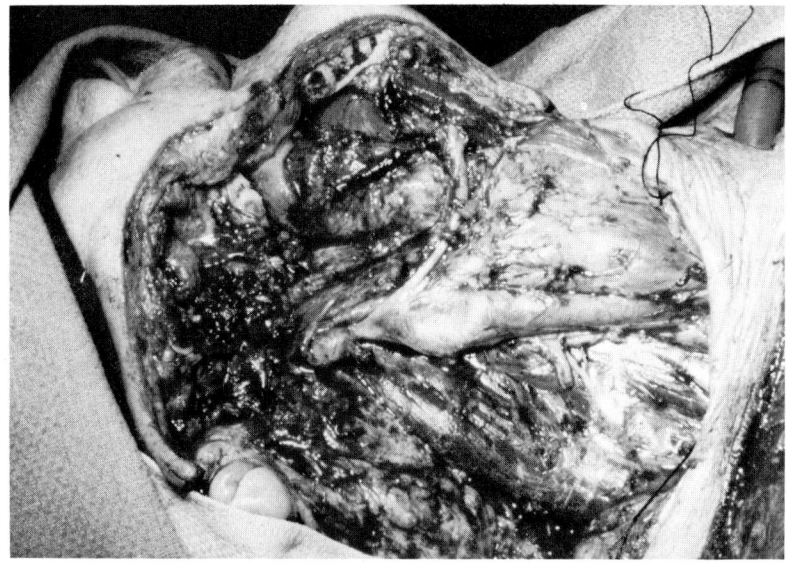

Figure 266. The extirpative portion of the procedure has been completed. The primary lesion, the overlying skin, and the mandible (from anterior to the mental foramen to the temporomandibular joint) have been excised en bloc with the radical neck dissection.

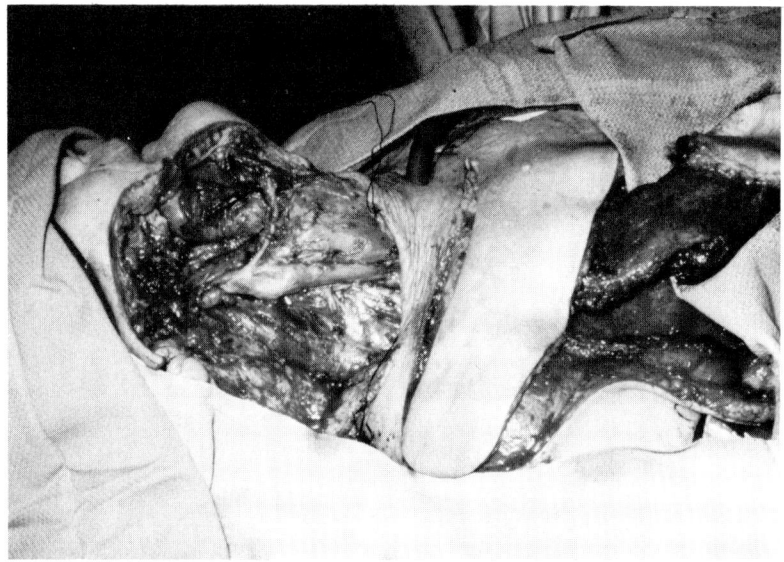

Figure 267. The deltopectoral flap and the pectoralis major myocutaneous flap have been elevated.

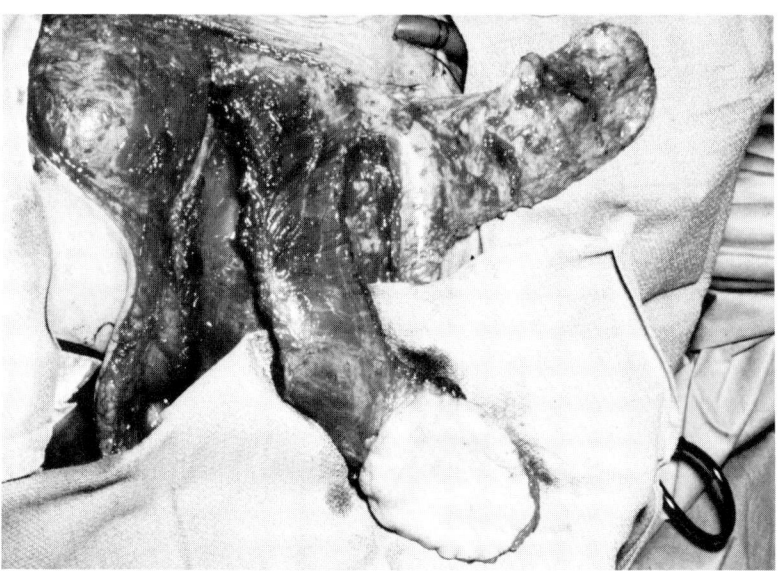

Figure 268. The deltopectoral flap is folded medially to show the pedicle of the pectoralis major myocutaneous flap.

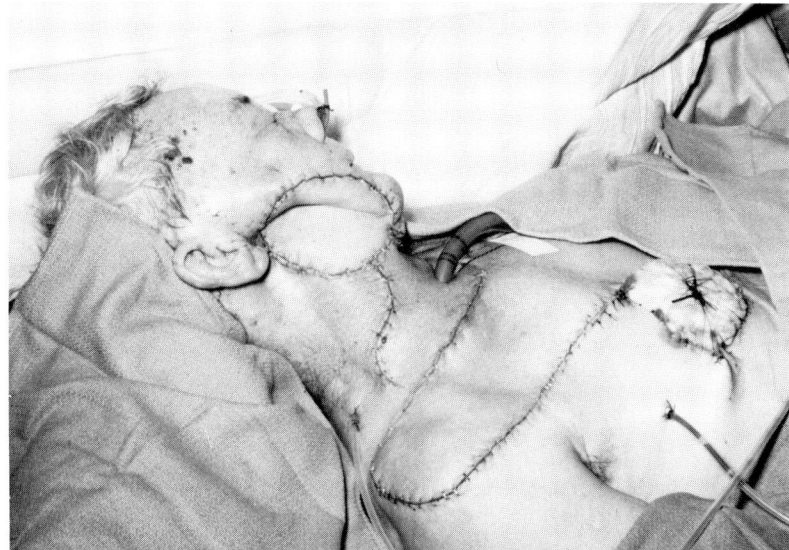

Figure 269. The defect is reconstructed using the pectoralis major myocutaneous flap. The deltopectoral flap is sutured back into place, and a cotton bolster is sutured in place over a split-thickness skin graft at the myocutaneous flap donor site.

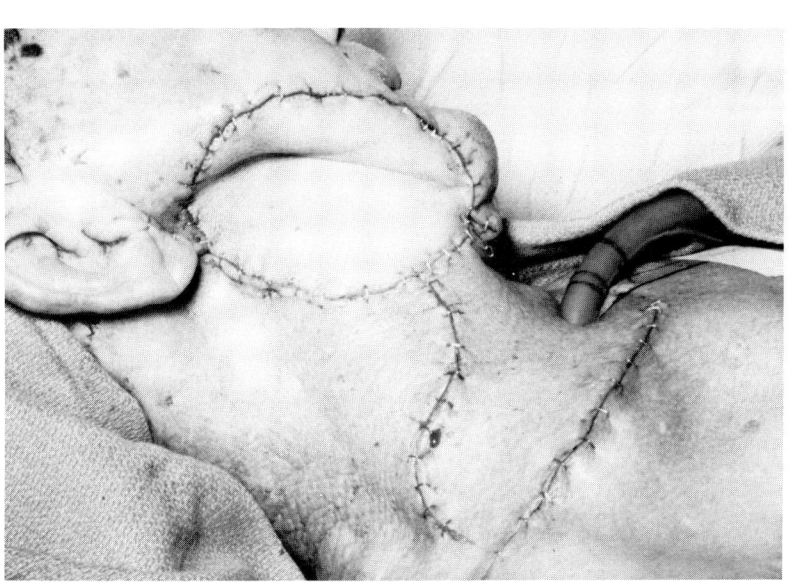

Figure 270. Close-up view of the pectoralis major myocutaneous flap and operative site. Note the use of staples for skin closure.

skin, and mandible en bloc with a radical neck dissection, the PMM flap is used to fill the tissue defect. In this instance the bulk of the myocutaneous flap is advantageous.

Mandibular Resection and Reconstruction Using Sternocleidomastoid Osteomyocutaneous Flap

Case 2. This 64-year-old woman had noted the presence of a tender swelling in her mouth for 5 months. Physical examination disclosed a 3 cm × 4 cm ulcerated lesion of the anterior floor of the mouth, adjacent to the mandible, and a 2 cm × 2 cm, mobile, firm, nontender lymph node in the right jugulodigastric region. Biopsy of the oral lesion provided a diagnosis of invasive, well-differentiated squamous cell carcinoma. No evidence of distant metastasis was present. A treatment plan consisting of surgical resection, postoperative radiation therapy, and chemotherapy was initiated.

The surgical procedure undertaken was local excision of the anterior floor of the mouth in continuity with the adjacent mandibular symphysis. A right radical neck dissection and a left modified neck dissection were performed to control neck metastasis. Reconstruction was accomplished using a sternocheidomastoid osteomyocutaneous flap.

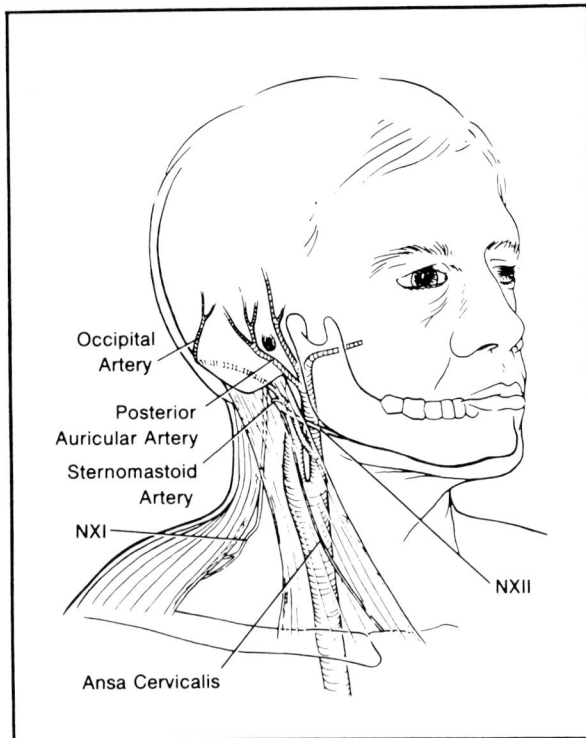

Figure 271. Bulk of blood supply to sternocleidomastoid muscle from external carotid system. Superior portion of muscle is supplied by occipital artery and middle portion by superior thyroid artery. Inferior supply is from thyrocervical trunk (not shown). Innervation is via spinal accessory nerve. (From Barnes DR et al.: Arch Otolaryngol 107:712, 1981. With permission.)

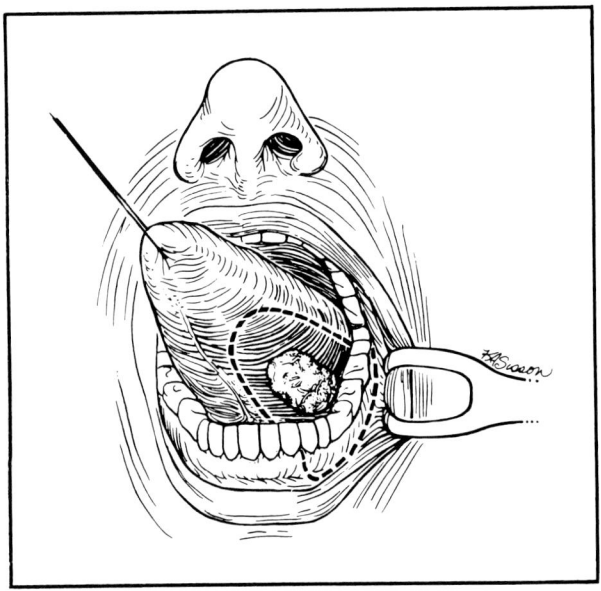

Figure 272. Radical neck dissection. Primary lesion and mandible are marked for resection. (From Barnes DR et al.: Arch Otolaryngol 107:712, 1981. With permission.)

The technique used in Case 3 resembled that described by Barnes and colleagues[21] and illustrated in Figs. 271–276. In Figures 277–281, we show the method used in this particular patient.

Several issues regarding this technique remain unresolved because the number of patients reported to date is small and the follow-up time is short. The dissection and handling of this flap must be precise if the blood supply to all three tissue com-

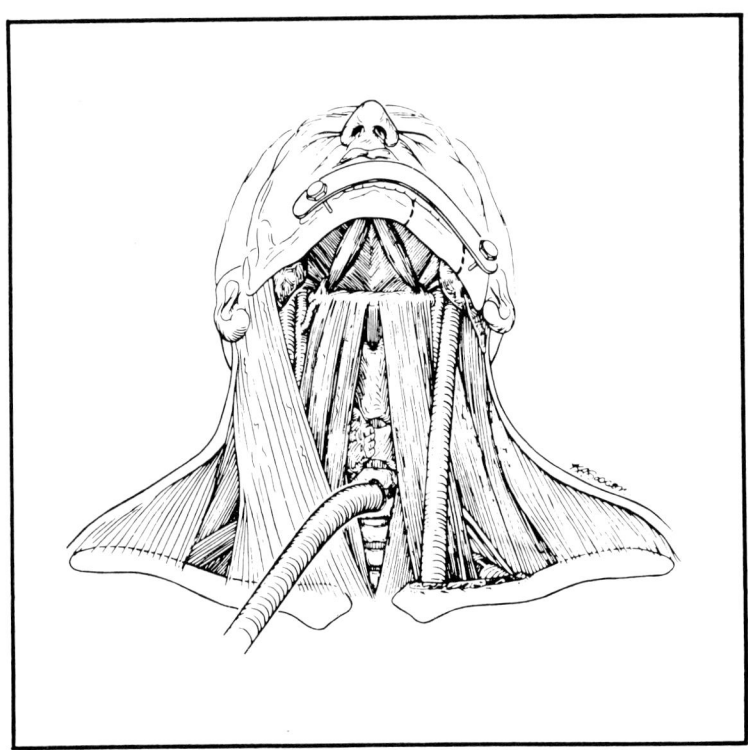

Figure 273. Mandible prepared for grafting after external fixation device has been applied. (From Barnes DR et al.: Arch Otolaryngol 107:712, 1981. With permission.)

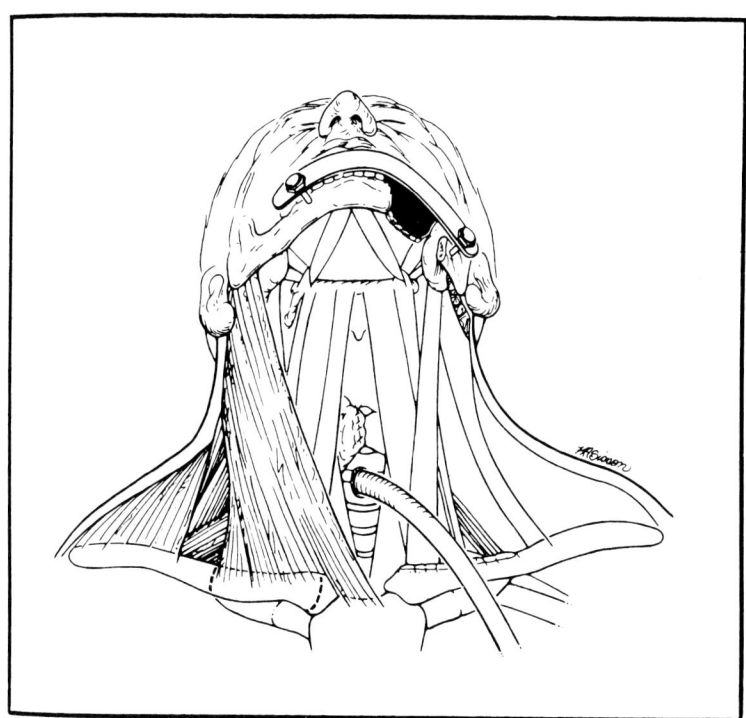

Figure 274. Mandibular defect. After careful measurement of defect, clavicle is marked to fit defect precisely. (From Barnes DR et al.: Arch Otolaryngol 107:713, 1981. With permission.)

ponents is to be preserved. Even with very careful surgery, the skin covering overlying the clavicle is lost about half of the time. Some surgeons feel that even though the skin is lost, it serves temporarily as a protective dressing during the reestablishment of oral epithelial continuity and prevents bone graft infection. If this is so, the surgeon must debride necrotic skin tissue so that it does not become a source of infection.

Mandibular Reconstruction Using Autogenous Mandible

Case 3 (provided by Charles Cummings, M.D.). This 66-year-old man presented with a T4N3BMO squamous cell carcinoma of the floor of the mouth. The surgical management consisted of resection of the floor of the mouth, bilateral modified neck dissections, and implantation of the mandibular

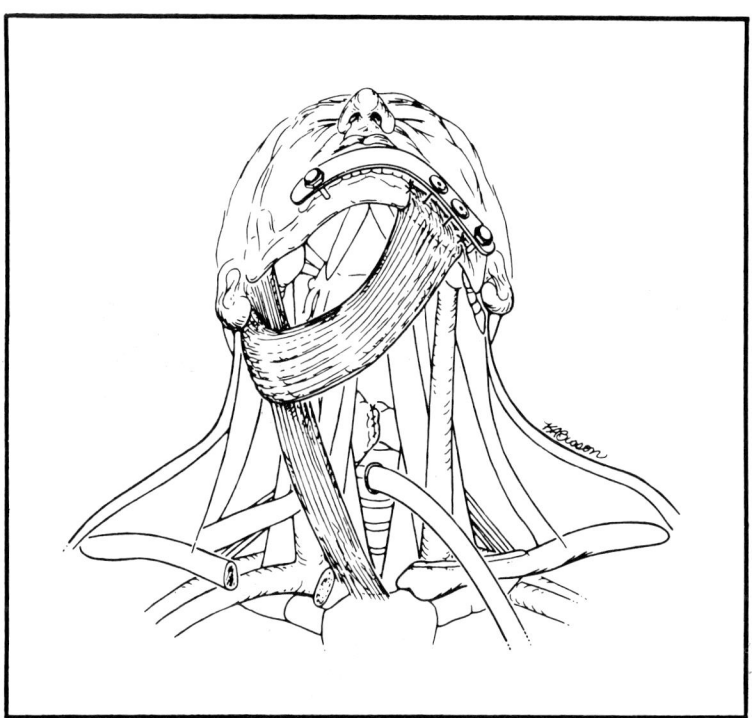

Figure 275. Carefully preserved sternocleidomastoid muscle. Blood supply from superior thyroid artery and occipital arteries has been preserved. Transosseous wires and a third set of bipahsic pins have been placed. (From Barnes DR et al.: Arch Otolaryngol 107:713, 1981. With permission.)

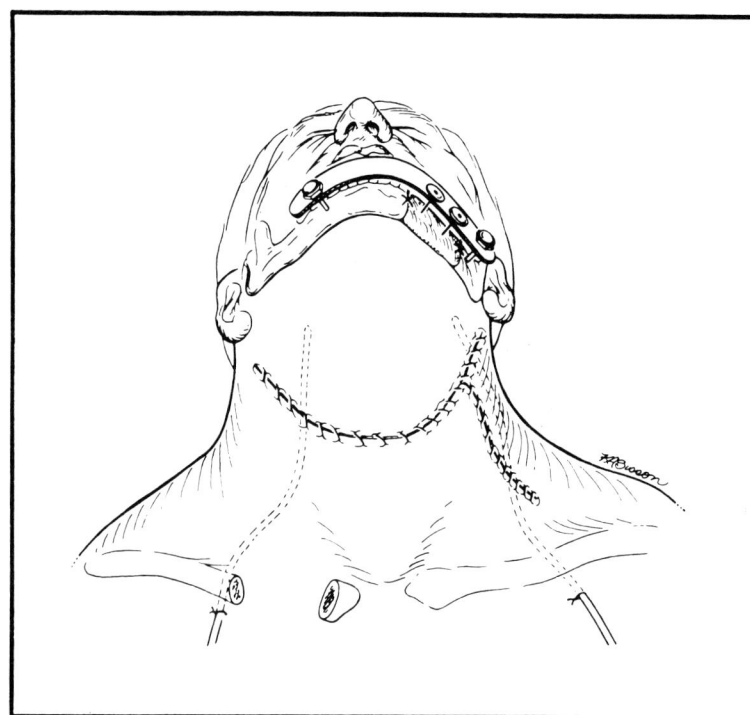

Figure 276. Closed intraoral incision. Wound is closed in standard two-layer fashion with suction drains placed. (From Barnes DR et al.: Arch Otolaryngol 107:713, 1981. With permission.)

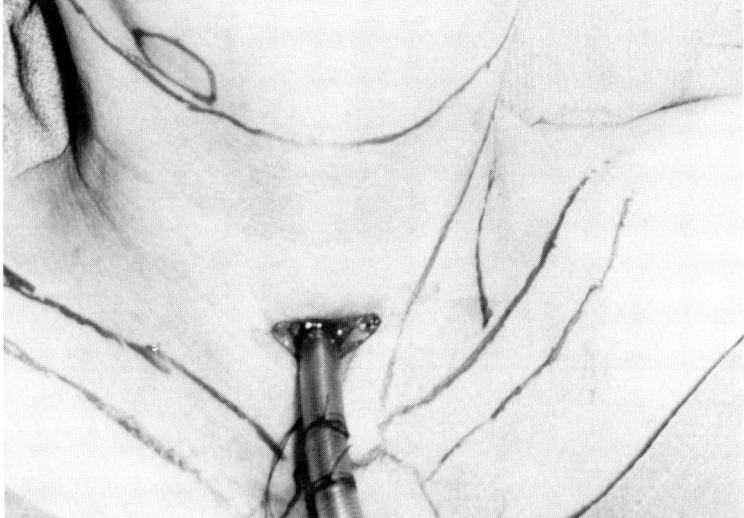

Figure 277. Patient prepped for surgery, with the sternocleidomastoid-clavicular flap region outlined on the skin.

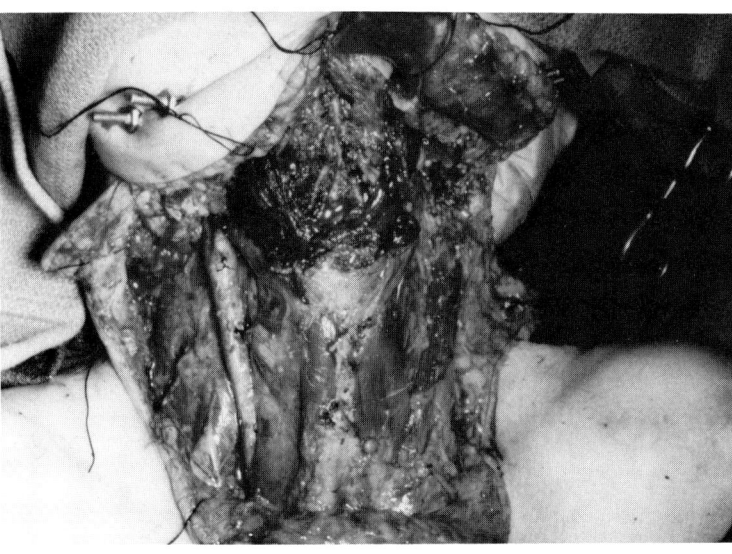

Figure 278. The tumor excision and neck dissection phase is completed. The mandibular symphysis and floor of mouth defect is prepared for reconstruction.

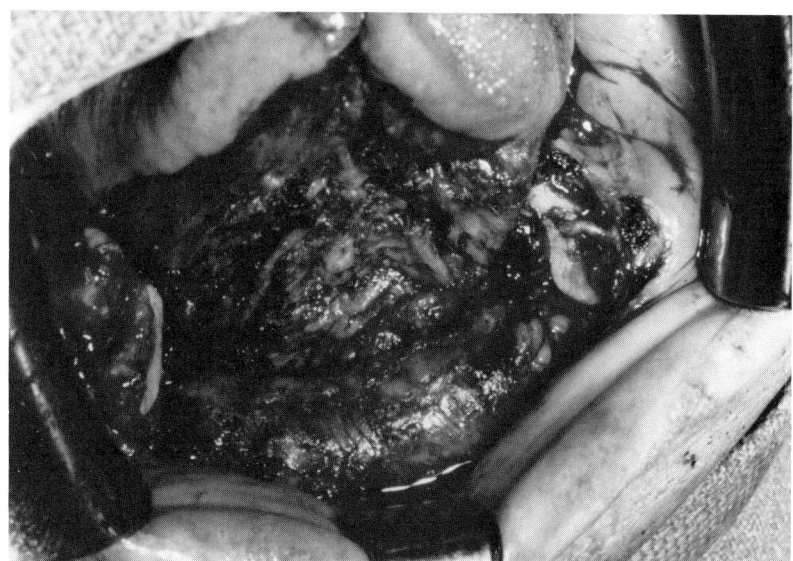

Figure 279. Intraoral view of the defect at the same point as in Figure 278.

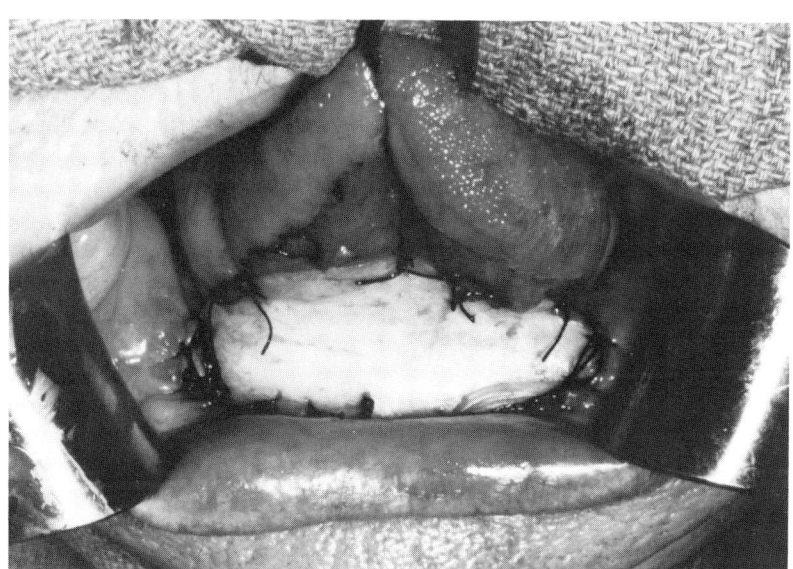

Figure 280. Intraoral view after the sternocleidomastoid osteomyocutaneous flap has been secured in position.

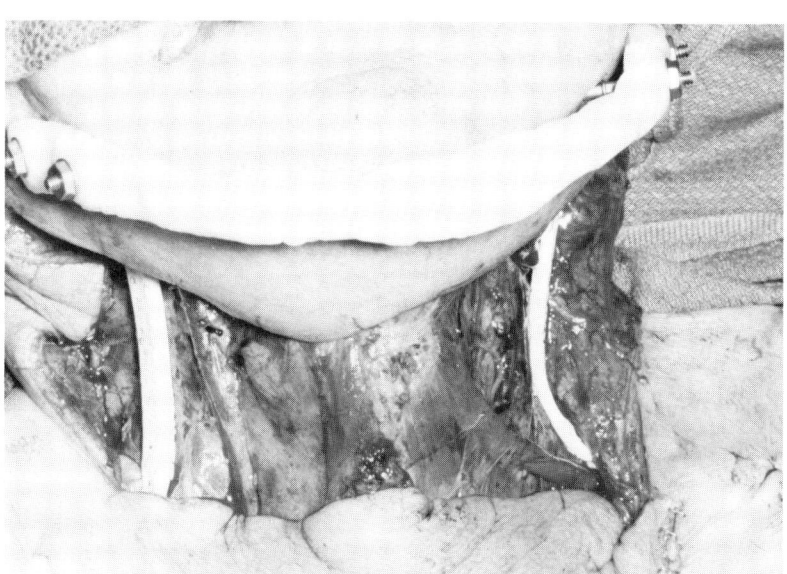

Figure 281. Biphase appliance for mandibular stabilization during the postoperative period. Suction drains are placed and the wound is ready for closure.

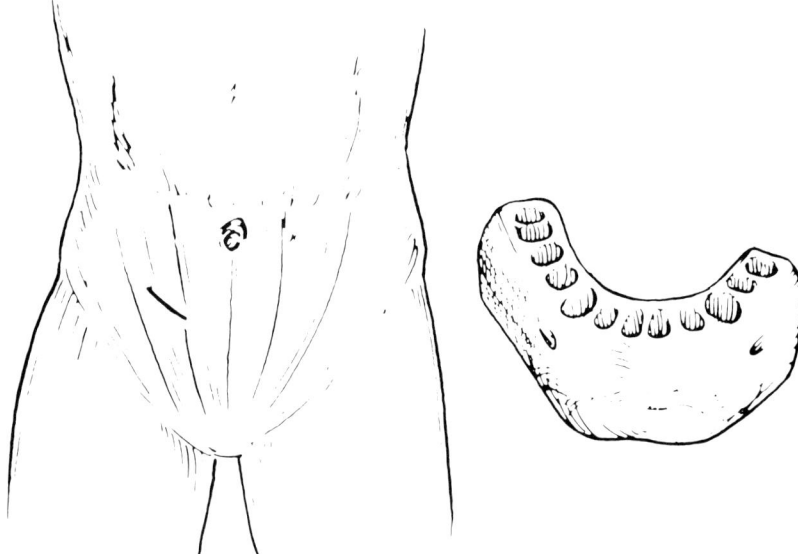

Figure 282. Mandibular segment is frozen and thawed, then implanted in the subcutaneous fat pad of the left lower quadrant of the abdomen.

segment (initially adjacent to the oral cancer) into the subcutaneous tissue of the left lower quadrant of the abdomen (Fig. 282). The surgical defect was reconstructed with a pectoralis myocutaneous flap and a plastic mesh mandibular tray prosthesis for the interim period.

Nine months later, the mandibular segment was harvested from the left lower quadrant and prepared for grafting (Fig. 283). Iliac bone marrow was placed in the graft and a Kirschner wire was incorporated for stabilization (Figs. 284–287).

Case 4 (provided by Charles Cummings, M.D.). This 62-year-old woman with T4NOMO squamous cell carcinoma of the floor of the mouth underwent surgical excision and reconstruction similar to that described in Case 3. Surgical management differed slightly in this patient in that the graft was harvested and reimplanted after 2 months (Fig. 288).

Two months after the autograft was replaced into the mandibular arch, a bone scan performed using Tc^{92m} showed evidence of partial revascularization of the reattached anterior portion of the mandible. The patient had been stabilized with an external biphase splint appliance; 2 months after surgery when the bone graft appeared to be solidly healed and was removed. The patient has functioned well and her appearance at 4 years is illustrated in Figure 289.

Frozen Autograft Without Staged Abdominal Wall Implantation

Case 5 (provided by Roger Crumley, M.D.). This 58-year-old man was found to have a T3N1MO squamous cell carcinoma of the anterior floor of

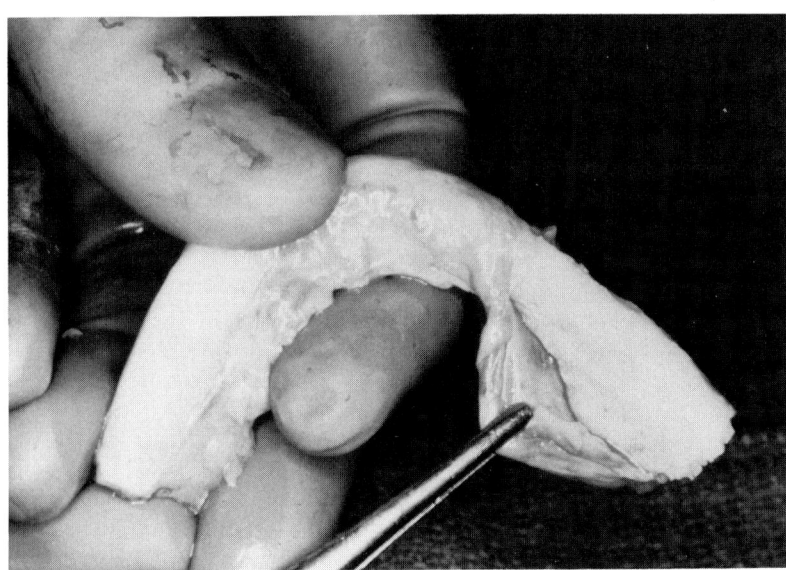

Figure 283. Appearance of the mandibular segment upon harvesting 9 months after implantation.

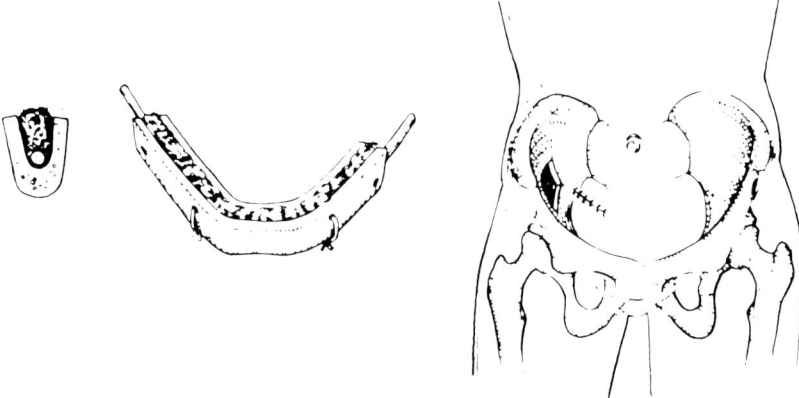

Figure 284. Iliac bone marrow is obtained and placed in the autograft.

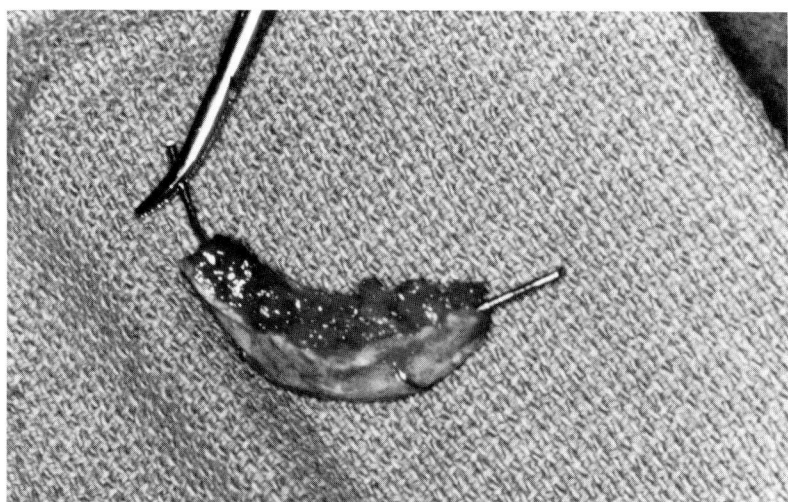

Figure 285. A Kirschner wire is incorporated to assist in stabilizing the bone graft.

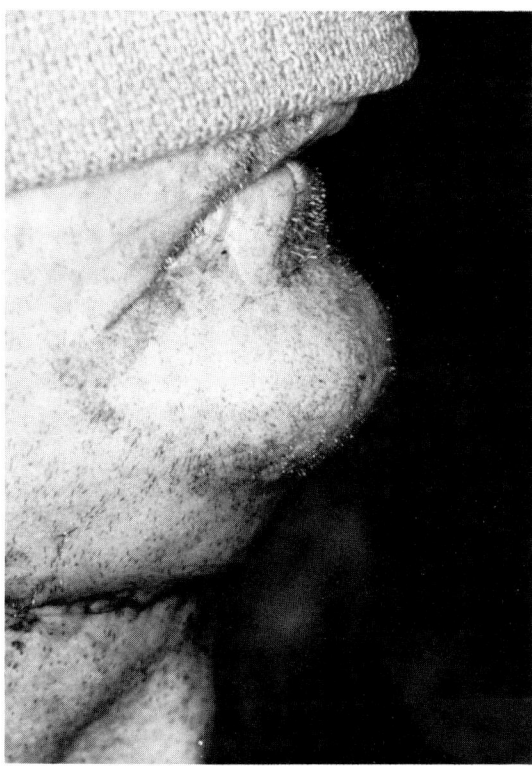

Figure 286. Patient appearance at the conclusion of the procedure.

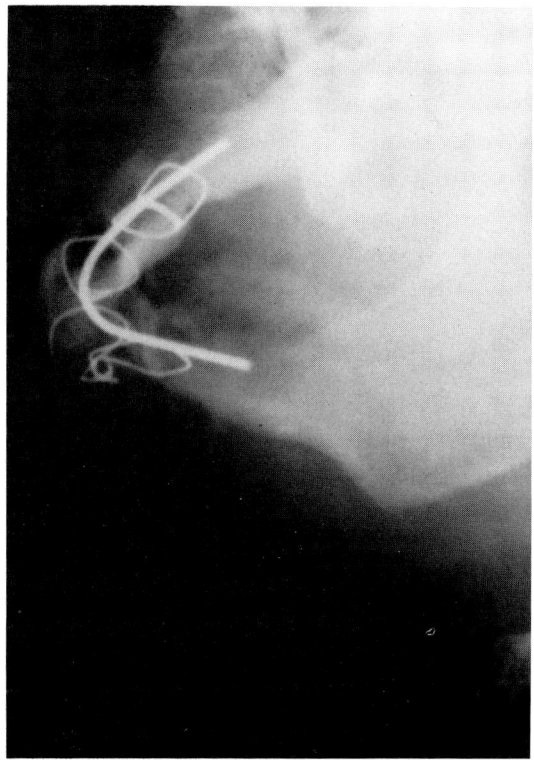

Figure 287. Postoperative radiograph of the reimplanted mandibular segment.

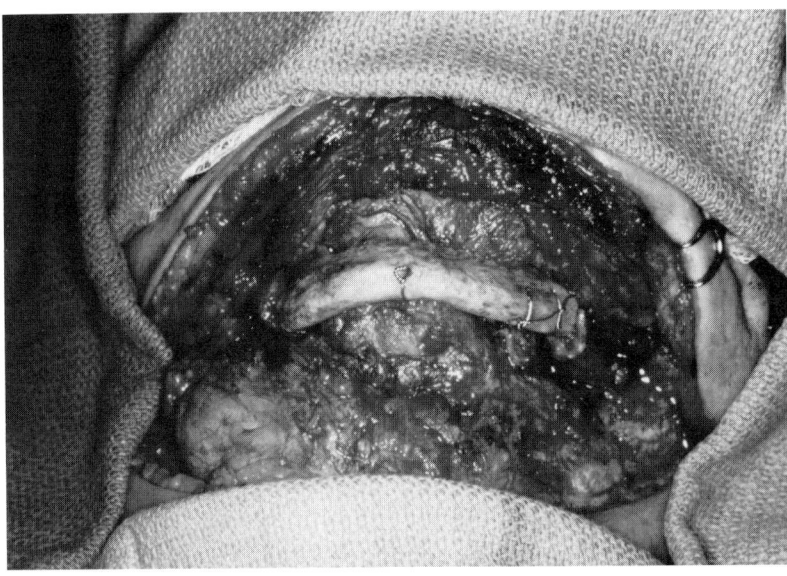

Figure 288. Mandibular segment has been harvested and reimplanted.

the mouth with evidence of mandibular involvement. Surgical management consisted of a composite resection including partial glossectomy, hemimandibulectomy (symphysis and right body), plus a right radical neck dissection.

Immediate (primary) reconstruction was elected. The mandibular segment that had been excised was cleaned of all covering soft tissue (Fig. 290). The segment was then frozen in liquid nitrogen (Fig. 291) and thawed.

The mandibular segment was wired into position, and a PMM flap was raised to reconstruct the soft tissue defect. Care was taken to include the external rib periosteum of two ribs on the deep surface of the PMM flap. These periosteal regions were sutured so that they overlaid the mandibular segment on its exposed surfaces; with the remainder of the flap wrapped around the mandibular reconstruction to separate the bone segment from the oral cavity (Fig. 292 and 293).

Postoperatively, the patient developed a wound infection, despite all reasonable efforts, the autogenous bone graft was ultimately lost to infection. The late postoperative result, however, was adequate in terms of function and appearance (Fig. 294). Presumably, the degree of tissue reaction and fibrosis was sufficient to provide rehabilitation in this particular patient.

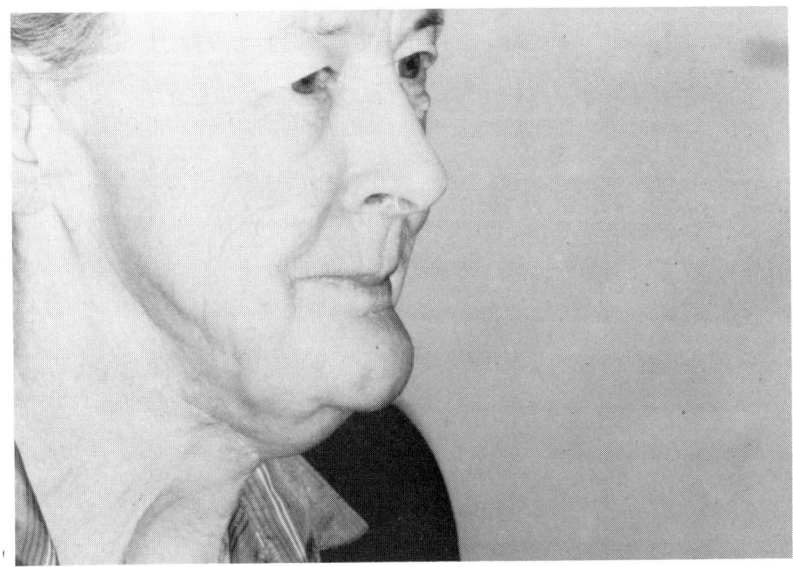

Figure 289. Postoperative appearance of patient at 4 years.

Principles and Preferences in Mandibular Reconstruction 203

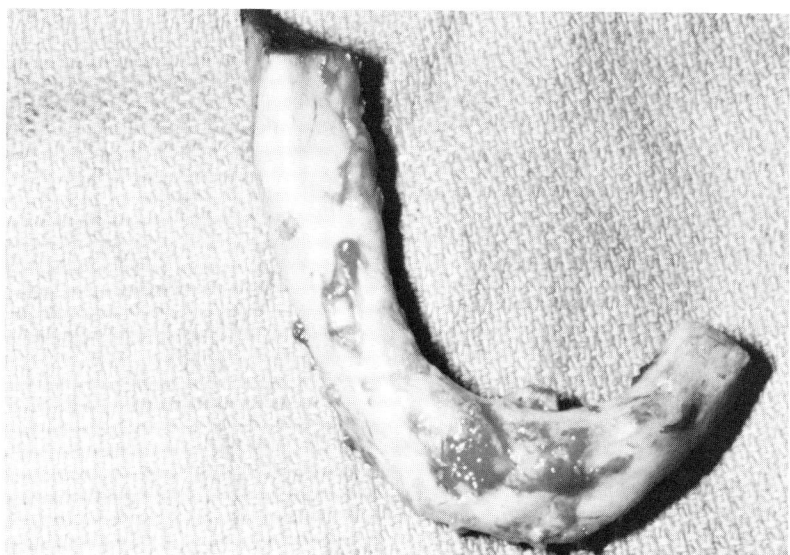

Figure 290. Mandibular segment with soft tissue covering removed.

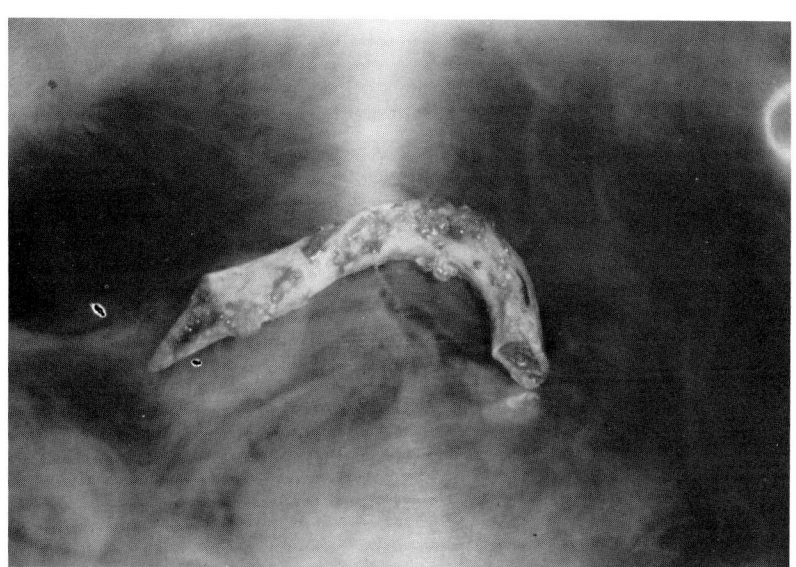

Figure 291. Mandibular segment being frozen in liquid nitrogen.

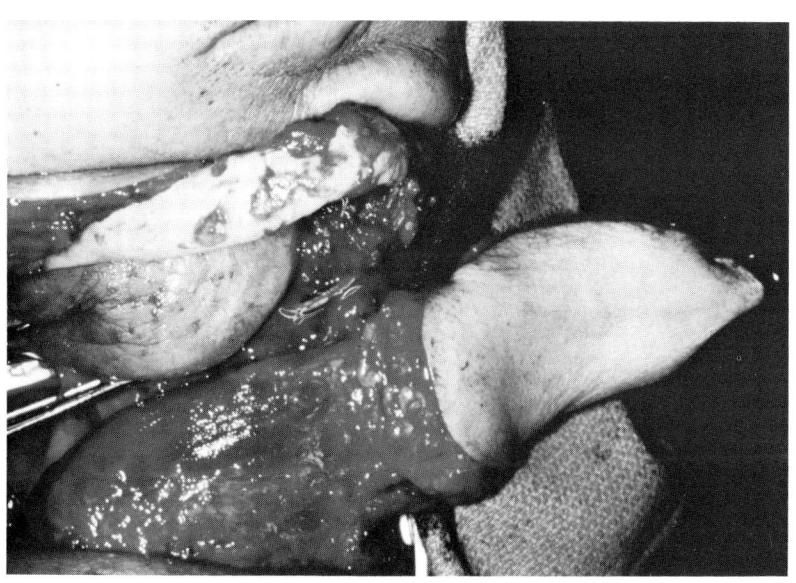

Figure 292. Mandibular segment wired in place.

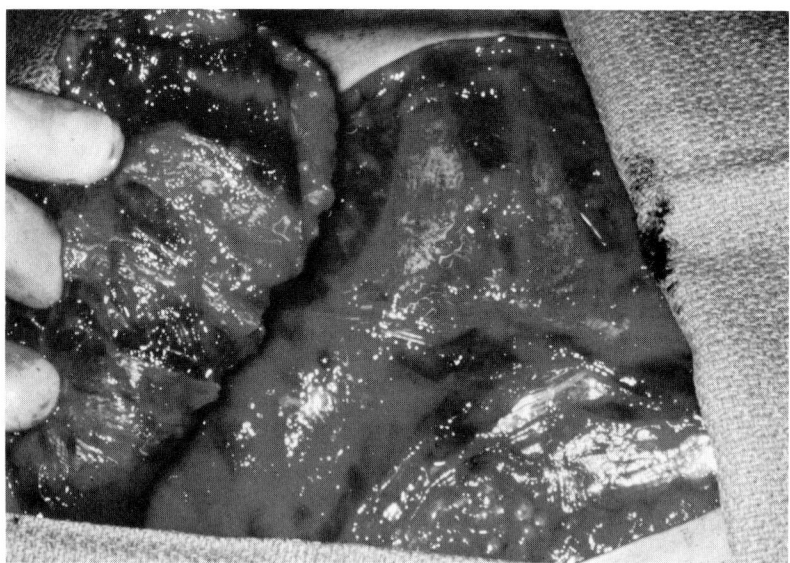

Figure 293. Pectoralis major myocutaneous flap is inset with rib periosteum placed in contact with frozen and thawed mandibular segment.

Reconstruction Using Trapezuis Osteomyocutaneous Flap that Incorporates the Spine of the Scapula

Case 6 (provided by Roger Crumley, M.D.). This 59-year-old man developed an extensive squamous cell carcinoma of the floor of the mouth and alveolar ridges, bilaterally. This lesion was staged T3N1MO and the patient was treated with radiation therapy. After recurrence followed an initial marked tumor regression, the patient underwent a composite resection with right radical neck dissection.

The mandibular defect extended from angle to angle (Figs. 295 and 296). The surgeon elected to perform a primary reconstruction of the opposite side using a free iliac crest bone graft.

The trapezuis osteomyocutaneous flap has been described recently by Panje,[4] who has had an excellent personal experience with it. The vascular supply and skin incisions must be carefully considered and accomplished. The scapular spine (Figs. 297 and 298) provides a viable bone segment for reconstructing long defects.

This flap also provides an extensive skin paddle for resurfacing. In this patient, the surgeon estimated that that nearly 400 cm^2 was available (Fig. 299).

Stabilization was achieved by use of an external biphase, splint (Figs. 300 and 301). The patient's appearance when the appliance was removed is shown in Figures 302 and 303.

The left hemimandibular defect was repaired with a free iliac crest bone graft (Fig. 304). Subsequent stabilization and elevation of the mandibular segments were accomplished by combining the standard biphase splint with a Mills head frame (Figs. 305 and 306).

SUMMARY

We have reviewed the principles of mandibular reconstruction designed to accomplish optimal postoperative function and appearance, while

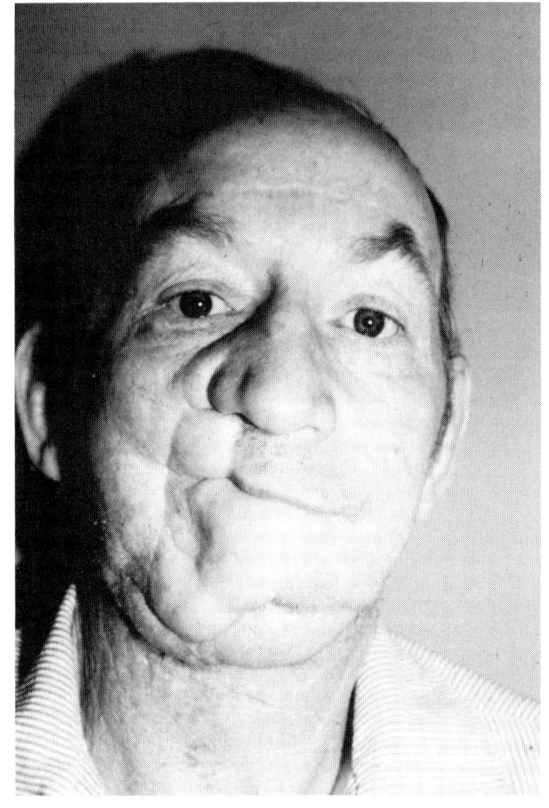

Figure 294. Late postoperative photograph of patient showing competence of orostome.

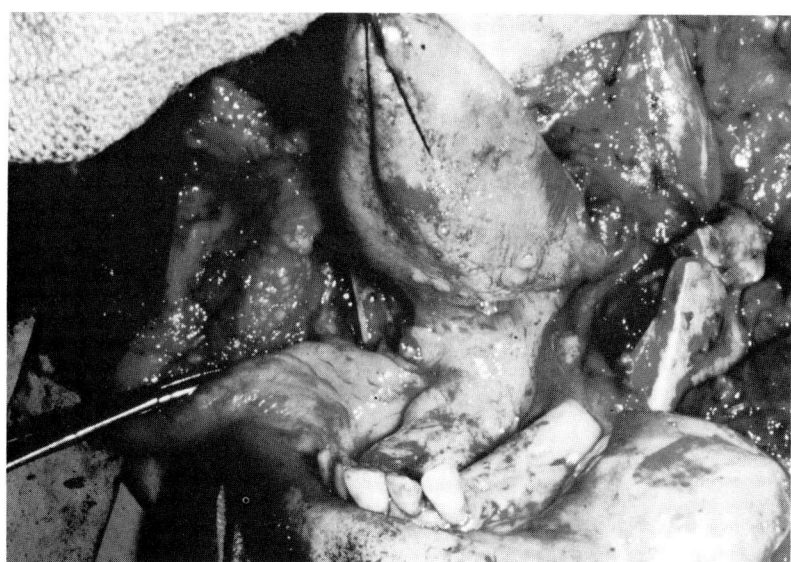

Figure 295. Intraoperative view of resection.

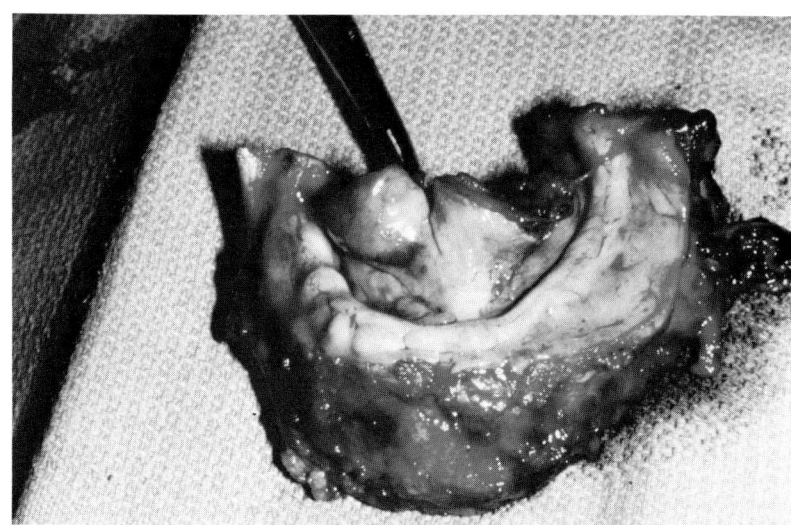

Figure 296. Surgical specimen from Case 8.

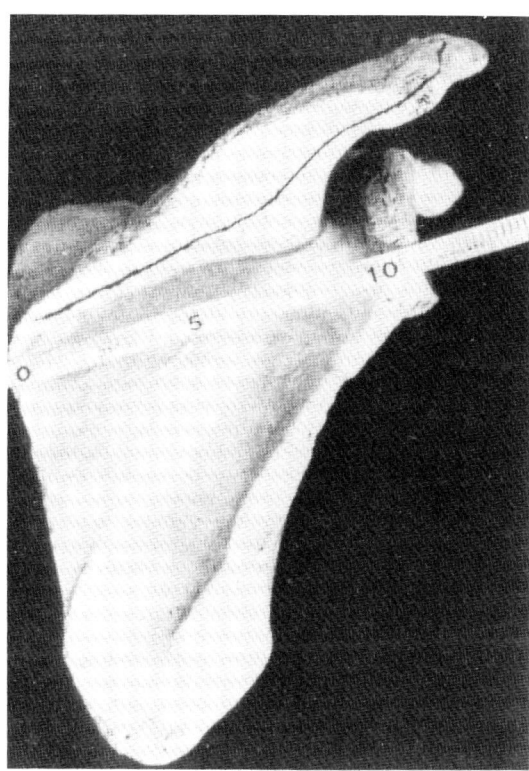

Figure 297. Scapula skeleton. Line indicates bone cut for obtaining maximum spine length. (From Panje WR: Arch Otolaryngol 111:228, 1985. With permission.)

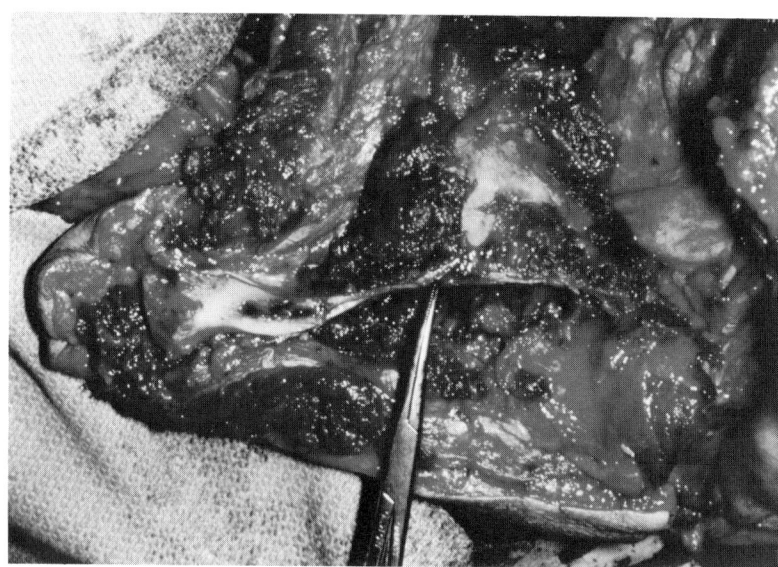

Figure 298. Patient's scapular spine as seen on the deep surface of the trapezius osteomyocutaneous flap.

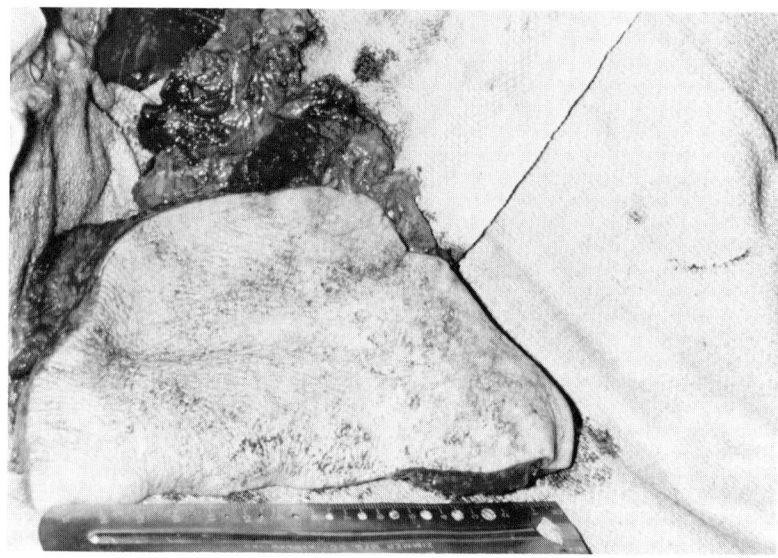

Figure 299. Skin paddle available on the trapezius osteomyocutaneous flap.

avoiding postoperative complications. Careful attention to basic general surgical principles and these specific principles will limit the degree of salivary contamination, infection, and wound breakdown. Spacing and bridging devices are proposed to limit mandibular drift and consequent postoperative malocclusion. When possible, the repair should be accomplished as quickly as possible and the patient returned to home and work as soon as possible.

Selection of the most appropriate technique to accomplish these goals rests on a series of decisions. The surgeon needs to make key decisions at more than a dozen points of possible divergence in the course of managing a particular patient. We have attempted to identify and list these decision points in the following questions that the surgeon must address during the course of the first operative procedure. These decision points are as follows:

1. Have I adequately resected the tumor?
2. Have I chosen the best method for tissue coverage in this patient?
3. Have I maintained the mandibular relationships adequately?
4. Is the reconstruction stable and immobile?
5. Is the reconstruction durable?
6. Is the reconstruction compatible with the use of radiation therapy?
7. Is the repair sufficiently strong to withstand postoperative function and stress?

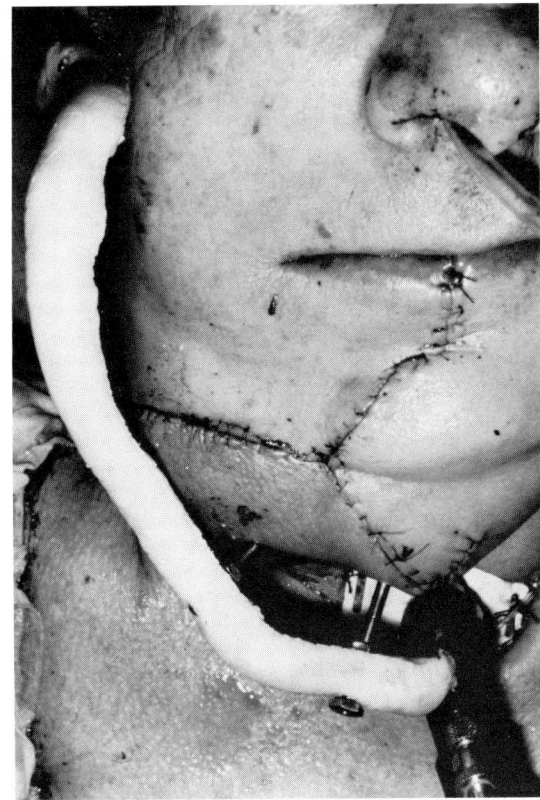

Figure 300. Biphase splint, anterior view.

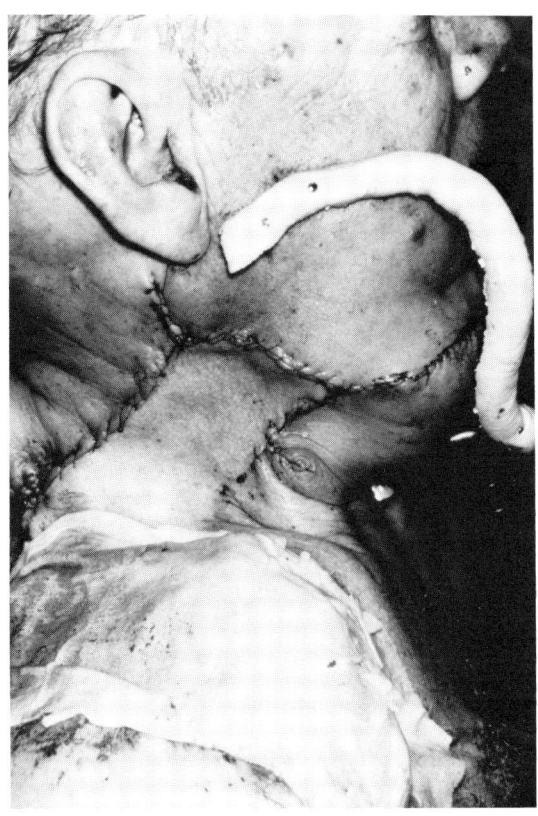

Figure 301. Biphase splint, lateral view.

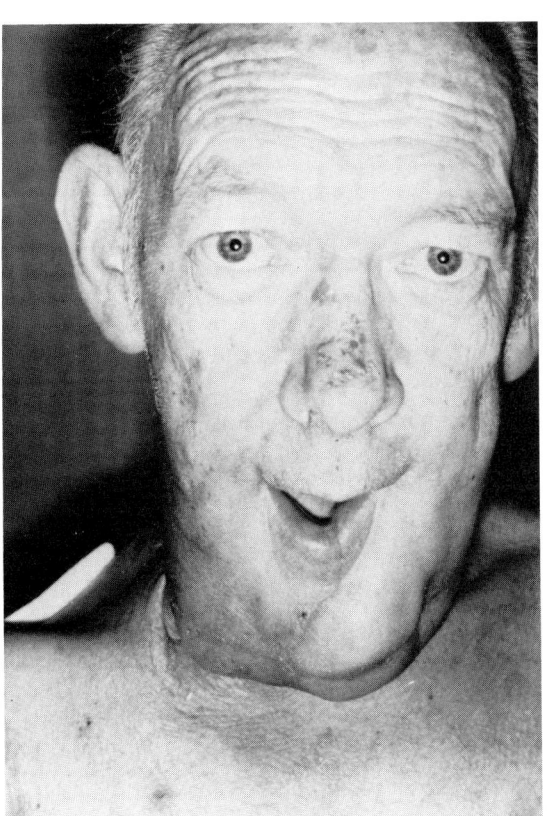

Figure 302. Anterior view of patient.

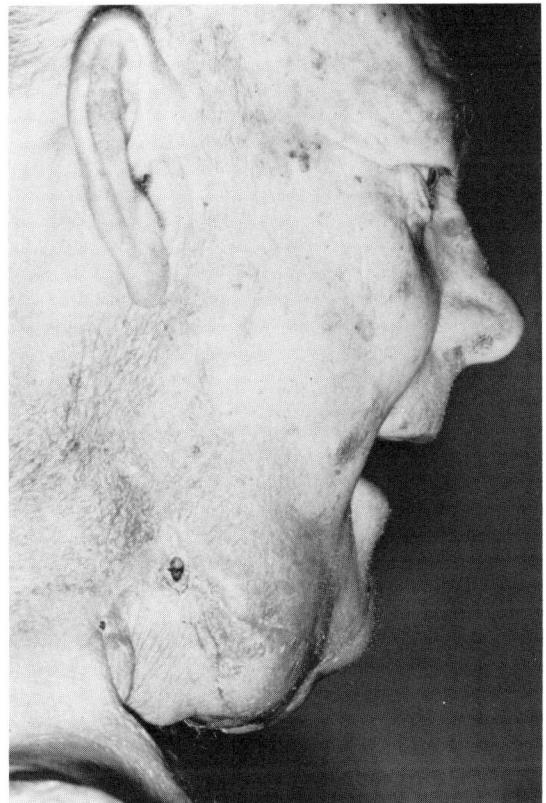

Figure 303. Lateral view of patient.

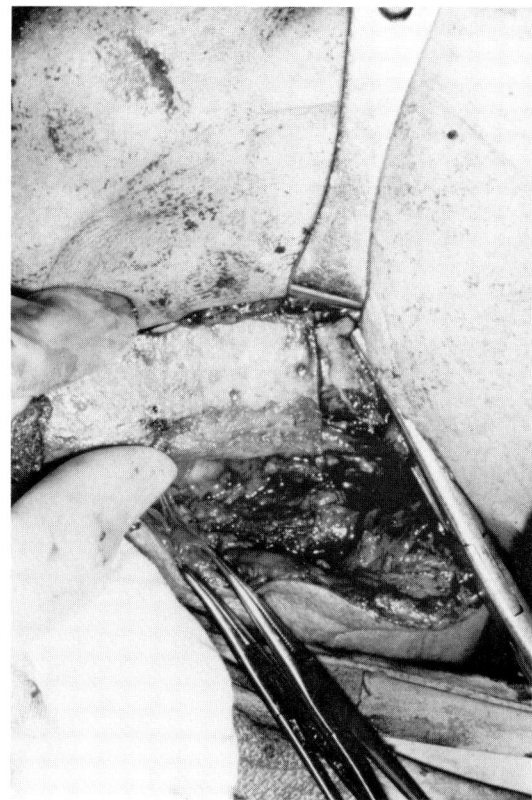

Figure 304. Iliac crest bone graft in place.

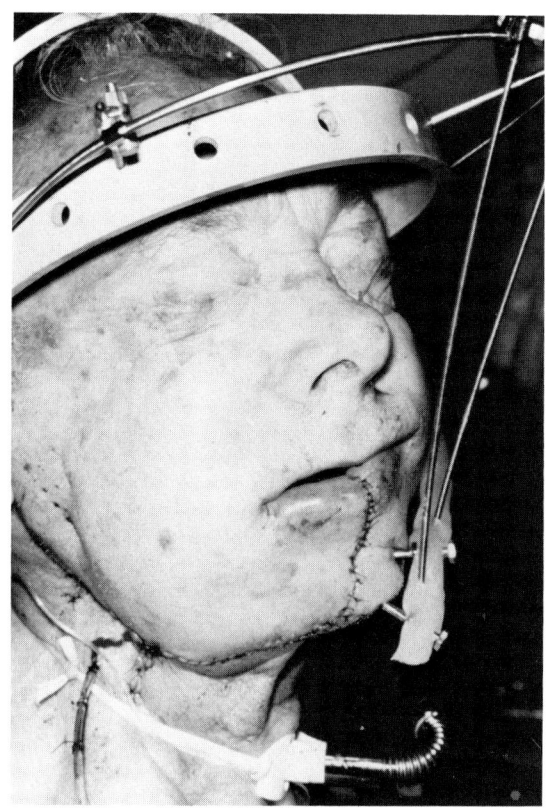

Figure 306. Biphasic splint secured to Mills head frame to provide elevation and support of graft during postoperative healing period.

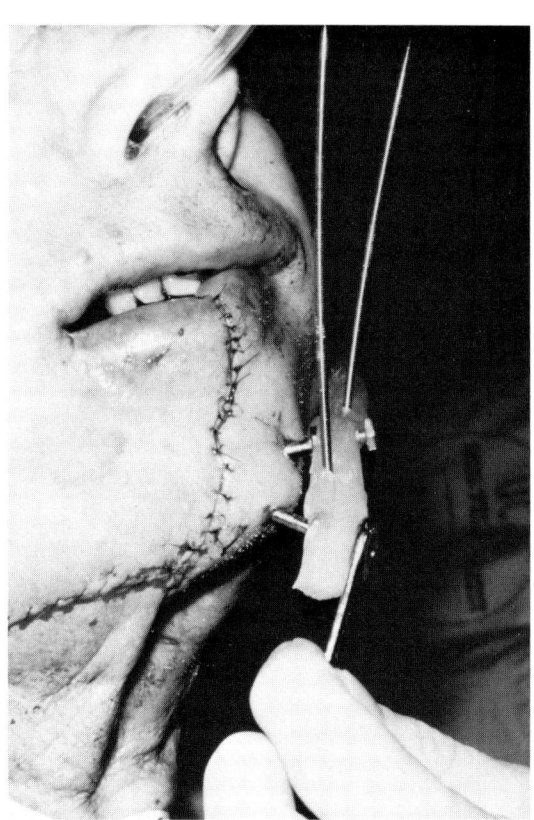

Figure 305. External biphasic splint for stabilization.

8. Is the reconstruction cosmetically satisfactory?
9. Do size, site, associated medical problems, or other issues call for special individual consideration in this patient?
10. Have I considered appropriately the factors of cost, time, number of stages, and postoperative morbidity?

As we clarify more of the answers to these questions, both as individuals and as a profession, we will be able to meet the needs and desires of our patients in a more satisfactory manner.

REFERENCES

1. Hilger PA, Adams, GL: Mandibular reconstruction with the A-O plate. Arch Otolaryngol 111:469–471, 1985
2. Strelzow VV: Mandibular reconstruction using implantable stabilization plates. Arch Otolaryngol 198:333–337, 1983
3. Berktold RE, Ossoff RH, Sisson GA, et al.: Chin reconstruction with pectoralis myocutaneous flap. Otolaryngol Head Neck Surg 94:181–186, 1986
4. Panje WR: Mandible reconstruction with trapezius osteomusculocutaneous flap. Arch Otolaryngol 111:223–229, 1985
5. Maisel RH, Adams GL: Osteomyocutaneous reconstruction of the oral cavity. Arch Otolaryngol 109:731–734, 1983
6. Wersall J, Bergstedt H, Korlof B, et al.: Split-rib graft for reconstruction of the mandible. Otolaryngol Head Neck Surg 92:270–275, 1984

7. Lawson W, Biller HF: Mandibular reconstruction bone graft techniques. Otolaryngol Head Neck Surg 90:589–594, 1982
8. Baker SR: Reconstruction of mandibular defects with the revascularized free tensor fascia lata osteomyocutaneous flap. Arch Otolaryngol 107:414–418, 1981
9. Panje WR: Free compound groin flap reconstruction of anterior mandibular defect. Arch Otolaryngol 107:17–22, 1981
10. Harrison TJ, Quillen CG: Free osteocutaneous groin flap in the reconstruction of large mandibular defects. Arch Otolaryngol 109:485–488, 1983
11. deFries HO: Reconstruction of the mandible: Use of combined homologous mandible and autologous bone. Otolaryngol Head Neck Surg 89:694–697, 1981
12. Cummings CW, Leipzig B: Replacement of tumor-involved mandible by cryosurgically devitalized autograft. Arch Otolaryngol 106:252–254, 1980
13. Schuller DE, Bardach J, Monteith CG, et al.: Titanium tray mandibular reconstruction. Arch Otolaryngol 108:174–178, 1982
14. Boyne PJ: Restoration of osseous defects in maxillofacial casualties. J Am Dent Assoc 78:765–776, 1969
15. Shrewsbury DW, Meyerhoff WL, Szachowicz EH: Repair of complicated mandibular defects. Arch Otolaryngol 108:162–166, 1982
16. Leake DL: Mandibular reconstruction with a new alloplastic tray. J Oral Surg 32:23–26, 1974
17. Albert TW, Smith JD, Everts EC, et al.: Dacron mesh tray and cancellous bone in reconstruction of mandibular defects. Arch Otolaryngol Head Neck Surg 112:53–59, 1986
18. McKee JC, Bailey BJ: Calcium sulfate as a mandibular implant. Otolaryngol Head Neck Surg 92:277–286, 1984
19. Stanley RB, Rice DH: Osteogenesis from a free periosteal graft in mandibular reconstruction. Otolaryngol Head Neck Surg 89:414–418, 1981
20. Wurster CF, Krepsi YP, Davis JW, et al.: Combined functional oral rehabilitation after radical cancer surgery. Arch Otolaryngol 111:530–533, 1985
21. Barnes DR, Ossoff RH, Pecaro B, et al.: Immediate reconstruction of mandibular defects with a composite sternocleidomastoid musculoclavicular graft. Arch Otolaryngol 107:711–714, 1981

14 Complications of Mandibular Surgery

G. Richard Holt, M.D.

While the overall goals of mandibular surgery are usually achieved to a high degree, there are certainly many patients in whom total or partial success is not achieved. This failure to achieve success is mandibular surgery is usually due to an untoward effect or to an actual complication of the surgery. Since mandibular surgery encompasses a wide variety of techniques, from fracture repair and orthognathic surgery to tumor resection and osseous reconstruction, there also exists a significant pool of potential complications.

Obviously the most frequent and disturbing complications of mandibular surgery are those that interfere with form and function. For most patients who have had mandibular surgery, the main difficulty is impaired speech and deglutition. Obviously the patient who has had a mandibular fracture and who is placed in intraoral or extraoral fixation must face 4 to 6 weeks of abnormal speech and swallowing. This same situation is also present in patients undergoing orthognathic surgery. During this period of time, the patient faces a temporary alteration of diet, usually undergoes weight loss, and has some alteration in gastrointestinal function due to a decreased food fiber intake. However, in the case of fracture healing and orthognathic surgery, the disabilities are short-lived and the patient can generally recoup the weight loss. It should be understood though, that the older patient, who may also be in marginal nitrogen balance, could develop serious nutritional problems in a short period of time. In order to lessen the risk of malnutrition, the surgeon can utilize the commercially available high-protein, high-caloric liquid drinks, which along with multiple vitamin supplementation, can adequately prevent this problem.

The real risk of inadequate nutrition develops during prolonged reconstructive procedures and multiple-staged operations. As a rule, patients undergoing these procedures are generally older, as in the case of the floor of the mouth-mandibular carcinoma patient, and tolerate the significant alteration in nutrition poorly. For this reason, the practitioner should consider using total parenteral nutrition (hyperalimentation) via a central line during crucial periods of healing to provide concentrated nutritional support. One drawback is the concomitant presence of tracheostomy and/or chest flaps which can cause contamination of the central line. It therefore appears prudent to utilize central parenteral nutrition during the preoperative time frame to best prepare the patient for the forthcoming surgical procedures.

Speech and communication difficulties have not been given important coverage in mandibular reconstruction literature, probably because not a great deal in available to improve these conditions. Almost any procedure involving the mandible will potentially affect speech, either temporarily or permanently. The presence of mandibular-maxillary fixation (MMF) or an external fixation device will cause some disruption of speech and will alter the clarity and enunciation of words. However, these patients can usually still be understood. On the other hand, patients who have extensive osteoradionecrosis (ORN) of the mandible, or who have undergone wide resection of the mandible with soft tissue collapse, will have very serious speech deficits. The worst form of this is the familiar "Andy Gump" appearance where there is essentially no anterior lower jaw projection, producing a nearly indistinguishable speech pattern. While most head and neck surgeons are insightful into the absence of speech after a laryngectomy and take responsible and definite steps to reestablish speech (tracheoesophageal puncture and prosthesis), very little work has been done in the area of mandibular-deficient speech. Unfortunately for the patient, no definitive assistance is available for the mandibular-deficient patient until the mandibular arch and anterior floor of the mouth have been reconstructed. An additional or compounding problem occurs when part of the tongue has been resected or lost or when a tongue flap has been utilized to cover an intraoral defect.

For the most part, surgeons have to rely on paramedical support personnel to assist their efforts to provide temporary or permanent speech rehabilitation to the mandibular-deficient patient. Psychologists and speech therapists can give support to the patient in terms of coping with diminished speech and communication. It is well known, anecdotally, that a large number of patients with cancer of the floor of the mouth (usually due to smoking and drinking) have preexisting communication problems, due either to diminished reading or verbalization skills or both. These individuals are uniformly frustrated after mandibular surgery due to their increased disability in communication and often respond by increasing their alcohol intake and becoming more withdrawn in their relationships with friends, family, and medical personnel. It is important, therefore, that the head and neck surgeon recognize and understand this potential problem and involve the support personnel in addressing it. Psychological evaluation and support, home nursing care, occupational therapy, and speech therapy all have a role in the management of this disability.

Another important aspect of the postsurgical alteration of the patient who has undergone mandibular surgery is the cosmetic deformity that often accompanies this problem. While perhaps not as devastating cosmetically as a maxillectomy or orbital exenteration, the loss of mandibular substance does cause a serious loss of body awareness and can cause the patient to become reclusive and introverted. Since the face has perhaps the most serious ramifications psychologically insofar as cosmetic alterations are concerned, the surgeon must counsel the patient and family and be aware of early signs of depression. Professional assistance can be obtained to help the patient deal with his response to the cosmetic deformity.

Thus, when considering the cosmetic and functional debilities that can be produced by some types of mandibular surgery, it is apparent from the author's experience that they can represent one of the worst type of morbidity for head and neck patients. The surgeon must be responsive to the total needs of the patient and give the patient the appropriate personal concern and empathy.

AIRWAY COMPROMISE

Depending on the location of the mandibular pathology or surgical procedure, some degree of airway obstruction can occur. It is well-known to the maxillofacial surgeon that when a patient is placed in MMF for either the repair of a fracture or after a reconstruction procedure, the patient is at increased risk of airway compromise and aspiration if vomiting should occur. For that reason, provision is always made to allow the patient the opportunity to remove any bands or wires securing the MMF. This principle was first developed during World War I when patients with wounds around the head and neck were dying of airway obstruction during transportation to a medical treatment facility. It is now common knowledge that a patient with a mandibular injury must be transported and/or cared for on the expectation that airway obstruction could and will occur. This includes the use of the prone position to allow oral secretions to be evacuated by gravity, the use of the extended neck position, and the placement of an oral airway if necessary.

While the use of a cervical collar is mandatory if there is a suspicion of neck injury, he must be cautioned that its use can also aggravate loss of airway due to floor of mouth or submandibular swelling. If necessary, an endotracheal tube or tracheostomy should be placed to secure the airway prior to any definitive surgical therapy. All personnel who will be providing care to the patient with a mandibular problem should be taught the basic principles of airway management.

Respiratory compromise can conceivably occur following any surgical procedure involving the mandible and floor of the mouth. By virtue of the texture and looseness of the soft tissue around the mandible, edema or hematoma can occur quite rapidly and airway compromise may develop within several hours postoperatively. Popowich and Samit[1] reported a case of respiratory obstruction following vestibuloplasty and lowering of the floor of the mouth and attributed it to postoperative bleeding. Although bleeding within the tissues of the sublingual and submandibular regions has a tendency to tamponade itself, it can lead to elevation of the base of the tongue and airway compromise before it ceases. In these circumstances it is always wise to perform a tracheostomy, preferably a controlled tracheostomy, with an endotracheal tube in place, and maintain the patient's airway in that manner until the swelling resolves.

In a later situation, loss of mandibular support may lead to chronic, low-grade airway compromise which may take the form of sleep apnea. Panje and Holmes[2] have reported that mandibulectomy without immediate reconstruction can cause sleep apnea. This may be particularly true for patients who have undergone extensive resection of the anterior mandibular segment. These authors recommend that all head and neck tumor patients having extensive composite anterior oral cavity resections should be elevated for sleep apnea by the appropriate sleep studies before decannulation of their tracheostomy tube. Also, if the anterior mandible is not feasibly reconstructed, a tracheostomy should be maintained in those patients in whom sleep apnea is present.

This condition is probably due to the loss of the soft tissue support in the suprahyoid region and its subsequent effect on the tongue and hypopharynx. Subsequent flap and/or rigid reconstruction of the lower jaw appears to prevent the development of sleep apnea.

EXTRUSION OF IMPLANT MATERIAL ON FOREIGN BODIES

A number of surgical procedures on the mandible require the implantation of foreign bodies (wire, tray, plate, or screw) or the onlay or interposition of autogenous or alloplastic graft material. While the majority of these materials either remains in place and cause no problems or are electively removed before they cause problems, there are also circumstances where the material will cause trouble.

In the case of metallic objects used to stabilize mandibular segments, several factors may be responsible for their extrusion, exposure, or the need to remove them. Obviously, the larger the size of the metallic device, the more likely it is to cause pain or erode overlying soft tissue. This is generally seen with larger compression plates or reconstruction bars which not only affect the soft tissues but are easily palpated by the patient and may serve as some stimulus to irritation or manipulation by the patient. Usually the first indication the surgeon has of problems with the bars or plates is the complaint of pain by the patient. Examination will determine whether the plate or metallic device is loose and causing painful movement or whether it is inciting a foreign body reaction of the surrounding soft tissue. It should be apparent that if the metallic object is the culprit in the discomfort then it should be electively removed, usually through the original healed incision.

The second condition that may lead to exposure or extrusion is the presence of a metallic foreign body beneath a thin mucosal or epithelial surface. Even a small figure-of-eight wire can be exposed if it is very close to the attached gingiva or lies beneath scarred or atropic skin. The single strand of the interosseous wire is less likely to cause problems than the rosette of twisted wire that is commonly inserted into one of the wire holes. When the wire is seen just beneath the skin or mucous membranes or if it is frankly exposed through the tissues, the best therapy usually is to remove the wire. This can be accomplished by injecting local anesthesia with a low concentration of epinephrine to diminish bleeding and removing the wire by grasping it with a hemostat or needle holder, pulling it away from the bone sufficiently to insert the jaws of a wire cutter. The wire segment that contains the twisted wire rosette should be pulled outward first and at the same time the mandible should be stablized to avoid damaging the healing segments.

Obviously, if the mandible is not yet healed or stable, the decision to remove an exposed wire must be made by weighing the benefits of removal against the risks of distracting healing mandibular segments. It is possible to conservatively treat the local tissue surrounding the wire with saline and hydrogen peroxide irrigation and dressing of the wound. In the case of a wire exposed through the attached gingiva, extensive local care and hygiene can be utilized to keep the area around the wire clean and free from infection until the mandible is stable enough to tolerate the wire removal. However, if the wire must be removed, even in the face of movable fragments of the mandible, several steps can be taken to lessen the risk of distraction. First, if the patient is still in MMF, the rubber bands can be removed and wire circles applied to immobilize the mandibular fragments; the wires can then be left on or can be replaced again by rubber bands, depending on the stability of the mandible. Second, if the MMF has been previously removed, or if the wire is securing a graft in place, it can be removed in segments by cutting its length several times along a wider exposure or with multiple incisions over its length.

Fortunately, there is a very low incidence of exposure or extrusion of graft material; however, if it does occur, steps need to be taken to ensure that the entire graft is not lost. In the case of exposure of an autogenous cortical onlay graft, the aim would be to remove the small amount of exposed bone if, and only if, the conservative local tissue management will not cause the subsequent overclosure of the tissues. Again, this local tissue therapy includes minimal but definitive debridement, cleaning with saline/peroxide irrigations, and the appropriate diet to decrease intraoral trauma. If the graft material is exposed through the skin incision or through a breakdown of the overlying skin, local skin care can be supplemented by the addition of topical antibiotics.

If local conservative tissue therapy does not cause the mucosa or skin to close over the graft, it will probably be necessary to drill or rongeur the exposed cortical bone segment, thus allowing the epithelial or mucosal surface to better close over the residual graft. Topical or local injectable anesthesia may be used on the surrounding tissue to assist the bone debridement process—the bone itself does not require any anesthetic medications. If the structural integrity of the mandible depends on the intact cortex, either the debridement must carefully avoid a through-and-through cortical disruption or one must apply MMF or external skeletal fixation to bypass the graft.

When cancellous bone chips have been used to reconstruct the mandible, in conjunction with some form of internal or external skeletal support, or have been utilized following autogenous bone grafting in conjunction with orthognathic surgery, they may have become exposed through the mucosal or epithelial incisions. In this case, the bone chips are readily removable in small pieces with a forceps, and the same local tissue care may be instituted. Since the structural integrity of the mandible is not dependent on these bone chips, removal of those exposed to the air or oral secretions will not affect the position of the mandibular segments. On the other hand, since the advantage of the use of cancellous bone chips is to provide a "bank" of osteoblasts to reossify the mandibular segment, an attempt should be made to minimize the debridement of bone chips. Obviously, intensive local tissue care is important in order to limit the amount of bone chips that have to be removed and to facilitate closure of the wound.

Although these materials are not commonly used in mandibular surgery, some surgeons have used other alloplastic materials such as silicone, Dacron, and plaster of paris for mandibular reconstruction. It is more likely that these foreign devices will cause problems of exposure, simply because of the past history of these materials when implanted in the body. While some authors have reported that if an alloplastic material is exposed only simple excision of the exposed material is adequate, it seems reasonable that the chance of arresting the exposure and effecting closure of the defect is low. However, the same care should be taken when alloplastic materials are exposed as when autogenous materials are involved.

The above discussion is pertinent to the exposed graft material when a significant infection is not present. If significant infection is present in and around the graft, more intensive therapy is indicated and will be discussed in Infection, below.

ABSORPTION OF GRAFT MATERIAL

One of the most discouraging complications of mandibular surgery involves the slow or rapid absorption of graft material which results in a failure to achieve mandibular continuity. In the normal, uncomplicated state, there is a physiologic absorption on the graft material at a cellular level, with reossification occurring through the action of autogenous osteoblasts laying down new bone matrix within the confines of the defect. On the other hand, the gross or macroscopic absorption of graft material without concomitant osteoneogenesis is pathological and will lead to loss of continuity of the mandible and failure of the intended purpose of the graft.

If the graft is not exposed to contamination by saliva or exposed to the air, the identification of graft absorption can be made primarily on the basis of the physical findings. While the patient is in MMF or external fixation, it is very difficult to determine the status of a bone graft clinically. While one can follow the graft site serially with radiographs, it is not known how this local irradiation will affect osteoneogenesis. Therefore, the use of serial radiographs is not routinely employed. At the time when the discussion is made to release the patient from MMF or remove the external fixation device, the mandible should be palpated for substantial motion at the grafted area, for tenderness on palpation, and for loss of bulk in the regions of the previously placed graft.

Unfortunately, when the graft begins a pathologic absorption there is no definitive or uniform therapy to perform at the time graft absorption is identified. However, if graft absorption is present concomitantly with mobility of the mandible, then the mobility may have contributed to the graft absorption. If some residual graft material is still present, either seen on a radiograph or by palpation, the mobility of the mandible should be stopped, either by rewiring with internal fixation or by applying external fixation.

If graft absorption is occurring in conjunction with infection in or around the mandible, aggressive measures must be taken in order to prevent total loss of the graft material (see Infection, below) and even more aggressive measures must be utilized if the graft has been placed in a previously irradiated area (see Osteoradionecrosis of the Mandible, below).

Graft absorption can also occur as a result of altered host factors and may be due to increased macrophage, enzymatic, and osteoclastic activity; it may also be due to the body's false interpretation of the graft material as being foreign. Another possible cause of pathologic graft absorption is the failure of the osteoblasts to be activated, leading to failure of osteoneogenesis to keep pace with the osteoclastic bone absorption.

If graft absorption has occurred to the extent that the grafting procedure is considered a failure, then the site must be stabilized until the mandible is again ready to receive a bone graft. Considerations should be given to ensuring that the mandible is properly immobilized, that no infection exists, that overlying soft tissues are adequately thick and vascularized, and that the host factors are positively maximized. Normally, the mandibular reconstruction site, especially when reconstructed with autogenous bone, is thinner and less bulky than the normal side. It may be necessary to supplement its bulk with a dermis-fat graft or with a deepithelialized myocutaneous flap (Figs. 307–313).

NONUNION AND MALUNION OF MANDIBLE

One of the most frustrating circumstances that can occur after mandibular surgery is the failure of the bone segments to unite completely *(nonunion)* or to unite in a malposition with respect to that which was intended *(malunion)*. This condition is upsetting to both the surgeon and the patient because of the probable requirement for future therapy directed toward producing a favorable osseous union. Nonunion and malunion are seen most commonly following treatment for mandibular fractures but can also occur after orthognathic surgery and cancer reconstruction. While there may be several common underlying factors producing both nonunion and malunion, these two complications also have separate antedating conditions that are likely to predispose the patient to one or the other.

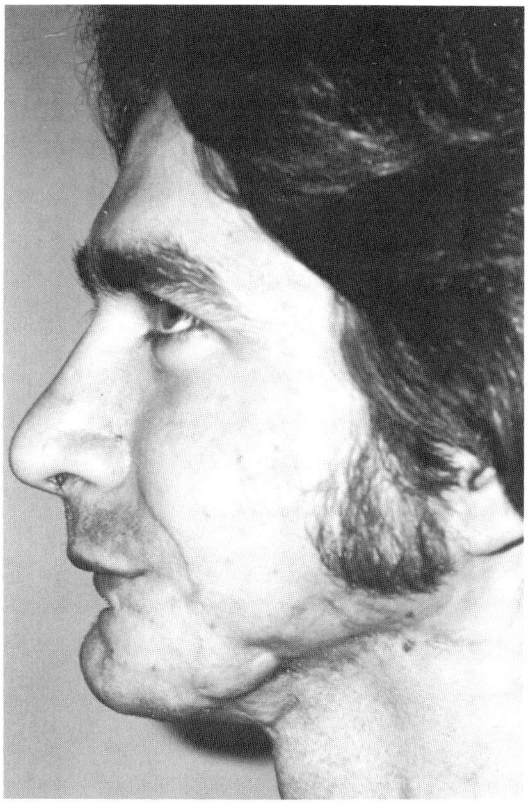

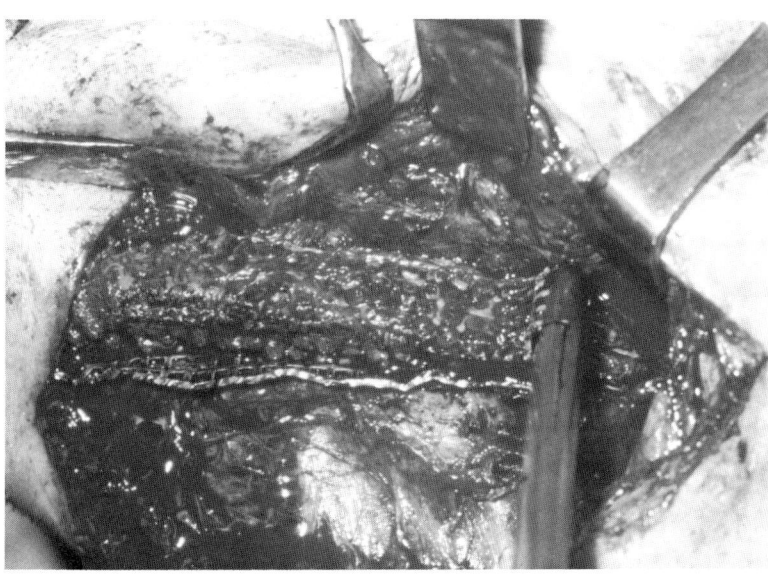

Figure 307. Patient after reconstruction of gunshot wound to left mandible using mesh tray and autogenous bone grafts.

Nonunion

The most common cause of this condition is failure to achieve proper immobilization of the bony segments or fragments. In the case of mandibular fractures, it is seen after "slippage" or loosening of the MMF and the subsequent movement or shearing that occurs between the fragments. Continual motion at the fracture site will not allow for adequate bony union and a nonunion will occur. Clinically, a nonunion will be seen as a painful area of the mandible that manifests relative motion of the fragments on chewing, talking,

Figure 308. Operative view showing removal of mesh tray; the mandibular segment is small (2 cm in height) but strong. However, it is noticeably less bulky than the right side.

216 Surgery of the Mandible

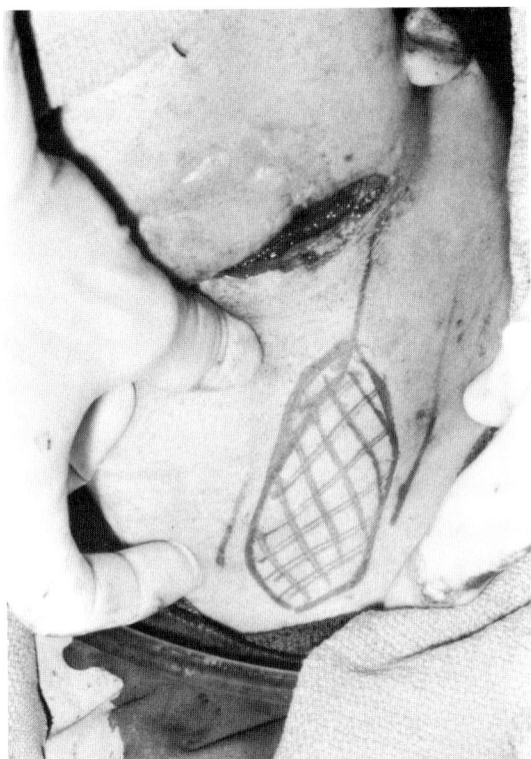

Figure 309. Outline of sternocleidomastoid myocutaneous flap on left neck to increase the bulk along the left mandible.

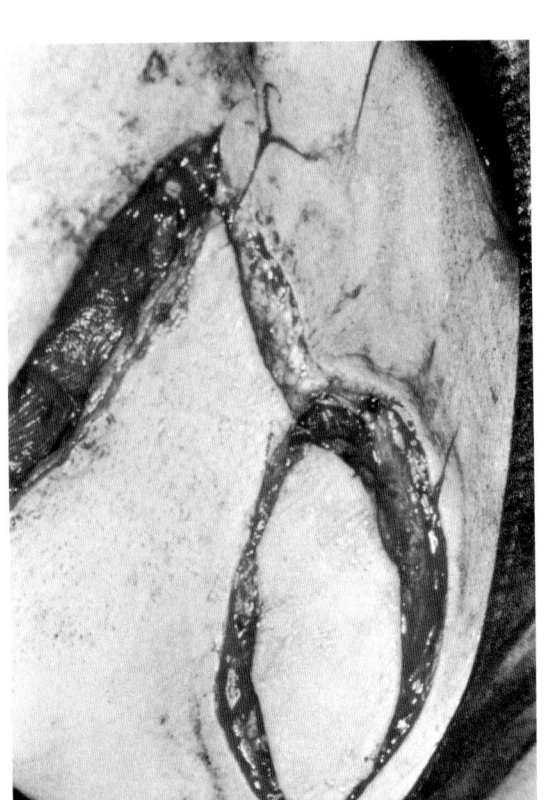

Figure 310. Sternocleidomastoid flap has been outlined and deepithelialized for transfer to subcutaneous tissues over the atrophic mandible.

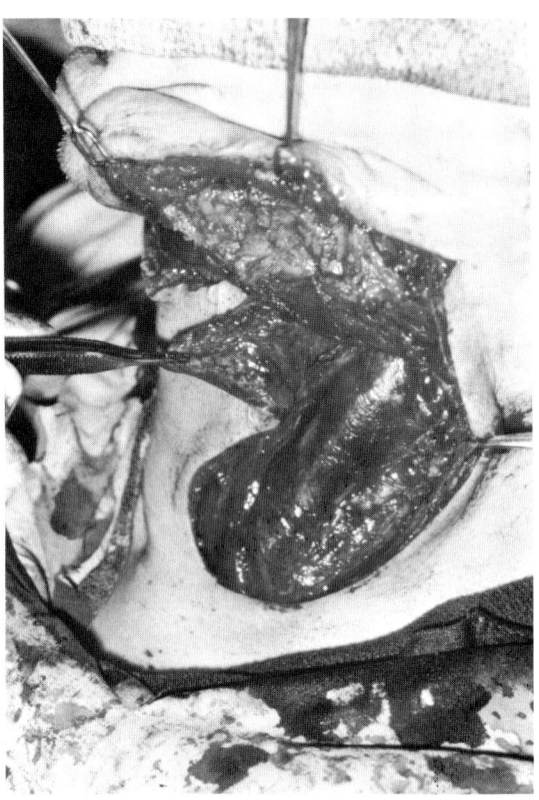

Figure 311. Rotation of deepithelialized myocutaneous flap over reconstructed mandible.

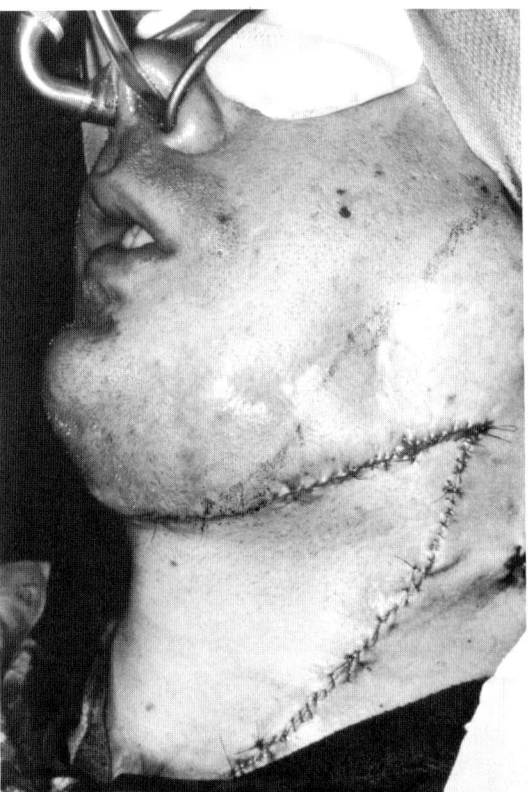

Figure 312. At end of operation following closure of both the tray removal incision and the sternocleidomastoid flap donor site. Note bulk increase in the mandibular region.

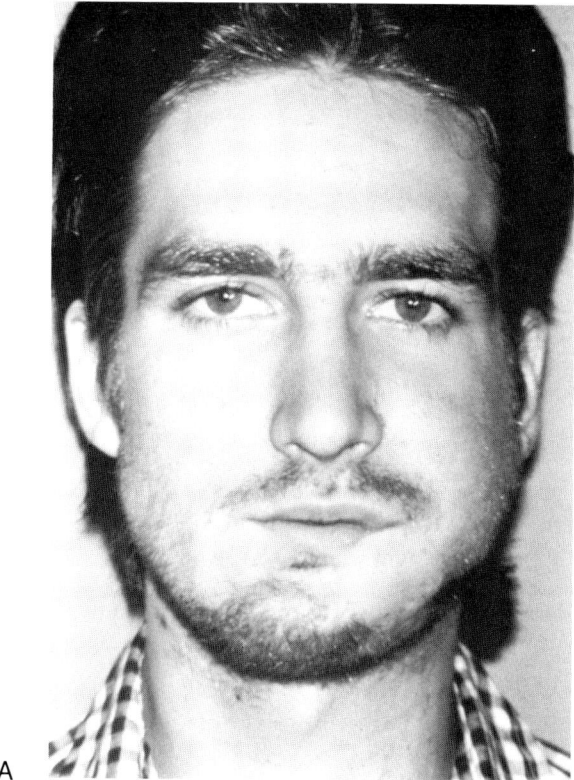 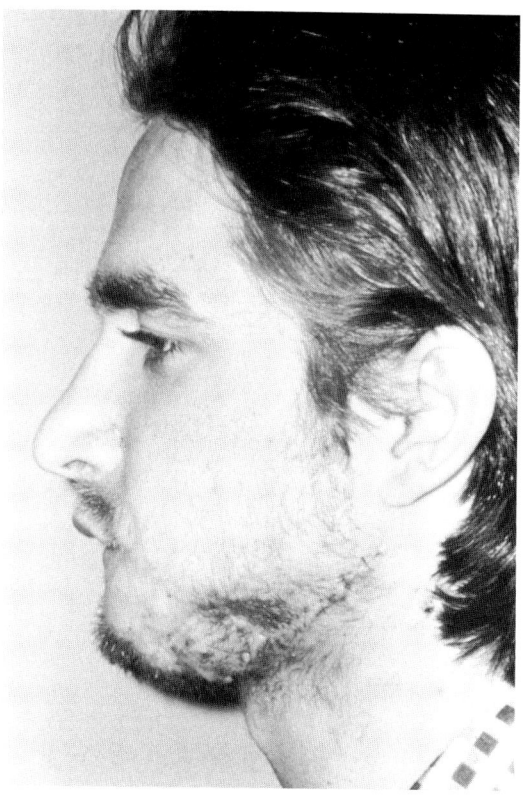

Figure 313. (A) Anteroposterior view; (B) lateral view of patient after removal of mesh tray and reconstruction of soft tissues using a sternocleidomastoid flap.

and so on by the patient and that can be palpated and moved by the examiner. If present on the anterior half of the mandible, the motion is readily visualized when inspecting the attached gingiva during bimanual palpation. However, it may be difficult to determine if a nonunion is present in the posterior segments of the mandible, including the ramus and the condyle. Here the motion of the nonunited fragments is very difficult to visualize and it will require bimanual palpation to appreciate the relative motion of the fragments. Typically, the most likely site for nonunion is in the symphyseal/parasymphyseal region, especially in edentulous mandibles, as this site is the most difficult to immobilize. The second most common site of nonunion is the body of the mandible. Although nonunion of the subcondylar region is not uncommon, it is usually not clinically significant as it may serve as a pseudoarthosis and function well. However, continued pain in the region of the movable subcondylar neck may necessitate reoperation. Nonunion of the ascending ramus of the mandible is uncommon, probably due to both the splinting effect and the high vascularity of the pterygoid and masseter muscles that surround that structure.

While failure to properly maintain MMF appears to represent the most common cause of mobility, other failed surgical techniques can also be potential culprits. The failure to properly place interosseous wires in mandibular fractures occurs frequently enough to warrant additional attention to the correct placement of these wires. If the wire is not placed at a 90 degree angle to the fracture site, the fragments can slip or shear and such frequent motion is likely to cause nonunion. The placement of Kirschner wires or steel rods across the fracture site will not adequately fix the fragments as rotation about the wire or rod can occur. Also, since these wires are placed transcutaneously, there is a greater chance for infection to occur at the wire-osseous interface. Certainly a broken wire, if weakened from undue stress during placement or twisting, will release the fragments from apposition and allow motion.

Other systematic factors such as poor oral hygiene, poor body nutrition, accidental fall or intentional blow, and inadequate local blood supply to the tissues surrounding the fracture or surgical site can also be significant. If nutrition, hygiene, and poor vascularity are felt to have contributed to the development of the nonunion, these factors must be improved or controlled before succcessful reconstruction can be attempted.

While a chance occurrence of trauma to the

mandible following surgery is difficult to avoid, the patient should be counseled and warned against exposing himself to situations where repeated trauma might occur, such as playing close to small children, participation in sports, or patronage of bars known for violent brawls. This is also important following revision surgery for nonunion.

Nonunion is normally diagnosed about 6 to 8 weeks after the initial surgery or fracture repair, which the patient is seen for removal of the MMF wires or bands. Bimanual palpation of the mandible is always performed *before* the decision to remove the arch bars or other fixation device is made. The diagnosis may be made earlier if the patient relates the feeling of motion in the mandible, or when there has been an identifiable episode of external trauma to the region.

The simplest form of therapy for nonunion of the mandible is to place the patient in MMF again, using either wire loops or multiple rubber bands to reestablish immobility of the jaws. Usually the patient is maintained in MMF for an additional 4 to 6 weeks before another examination is performed to determine if healing has occurred. It is also wise during this time to ensure that the patient has adequate nutritional intake of calories as well as vitamin and mineral supplements. If the mandible heals within this time frame of 4 to 6 weeks, then the MMF may be removed.

Plain radiographs of the mandible may not yet be diagnostic of nonunion at the time the clinical diagnosis is made. Unfortunately, the healing mandible does not lay down callus similar to a healing long bone; therefore, a dynamic study such as radionuclide bone scan is required to ascertain the degree of bone healing activity. However, if the nonunion is a result of bone resorption at the fracture or surgical site, a radiograph may be interpreted as positive by a knowledgeable reader.

If maintenance of the patient in MMF for a longer period of time does not cause bony union, an open surgical procedure is probably indicated. Here the MMF is left in place and the fracture site explored or reexplored in the standard fashion. Some surgeons prefer to keep this exploration and revision extraoral while others do not hesitate to repair nonunion through an intraoral approach. Whatever the choice, the surgical plan is to expose the fracture site, debride and clean out all fibrous and granulation tissue between the bony segments, and reapproximate these segments again to achieve immobility at the site of injury. This can be achieved either by using interosseous wires or by attaching a dynamic compression plate. These two techniques cause bone healing by different means; each has its respective advantages and disadvantages. Interosseous wiring is simple, effective, and does not cause wide stripping of the periosteum from the site of injury. However, bone union by wiring does not accomplish results as quickly as using a compression plate. The dynamic compression plate requires wide bone cortex exposure, is bulky, and usually requires elective removal at a later date. The use of external fixation devices at the stage of repair is normally not necessary.

Following reestablishment of adequate immobilization, the patient should be followed closely for another 6 to 10 weeks, depending on the problem, before determining success or failure of the secondary healing attempt. Failure to achieve union usually means that an autogenous bone grafting procedure will be required at this stage. It is typical for bone resorption to have occurred after two attempts to repair the mandibular injury area, and an autogenous bone graft will be used as both an onlay graft and an interposition graft between the two bony segments. The best source of bone graft is the cancellous portion of the iliac crest. The bone graft chips are placed between, and packed around, the freshened ends of the mandible, and the mandible is stablized. Stabilization at this stage usually involves the continued use of MMF as well as some sort of reconstruction plate, or, in some patients, an external fixation device. The external fixation device is the author's choice for utilization with autogenous bone grafting for nonunion because of its immobilization properties and the fact that no foreign body hardware is used in the region of the osseous discontinuity (Figs. 314–316). However, the use of a compression plate with cancellous bone packed around the remainder of the exposed injury site is also acceptable.

Malunion

The most common cause of malunion of the mandible is failure of the fixation efforts to hold the mandibular segments in proper alignment. This could include slippage of an incorrectly placed interosseous wire, failure to keep adequate tension on MMF bars, and failure to use open reduction and internal fixation in an unfavorable fracture. In the case of malunion, as opposed to nonunion, the patient's healing properties are usually normal and the local tissue blood supply is adequate. The circumstances surrounding nonunion usually involve some compliance failure on the patient's part, such as not keeping routine follow-up appointments. This is an important consideration because most pending malunions can be identified on physical examination, especially in fully denturous patients where abnormal dental occlusion would be the first sign of a malunion. Malunion is more

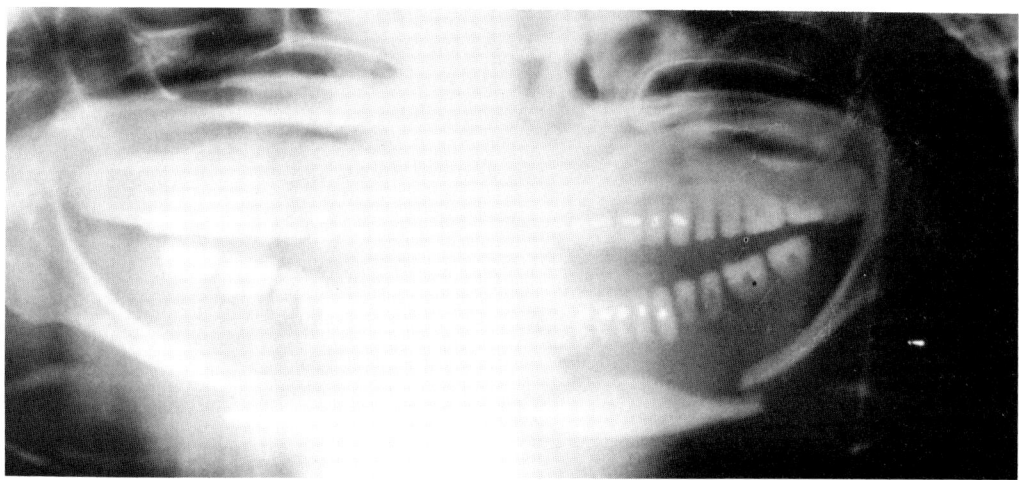

Figure 314. Elderly patient with edentulous mandible and nonunion of bilateral body fracture. Note thin, atrophic mandible on Panorex.

difficult to detect in partially dentulous patients as well as in edentulous patients, especially when inexact splints were used. In the case of patients who have very few teeth to which to attach arch bars, slippage of fragments can occur with mascular action during chewing and yawning; indeed, without the appropriate buttressing effect of the dentition, slippage will occur. A major difference between nonunion and malunion is that in the latter, the fragments are usually relatively well immobilized, and the slippage is a one-time event or a very slow process, neither of which continuously disturbs osteoblastic activity. The proof of this hypothesis is the fact that bony healing does occur (Fig. 317).

Malunion is best treated by open exposure of the area of malunion and performing an osteotomy using a power saw; the chisel or osteotome is not as useful as the power saw because of the transmission of forces to the temporomandibular joint (TMJ). However, it is very important to cool the area of the osteotomy with saline irrigation while drilling so as not to damage the bone. Following establishment of a surgical osteotomy, granulation tissue and scar tissue around the area are removed to achieve a clean site for maximal healing. The choices for initial internal fixation of the new osteotomy site include interosseous wiring and compression plate fixation. With both procedures, some form of MMF must be employed to initially achieve good occlusion—it should be maintained, however, throughout healing in the patient treated with interosseous wiring. If a malunion has occurred in an edentulous patient, it is not always necessary to perform an osteotomy; a small stepoff of the body of the mandible can either be offset

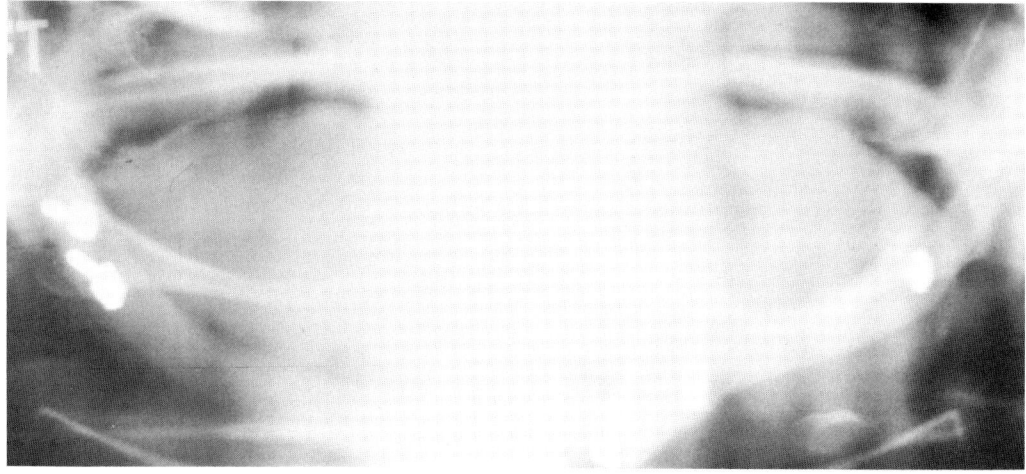

Figure 315. Panorex showing placement of external fixation devices preparatory to insertion of autogenous bone grafts.

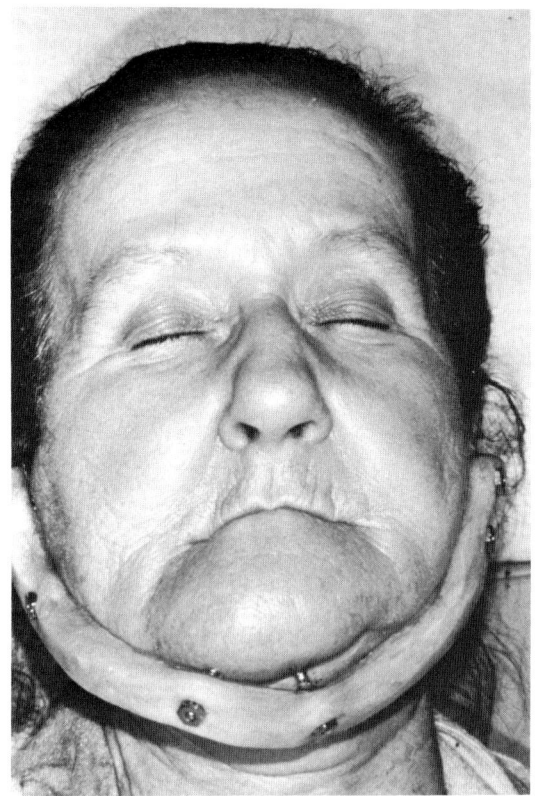

Figure 316. Patient after autogenous bone grafts of iliac crest with external fixation device in place. Stabilization should be maintained for approximately 6 months.

during denture fabrication or drilled down level through an intraoral incision. However, for significant deformities in an edentulous patient resulting from malunion, some form of onlay splint or modified denture will be required to achieve healing with an appropriate vertical height to the occlusion plane. Such splints can be wired circum-mandibularly to hold them in place. It has been the author's experience that nearly all cases of malunion will respond to open reduction and internal fixation, with the practioner paying strict attention to correcting the deficiencies in fixation and stabilization that produced the malunion. Any patients who do not respond to this therapy should be treated as described above for a nonunion of the mandible.

One final area to consider is a malunion of the region of the TMJ. As with other areas of the mandible, but to a much greater degree, bone remodeling will occur in the subcondylar and ramus regions, thus alleviating the need for reconstructive surgery in these malunions except in very serious and recalcitrant cases. In fact, some patients in whom occlusion is affected will require management by prosthodontic or orthodontic therapy.

COMPLICATIONS OF THE INITIAL DISEASE PROCESS

Since much surgery on the mandible performed currently is for repair of fracture, infection secondary to initial contamination is the most common complication. This topic will be discussed in the sections Infection and Osteoradionecrosis of the Mandible, below. Probably the second most common type of mandibular surgery is that related to orthognathic surgery. Failure to achieve a satisfactory result, either in occlusion or cosmesis, is the most frequently seen complication of this surgery.

Unfortunately, in some cases of mandibular reconstruction following cancer ablation, a recurrent or residual tumor can occur at the reconstruction site. This has occurred in the author's practice as early as 6 weeks postoperative when tumor grew

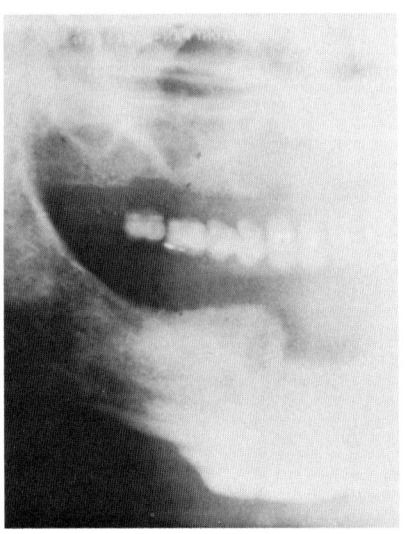 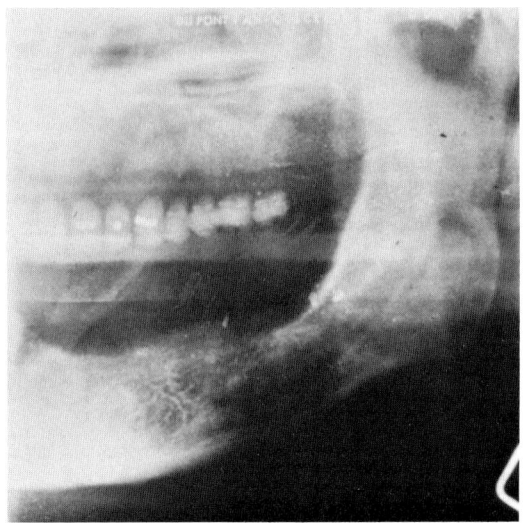

Figure 317. Panorex radiograph of malunion of edentulous mandible. Note firm callus formation at fracture site indicating normal bony healing ability.

out around the pins used to secure a biphase external fixation device used for proper spacing. Friedman and Vernon[3] reported a case of squamous cell carcinoma occurring in conjunction with reconstruction attempts using a mandibular staple bone plate. It is very important to wait at least 6 to 12 months to reconstruct a mandible that was resected for cancer, because of the high likelihood that a recurrence or regrowth of residual tumor will occur within that time frame. Any granulation tissue that tends to grow or flourish at the sites of bone ends or skin-penetrating pins should be biopsied and a high index of suspicion maintained through the entire course of reconstruction.

In the author's opinion, when a cancer does recur at the site of resection, further reconstructive efforts are not indicated, and efforts must be directed toward extirpation of the tumor. Salvage surgery for tumor recurrence at the site of mandibular resection must be aggressive if undertaken, and usually involves radical resection of the remaining mandible and its surrounding soft tissues. If radiation therapy has not been previously utilized, it may be considered, although in light of the fact that cancerous bone is usually resistant, it is often not effective. Radiation therapy is more effective against soft tissue involvement and as a modality against residual microscopic disease or nodal disease left behind after radical surgery.

The cancer itself may not manifest itself obviously in and around the operative or reconstructive site; rather, it may be manifested by signs and symptoms of base of the skull involvement due to tumor invasion of this region along nerve pathways. Although base of skull surgical techniques have progressed greatly over the past 5 years, cancer recurrence in this region carries a poor prognosis.

INFECTION

It is considered by some surgeons that operating on the mandible is inviting is "an infection just waiting to happen." This feeling is due to the high incidence of contamination of the operative site by intraoral bacteria and by the relatively tenuous blood supply to the bone under conditions of some types of mandibular surgery. Because of the high risk for infection following mandibular surgery, certain steps or conditions are important to consider in an attempt to decrease the risk of infection.

The utilization of elective antibiotics in "clean contaminated" surgery of the mandible (such as in orthognathic surgery) is widespread and clear-cut choices are present. In a prospective, randomized, double-blind study in 40 patients undergoing intraoral orthognathic surgery, Ruggles and Hann found that the use of perioperative penicillin did not produce any wound infections, while three were seen when no antibiotics were utilized.[4] These authors felt that the initial contamination of such a surgical wound with aerobic organisms probably provides an environment in which anaerobes can grow because of the removal of oxygen or the addition of reducing substances that lower the oxidation-reduction potential. Ruggles and Hahn also felt that the short-term use of perioperative antibiotics was as effective as long-term use and that resistance to penicillin probably would not develop with short-term antibiotics. Most surgeons performing mandibular surgery utilize some combination of aqueous and procaine pencillin G, beginning preoperatively and continuing intravenously during the surgical procedure and for up to 3 days postoperatively. In patients allergic to penicillin, effective alternatives might be a second-generation cephalosporin or erythromycin-sulfa. Since the patient will normally be hospitalized during the postoperative antibiotic period and since cross-sensitivity to pencillin with cephalosporin is very low, it appears to be an effective and safe agent for this purpose. While the duration of delivery of antibiotics appears to be most effective in terms of 3 to 4 days after the initial preoperative dose, the surgeon must individualize the antibiotic therapy for each patient depending on the circumstances of the surgery and the condition of the tissues.

If the patient develops a wound infection either while on a certain antibiotic or shortly after ceasing antibiotic therapy, a wound culture should be taken, either by direct swab or by needle aspiration. Needle aspiration is the preferable method, even with an open wound, because of the need for anaerobic culture techniques. There is a high likelihood of secondary infection by anaerobic or microaerophilic organisms and consideration must be given to their presence when deciding on the next course of antibiotics. While Gram stain will give an immediate indication of what organisms are present in the wound infection, formal cultures and antibiotic sensitivities provide the most reliable data. However, for the 48-h period during which the culture results are being awaited, an empirical initiation of antibiotics is in order. A combination of ampicillin and clindamycin or metronidazole (Flagyl) is effective against most likely culprits in wound infections around the mandible. If enteric gram-negative organisms are found on culture, gentamycin and/or carbenicillin or azlocillin can be used.

Fascial space infections can occur following surgery of the mandible and usually involve the masseteric, sublingual, submandibular, and mandibular spaces (Figs. 318 and 319). Since all fascial planes

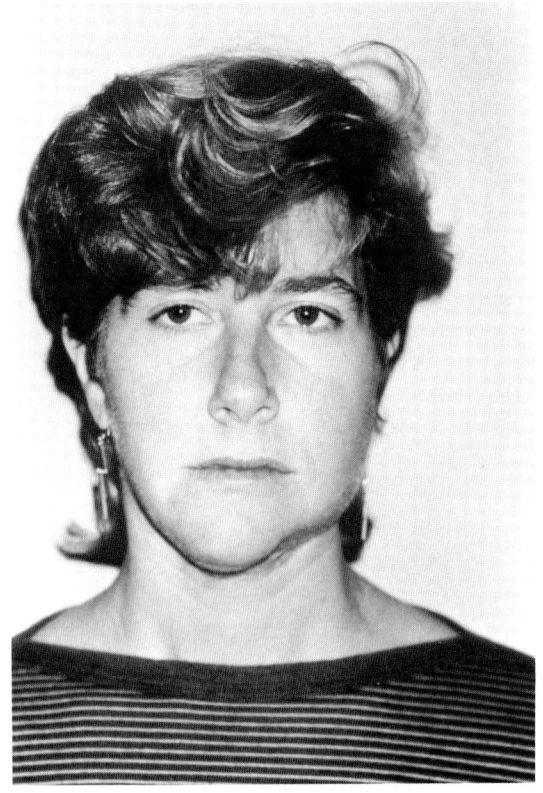

Figure 318. Patient after resection of ameloblastoma and immediate reconstruction using bone plate and cancellous bone graft (see Chapter 12). Note shifting of symphysis to right, and left lower cheek edema.

of the deep neck converge at the hyoid bone to form part of the carotid sheath, progression of a deep neck abscess to this location must be accounted for. The completed tomography scan can usually indicate the location and extension of deep space abscesses so that a surgical drainage procedure can be anatomically directed. Copious irrigation of the fascial space and the use of long-dwelling (3 to 5 days) surgical drains will be a necessary part of the drainage procedure. If possible, it is best to drain the perimandibular abscess extraorally so as not to further contaminate the operative site with extended intraoral contamination.

OSTEORADIONECROSIS OF THE MANDIBLE

Osteoradionecrosis of the mandible usually occurs after extensive radiation therapy (XRT) for perioral tumor that have invaded the periosteum or for the postsurgical patients in whom radiation therapy is given to control residual gross or microscopic disease. Extensive irradiation results in devitalization and devascularization of the bone due to obliteration of the fine vasculature, progressive fibrosis, loss of normal cellular elements, and fatty and fibrous degeneration of the medullary bone.[5] While all irradiated mandibles undergo these changes, certain precipitating factors are felt to precipitate the events leading to ORN. These factors include postirradiation extraction, severe periodontal disease, and loss of attached gingiva. Beumer and colleagues found that the episodes of ORN that were initially located within the zone of attached mucosa fared well with conservative measures, while those located primarily beyond the zone of attached mucosa fared poorly.[5] Most cancer surgeons and their dental colleagues recommend that all questionable teeth be removed prior to radiation therapy because dentition with significant periodontal disease is difficult to maintain and is quite susceptible to caries as well as periodontal infection after XRT. It also is well agreed that teeth

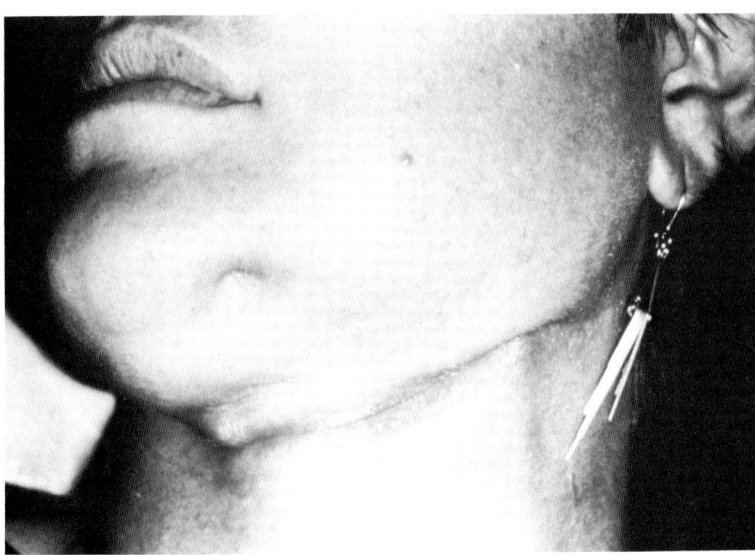

Figure 319. Closeup of patient in Figure 318 demonstrating localized submandibular wound abscesses 2 weeks after mandibular reconstruction. Infection responded to incision and drainage and appropriate antibiotic therapy.

should not be extracted after XRT has been given. When pre-XRT extraction is performed, a concomitant alveoloplasty is recommended and a minimum 10-day period of healing is allowed before radiation is begun.[6] During and after XRT, an aggressive program to prevent radiation caries should be followed, including oral lavage and application of topical fluoride gel.

However, if ORN occurs, the clinical picture is one of severe and unrelenting manibular pain, erythema, and swelling of the perimandibular tissues and possible exposure of the mandibular bone itself. Radiologic findings in ORN include increased radiodensity and periosteal thickening in some areas with other areas demonstrating diffuse radiolucency. Radionuclide bone scans should demonstrate increased areas of uptake in the pathologic portions of the mandible.

Baker found that, of 15 cases of ORN reported in 1983, all 15 occurred greater than 1 year after irradiation, most were in dentulous patients, and that all patients had received more than 6500 rad.[7] He felt that the basic principle of the aggressive surgical management of ORN of the mandible lies in the excision of all necrotic and heavily scarred tissue and replacement with nonirradiated skin or a flap. Thus, the therapy of ORN of the mandible ranges along a continuum, from initial conservative therapy to a much more aggressive surgical approach, based on the response of the disease process to the level of therapy.

The initial conservative measures to be taken include the initiation of broad-spectrum, culture-specific antibiotics (preferably intravenous), debridgement of the necrotic soft tissue and bone, and warm saline oral lavage. When available, the use of hyperbaric oxygen (HBO) is a successful adjunct to the management of ORN, especially when conservative measures have failed and radical surgical resection appears to be the only remaining therapeutic alternative. According to Triplett and associates, the rationale for the use of HBO in the treatment of ORN is based on the favorable events that occur when the partial pressure of oxygen is raised in the tissue.[8] These include increased capillary budding, esteoclastic and osteoplastic activity to remodel bone, callus formation and mineralization, and enhanced bacteriocidal activity of leukocytes in the wound. Thus, it is felt that increasing the partial pressure of oxygen in a hypoxic (infected) wound may enhance leukocyte killing and improve the local environment, thus favoring neovascularization, epithelialization, collagen synthesis, and eventual osseous repair. Much of the early work in the use of HBO in treating ORN is attributable to Davis and Dunn through their work in developing the clinical applications of the hyperbaric chamber while these authors were in the U.S. Air Force.[9] Hyperbaric oxygen protocols are available to the interested reader; these include the Wilford Hall Air Force Medical Center Protocol by Marx.[10]

It appears, however, that HBO therapy alone is usually not sufficient to control the process to the point of complete healing. The authors feel that it is an excellent adjunctive measure and should be utilized prior to and following surgical excision of the involved soft tissues and bone and the placement of a regional flap for new coverage. The usual method to accomplish this task is to send the patient to HBO therapy for several weeks to assist in clearing up the local infection, following by surgical excision of remaining marginal or nonviable tissue and insertion of a major myocutaneous flap such as the pectoralis, trapezius, or latissimus dorsi into position. No attempt is made to perform osseous reconstruction at this time. Hyperbaricoxygen therapy is reinitiated within several days after surgery and continued for several more weeks until flap viability and wound healing is assured. Since the majority of cases of ORN of the mandible come to aggressive surgical therapy, the author has found this combined technique to be clinically effective.

The patient is not allowed to wear dentures after healing, and secondary bone reconstruction is not attempted before 1 year after resolution of the ORN and is postponed indefinitely in patients who are maintained their nutrition well with only soft tissue reconstruction. Marx has estimated the cost of HBO plus surgery to be approximately $24,000 compared to non-HBO therapy ($62,000) and HBO without surgery ($56,000).[11] It should also be stated that the HBO plus surgery therapy is nearly always successful in relieving pain and returning the patient to near-normal functioning.

UNUSUAL COMPLICATIONS OF MANDIBULAR SURGERY

While the complications reported in this section are infrequent or rare, they are presented for interest and completeness and to make the mandibular surgeon aware of such occurrence when counseling the patient preoperatively.

As reported in Chapter 12, the main branch of the facial nerve is in jeopardy of injury when reconstruction is attempted high in the region of the condyle or the TMJ, as the facial nerve is only about 1 cm from the operative site and may be injured during surgery. If the paralysis occurs immediately postoperatively, the patient should be returned to the operating room and the facial nerve explored in the usual preauricular fashion and repaired. If, however, the paralysis develops slowly over several days after surgery and is not complete, then neuroproxia is likely and the therapy is expectant and medical in nature. If any residual weakness occurs, secondary revisions or reconstruction may be required (Figs. 320–322).

Tuinzing and Van Der Kwast reported the case of Frey's syndrome occuring after an uncontrolled sagittal split of the mandibular ramus that resulted in a horizontal ramus osteotomy. These authors felt that the auriculotemporal nerve was injured which resulted in facial sweating and flushing during eating (auriculotemporal syndrome).[12] Baddour and co-workers reported a successful repair of this condition that was accomplished by interposing a fascial graft between the skin and the underlying tissues to reduce innervation to the sweat glands of the skin.[13] In an associated surgical maneuver, Dendy related a case of facial nerve paralysis following a sagittal split of the mandible.[14] This event can be managed conservatively if neurapraxia exists, but must be surgically corrected if the nerve has been physically disrupted.

Sanni and associates reported the case of a 48-year-old woman who developed internal carotid artery occlusion following bilateral mandibular osteotomies.[15] She had an uneventful postoperative course until the third day when she developed a

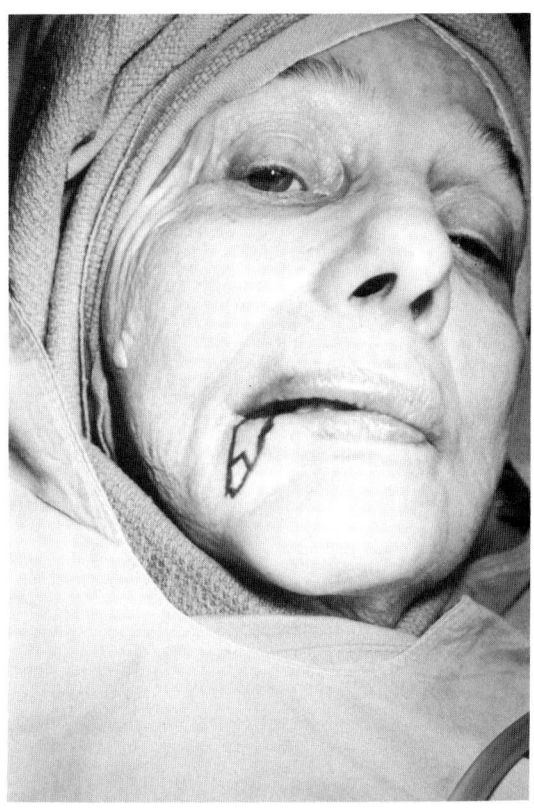

Figure 321. Wedge resection of right lower lip designed to overcome incompetent right oral sphincter.

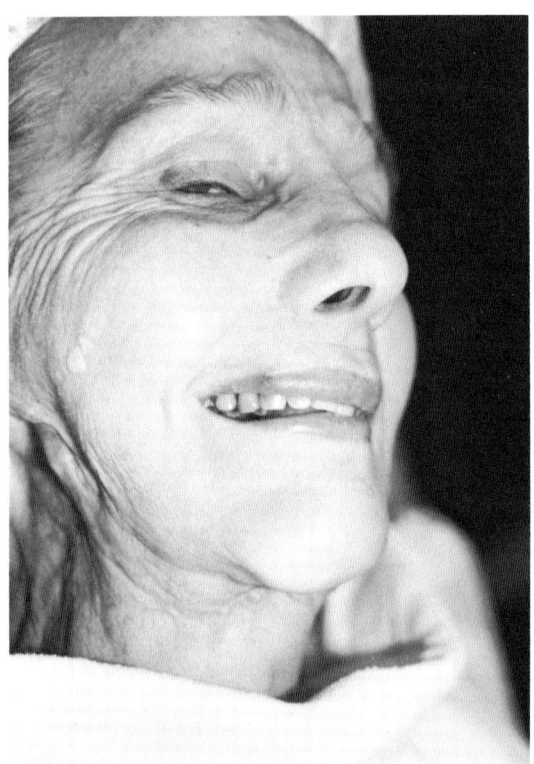

Figure 320. Patient seen in Chapter 12 who sustained a temporary right facial paralysis after reconstruction utilizing split rib and autogenous bone grafts. Patient had residual atrophy and weakness of right oral commissure.

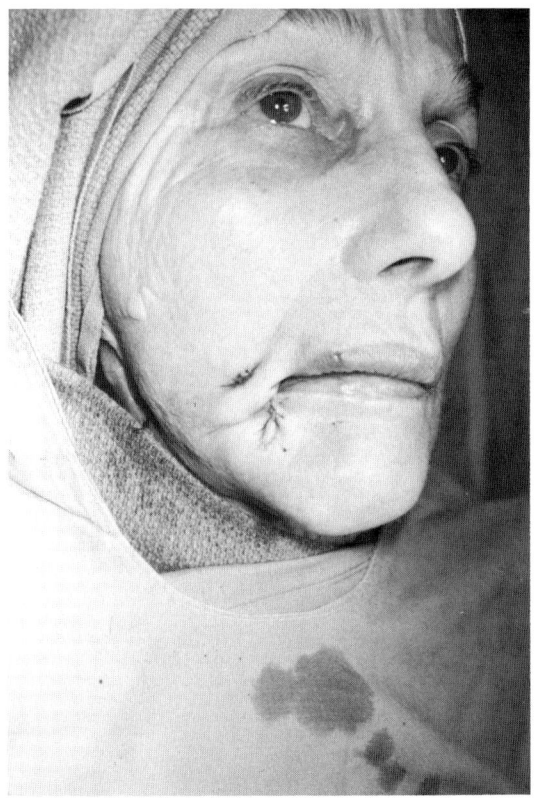

Figure 322. Reconstruction of right oral commissure by wedge resection of commissure and Prolene suspension of orbicularis oris muscle to close muscular defect.

Horner's syndrome, hemiplegia, and central facial nerve palsy. An arteriogram confirmed the occlusion. Unfortunately, the patient subsequently died.

Condylar dislocation can occur after subcondylar osteotomies with fairly insignificant or minor trauma to the mandible.[16] If the patient is already in MMF, however, conservative therapy will generally allow the bone to remodel acceptably. Storum and Bell found that many patients after mandibular osteotomies will exhibit a limitation of the mandibular-maxillary opening which may be iatrogenic or may occur as a consequence of a preexisting internal derangement of the TMJ.[17] The mandibular surgeon should be cognizant of this possibility and initiate a systematic regimen of rehabilitation as soon as possible to restore not only muscle function but also TMJ translation and mandibular range of motion.

Because of the tenuous blood supply and the possibility of contamination from intraoral secretions, surgery of the mandible is at high risk for the development of infection and bone necrosis. New therapy is available that can result in a high rate of success. Other complications include loss of fixation and stabilization of the mandible with imperfect occlusion. Correction of this problem may be simply involve reapplying rubber bands to the MMF or may require surgical reintervention. Unusual complications can occur; these may be related to either impaired function of the mandible or damage to surrounding neurovascular structures. Since the mandible is an extremely important dynamic bone, close attention must be paid to function as well as form in its reconstruction and surgery, in addition to the prevention and/or treatment of complications.

REFERENCES

1. Popowich L, Samit A: Respiratory obstruction following vestibuloplasty and lowering of the floor of the mouth. J Oral Maxillofac Surg 41:225–257, 1983
2. Panje WR, Holmes DK: Mandibulectomy without reconstruction can cause sleep apnea. Laryngoscope 94:1591–1594, 1984
3. Friedman KE, Vernon SE: Squamous cell carcinoma developing in conjunction with a mandibular staple bone plate. J Oral Maxillofac Surg 41:265–266, 1983
4. Ruggles JE, Hann JR: Antibiotic prophylaxis in intraoral orthognathic surgery. J Oral Maxillofac Surg 42:797–801, 1984
5. Beumer J, Harrison R, Sanders B, et al.: Osteoradionecrosis: Predisposing factors and outcomes of therapy. Head Neck Surg 6:819–827, 1984
6. Zarem HA, Carr R: Salvage of the exposed irradiated mandible. Plast Reconstr Surg 72:648–653, 1983
7. Baker SR: Management of osteoradionecrosis of the mandible with myocutaneous flaps. J Surg Oncol 24:282–289, 1983
8. Triplett RG, Branham GB, Gillmore JD, et al.: Experimental mandibular osteomyelitis; therapeutic trials with HBO_2. J Oral Maxillofac Surg 40:640–646, 1982
9. Davis, JC, Dunn JM, Gates GA, et al.: Hyperbaric oxygen: A new adjunct in the management of radiation necrosis. Arch Otolaryngol 105:58–61, 1979
10. Marx RE: A new concept in the treatment of osteoradionecrosis. J Oral Maxillofac Surg 41:351–357, 1983
11. Marx RE: Letter to Editor (response): Treatment of osteoradionecrosis. J Oral Maxillofac Surg 42:141, 171, 1984
12. Tuinzing DB, Van Der Kwast WAM: Frey's syndrome: A complication after sagittal splitting of the mandibular ramus. Int J Oral Surg 11:197–200, 1982
13. Baddour HM, Ripley JF, Cortez EA, et al.: Treatment of Frey's syndrome by an interpositional fascia graft. J Oral Surg 38:778–781, 1980
14. Dendy RA: Facial nerve paralysis following sagittal split mandibular osteotomy. Br J Oral Surg 11:101–105, 1973
15. Sanni KS, Campbell RL, Rosner MJ, et al.: Internal carotid artery occlusion following mandibular osteotoma. J Oral Maxillofac Surg 42:394–399, 1984
16. Weinberg S, Chu A, Tabano A: Condylar dislocation: An unusual complication observed after mandibular osteotomy. Oral Surg 56:581–583, 1983
17. Storum KA, Bell WH: Hypomobility after maxillary and mandibular osteotomies. Oral Surg 52:7–12, 1984

Index

Absolute stability, concept of, 90
Absorption of graft material, 214–15
Adenoameloblastoma, 43
Adenoidcystic carcinoma, 58
Adjunctive prosthetic devices, 184–86, 191, 192
Aesthetics, facial, 107
Airway compromise, 212–13
Alloplastic prostheses, 8, 57–60, 150–51, 157–60, 180–82, 189, 190
Alveolar process, 2
Ameloblastic odontoma, 42
Ameloblastoma, 40, 43, 58, 161–64
American Burkitt's lymphoma, 58
Anastomosis, microvascular, 176
Anatomy, 3–6
"Andy Gump" appearance, 211
Aneurysmal bone cysts, 41
Antibiotics, 221
Apnea, sleep, 212
Arch bars
    application of, 66–67, 72
    preformed, 26–27
Arch cartilages, 2
Arteriovenous malformation, 154–57, 158
Asymmetry, facial, 111
Augmentation mentoplasty, 139–48; see also Alloplastic prostheses; Implants; Prostheses
Autogenous bone, 121
    grafts, 149–50, 152–57
Autogenous cartilage, 121
Autograft, frozen, 200–204

Balance, facial, 107–16
Bars, reconstruction, 150
Benign ("true") cementoblastoma, 42
Body osteotomy, 114
Bone
    autogenous, 121
    cancellous, 149–50, 180
    fibrous dysplasia of, 41
    formation of, 7
    healing of, 7–8, 90–91
    scans, 46
    structure and composition of, 1
    tap, 91, 93
Bone banks, 177–78, 179
Bone grafts, see Graft(s)
Bone plate, exposure of, 101–3

Bone plate osteosynthesis, see Osteosynthesis, bone plate
Bridging plates, 33–34, 173–74
"Brown tumor," 41

Cancellous bone, 149–50, 180
Cancer staging, 45–46
Cap splint fixation, 35–37
Carcinoma involving the mandibular alveolus, 18–19; see also Tumor(s)
Cartilage
    arch, 2
    autogenous, 121
Cementifying fibroma, 42
Cementomas, 42
Cephalometry, 108
Cetacaine, 64
Cherubism, 41
Chin, 3
    splinting of, 143
    surgery, 117–37
        anatomic considerations, 118
        case reports of, 125–35
        general considerations, 117–18
        implant materials for augmentation, 118–21
        planning new chin position, 121–23
Chondroma, 43
Clamp, bone-holding, 91, 92
Communication difficulties, 211
Complications, surgical, 211–25
    absorption of graft material, 214–15
    airway compromise, 212–13
    extrusion of implant materials on foreign body, 213–14
    infection, 221–22
    malunion, 218–20
    nonunion, 215–18
    osteoradionecrosis, 222–23
    from osteotomy, 23–24
Composite grafts, free, 151, 165–68
Compression plates, see Plates, compression
Condylar cartilage, 1–2
Condylar dislocation, 71–74, 225
Crossbite, 64
Cysts
    aneurysmal bone, 41
    hemorrhagic (traumatic) bone, 41

nonodontogenic, 40
odontogenic, 40

Dacron-urethane prosthesis, 160, 180–82
Debridement, soft tissue, 101
Dentition, 5, 77–78, 95
Dentures, 68–70
Depth gauge, 91, 93
Dislocation, condylar, 71–74, 225
Dissection, neck, 49–50
Dressings, supportive, 25
Drill guide, 91, 93
Dynamic compression plates, 31–33, 87, 88, 89
Dynamic plate compression (DC), 31–33, 87, 88, 89
Dysplasia, periapical cemental, 42

Eccentric dynamic compression plates, 31, 33, 87
Edema, 212
Elevators, 5
Endosteum, 1
Enostoses, 42
Epithelial tumors, calcifying, 43
Essig wiring, 25
Exostoses, 42
Extensive radiation therapy (XRT), 222
Extra-oral incision, 141

Facial balance, 107–16
Facial nerve, injury to the marginal branch, 24
Familial multiple (gigantiform) cementoma, 42
Fibroma, odontogenic, 42
Fibrous dysplasia of bone, 41
Fixation, mandibular, 29–37
    cap splint, 25–37
    by direct osseous wiring, 29–31
    external pin, 34, 35, 36
    intermaxillary, 20–23, 25–28
    mandibular-maxillary (MMF), 211, 218
    rigid internal, 31–34
Flap, see Graft(s)
Forceps, bone-plate-holding, 92
Fossae, incisive, 118

Fractures, 61–86
  of atrophic-edentulous mandible, 78–81
  in children, 81–82
  of condylar neck, 71–74, 225
  dental arch application, 66–67, 72
  from gunshot wound, 76
  inadequate dentition with, 77–78
  late repair of malunion of, 82–85
  left-angle, 98
  management principles, 63–64
  of mandibular angle, 75
  of mandibular body, 70–71
  of mandibular symphysis, 75
  nonunion of, 103–4, 215–18
  parasymphyseal, 68, 75, 96–97, 98
  pathologic, 23–24
  patient assessment, 61
  planning treatment for, 61–63
  severely comminuted, 76–77, 78
  surgical technique, 64–65
  wiring of, 67–70, 72–74
    circumferential, 68–70, 72, 74, 80
    interosseous, 67–68, 74
    open reduction, 67–68, 71, 74
  see also Osteosynthesis, bone plate; Prostheses
Frey's syndrome, 224

Genioplasty, 111
  asymmetrical, 115
Giant cell tumors, 41, 43
Gigantiform cementoma, 42
Graft materials, absorption of, 214–15
Graft(s), 8–9, 193–95
  autogenous, 149–50, 152–57
  free composite, 151, 165–68
  free periosteal, 182–84, 191
  free rib, 174–77, 183
  iliac crest, 176–77, 183, 184, 185, 186
  myocutaneous, 174, 179, 180
  osteocutaneous, 187
  osteomyocutaneous, 168, 181, 182, 195–97, 198, 204
  pedicled composite, 151
Granuloma, giant cell reparative, 41
Gunning splints, 28
Gunshot wounds, 76, 151–52

Haversian canal system, 1
Healing, bone, 7–8, 90–91
Hemangiomas, 42
Hematoma, 212
Hemimandibulectomy, 47, 48
Hemorrhagic (traumatic) bone cyst, 41
Hohmann retractors, 91, 92
Homografts, autogenous frozen or irradiated, 177–78, 179
Hydroxylapatite calcium sulfate, 121, 182–84, 191
Hyperbaric oxygen (HBO), 57, 223

Iliac crest grafts, 176–77, 183, 184, 185, 186

Implants
  alloplastic, 8, 57–60, 150–51, 180–82
  chin
    hydroxylapatite, 121
    Proplast, 120–21, 139
    Silastic, 118–20, 139, 140
  extrusion of, 213–14
  see also Alloplastic prostheses; Implants; Prostheses
Infection, 221–23
  soft tissue, 97–98
Intermaxillary fixation, 25–28
Internal carotid artery occlusion, 224–25
Intraoral incision, 141
Irons, bending, 91

Kirschner wire, 173, 175, 176

Lacunae, 1
Lag screws, 34
Laser therapy, 56–57
Lateral pterygoid muscle, 5
Lesions
  benign, 39–43
  laser excision of, 56–57
  low-grade malignant, 39–43
  neoplastic, 42–43
  non-neoplastic, 40–42
Lidocaine, 64
Ligation of teeth, simple, 25
Lingual splint, 28–30, 78
Lingula, 4
Load guide, 93
Lymphoma, American Burkitt's, 58

Malignant tumors, see Tumor(s)
Malunion of fracture, 218–20
  late repair of, 82–85
  osteotomy and, 82–84, 219
Malocclusion, 104–5
Mandibular angle, fracture of, 75
Mandibular body
  fracture of, 70–71
  surgery, 109–11
Mandibular-maxillary fixation (MMF), 211, 218
"Mandibular swing," 12
Mandibular symphysis, fracture of, 75
Mandibulectomy
  marginal partial, 55–56
  segmental partial, 47, 48
  total, 47, 49
Mandibulotomy
  lateral, 17–18
  midline, 53–55
Marcaine, 140
Masseter muscle, 5
Meckel's cartilage, 1
Medial pterygoid muscle, 5
Melanoameblastoma, 43
Mentoplasty, 127
  augmentation, 139–48
  see also Alloplastic prostheses; Implants; Prostheses

Mesh tray, 164–67
Metal cage/crib prostheses, 178–79, 188
Metastatic carcinoma, 58
Mini-compression plates, 91
Mucoepidermoid carcinoma, 58
Muscles, mandibular, 4–5
Myeloma, multiple, 57
Mylohyoid groove, 4
Myocutaneous flaps, 174, 179, 180
Myxoma, 43

Natural head position, 108
Neck dissection, 49–50
Neoplasms, 40; see also Tumor(s)
Nerve injury, 104–5
Nerves, mandibular, 5
Neuropraxia, 223–24
Nonodontogenic cysts, 40
Nonunion of fracture, 103–4, 215–18
Nutrition, inadequate, 211

Occlusal wafer, 29
Odontogenic cysts, 40
Odontomas, 42
Osseomyocutaneous pedicle flaps, 168
Osteitis, 98–101
Osteoblast, 1
Osteoblastoma, 43
Osteoclast, 1
Osteocutaneous groin flap procedure, 187
Osteocyte, 1
Osteomas, 42, 43
Osteomyelitis, 98–101
Osteomyocutaneous flap, 168, 181, 182, 195–97, 198, 204
Osteon, 1
Osteoradionecrosis (ORN), 23, 211, 222–23
Osteosarcoma, 57–58
Osteosynthesis, bone plate, 87–106
  application technique, 93–95
  bone healing and, 90–91
  dynamics of, 87–90
  exposure of plate from, 101–3
  indications for use, 95–97
  instrumentation, 91–93
  malocclusion complication, 104–5
  nerve injury from, 104–5
  nonunion complication, 103–4
  objectionable scarring from, 105
  osteitis from, 98–101
  soft tissue infection from, 97–98
Osteotomy, 11–24, 54, 127
  anterior, 12–14
  body, 114
  complications of, 23–24
  lateral mandibulotomy, 17–18
  for malunion, 82–84, 219
  with marginal resection, 18–19
  posterior, 14–17
  rationale for, 11–12
  site stabilization and fixation, 20–23
  subapical, 110, 111, 112
  for surgery at base of skull, 20
Oxygen hyperbaric (HBO), 57, 223

Paralysis, 223–24
Parasymphyseal region, fracture of, 75
Pedicled composite flaps, 151
Penicillin G, 221
Periapical cemental dysplasia, 42
Periosteum, 1
Photodynamic therapy, 57
Pindborg tumor, 43
Plates, compression, 33–34, 81, 87–90, 160–65, 176, 177
   dynamic (DC), 31–33, 87, 88, 89
      eccentric (EDC), 31, 33, 87
   static fixation (SF), 87, 88
   see also Osteosynthesis, bone plate
Pliers, bending, 91
Pliers, reduction-compression, 91
Primary intention healing, 7–8
Profile, 107–8
Proplast, 120–21, 139
Prostheses, 169–71
   adjunctive, 184–86, 191, 192
   alloplastic, 8, 57–60, 150–51, 157–60, 180–82, 189, 190
   dacron-urethane, 160, 180–82
   metal cage/crib, 178–79, 188
   palatal, 192
   see also Alloplastic prostheses; Implants; Osteosynthesis, bone plate
Protrusors, 5
"Pull-through" operative procedure, 55

Radiation therapy, 57
   extensive (XRT), 222
Ramus surgery, 4, 109
Reconstruction, mandibular, 149–209
   alloplastic materials, 8, 57–60, 150–51, 157–60, 180–82
   autogenous bone grafts, 149–50, 152–57
   autogenous frozen or irradiated homograft replacements, 177–78, 179, 197–200
   bone banks and, 177–78, 179
   with bridging plates, 33–34, 173–74
   free composite bone flaps, 151, 165–68
   free periosteal grafts, 182–84, 191
   grafts, 79, 168, 174–77, 180, 183–86, 193–95, 204
   hydroxylapatite calcium sulfate and, 182–84, 191
   immediate vs. delayed, 151–52
   investigation, 192–93
   with Kirschner wire, 173, 175, 176
   plates and trays, 81, 87–90, 160–65, 176, 177
   principles of, 186–92
   resection and, 195–97, 198
   soft tissue closure, 173, 174
   "split-rib" technique, 56
   standardization of case reports, 192–93
   surgical preferences, 193–204
   see also Implants; Osteosynthesis, bone plate; Prostheses
Reconstruction bars, 150
Reconstruction plates, see Plates, compression
Retractors, 5
   Hohmann, 91, 92
Risdon wiring, 25

Sagittal split ramus osteotomy, 109
Sarcoma, osteogenic (osteosarcoma), 57–58
Scarring, objectionable, 105
Screwdriver, 93
Screws, lag, 34
Secondary intention healing, 7–8
Segmental surgery, 11, 108–9
Silastic chin implants, 118–20, 139, 140
Silicone rubber, 160
Skull, osteotomy for surgery at the base of, 20
Sleep apnea, 212
Soft tissue closure, 173, 174
Soft tissue infection, 97–98
   debridement, 101
Speech difficulties, 211
Spherical gliding principle, 87
Splints, 27–29, 30, 68–70, 78
   cap, 35–37
   for chin, 143
   lingual, 78
   mandibular labial-lingual, 79
   maxillary acrylic palatal, 79
   "Split-rib" mandibular reconstructive techniques, 56
Stability, postoperative, 112–16
Stabilization
   intermaxillary, 20–23, 25–27
   mandibular, 25–29
Standardization of reconstruction reports, 192–93
Stress shielding, 90
Stylohyoid pain syndrome, 23
Supportive dressings, 25
Supramid, 139

Synthes Maxillofacial Bone Plating System, 161

Teeth, simple ligation of, 25
Templates, malleable, 91
Temporomandibular joint, 4
Titanium prostheses, 169–71
Tooth bud, 2
Tori, 42
Trapezius osteomyocutaneous flap, 204
Trays, 160–65
   Dacron mesh, 180–82
   vitallium crib, 166–67
Tumor(s)
   "brown," 41
   calcifying epithelial, 43
   malignant, 152
      adenoidcystic and mucoepidermoid carcinoma, 58
      ameloblastoma, 40, 43, 58, 161–64
      American Burkitt's lymphoma, 58
      assessment of, 46–47
      cancer staging, 45–46
      contemporary surgical trends, 53–57
      dental issues in radiotherapy, 57
      earlier treatment patterns, 46
      factors associated with, 46
      giant cell, 41, 43
      metastatic, 58
      osteosarcoma, 57–58
      resection, 47–52
   odontogenic, 42–43
   Pindborg, 43
   see also Reconstruction, mandibular

Vessels, mandibular, 5
Vitallium crib (mesh) tray, 166–67

Wafer, occlusal, 29
Wiring
   circumferential, 68–70, 72, 74, 80
   continuous loop, 26–28
   direct dental, 26
   direct osseous, 29–31
   displaced direct, 81
   Essig and Risdon, 25
   horizontal, 25
   interosseous, 67–68, 74
   noncontinuous loop, 26–27
   open reduction, 67–68, 71, 74
Wolff's law of bone remodeling, 90